Other monographs in the series, *Major Problems in Clinical Pediatrics:*

Avery and Fletcher: *The Lung and Its Disorders in the Newborn Infant* — Third Edition published in January 1974

Bell and McCormick: *Increased Intracranial Pressure in Children* — published in July 1972

Cornblath and Schwartz: *Disorders of Carbohydrate Metabolism in Infancy* — published in February 1966

Oski and Naiman: *Hematologic Problems in the Newborn* — Second Edition published in March 1972

Rowe and Mehrizi: *The Neonate with Congenital Heart Disease* — published in June 1968

Brewer: *Juvenile Rheumatoid Arthritis* — published in January 1970

Smith: *Recognizable Patterns of Human Malformation* — published in February 1970

Markowitz and Gordis: *Rheumatic Fever* — Second Edition published in October 1972

Solomon and Esterly: *Neonatal Dermatology* — published in January 1973

Scriver and Rosenberg: *Amino Acid Metabolism and its Disorders* — published in October 1973

PEDIATRIC NEPHROLOGY

Pierre Royer, M.D.

Professor of Pediatrics, Faculté de Médecine de Paris.
Hôpital des Enfants Malades, Paris.

Renée Habib, M.D.

Professor of Research. Institut National de la Santé et de la Recherche
Médicale (INSERM). Hôpital des Enfants Malades, Paris.

Henri Mathieu, M.D.

Professor of Pediatrics, Faculté de Médecine de Paris.
Hôpital Bretonneau, Paris.

Michel Broyer, M.D.

Associate Professor of Pediatrics, Faculté de Médecine de Paris.
Hôpital des Enfants Malades, Paris.

Translated by
Anthony Walsh, F.R.C.S.I.

Urologist, Jervis Street Hospital, Dublin

Volume XI in the Series
**MAJOR PROBLEMS IN
CLINICAL PEDIATRICS**

ALEXANDER J. SCHAFFER
Consulting Editor

W. B. Saunders Company, Philadelphia, London, Toronto

W. B. Saunders Company: West Washington Square
Philadelphia, Pa. 19105

12 Dyott Street
London, WC1A 1DB

833 Oxford Street
Toronto, Ontario M8Z 5T9, Canada

Library of Congress Cataloging in Publication Data

Main entry under title:

Pediatric nephrology.

(Major problems in clinical pediatrics, v. 11)

Translation of Nephrologie pediatrique.

1. Pediatric nephrology.   I. Royer, Pierre, 1917–
   [DNLM: 1. Kidney diseases – In infancy and childhood.
   W1 MA492N v. 11 / WS320 N439]

RJ466.N4613   618.9′26′1   74–4585

ISBN 0–7216–7776–2

Pediatric Nephrology   ISBN 0-7216-7776-2

Title of original French Edition: P. Royer et al. NEPHROLOGIE PEDIATRIQUE.
Published and © 1973, by Ernest Flammarion, Paris, France.

English translation published by W. B. Saunders Company, Philadelphia, London and Toronto, 1974. Made in the United States of America. Press of W. B. Saunders Company. Library of Congress catalog card number 74-4585.

Last digit is the print number: 9   8   7   6   5   4   3   2

Contributors

ETIENNE BOIS, M.D. Research Associate, Institut National de la Santé et de la Recherche Médicale (INSERM). Hôpital des Enfants Malades, Paris.

MICHEL BROYER, M.D. Associate Professor of Pediatrics, Faculté de Médecine de Paris. Hôpital des Enfants Malades, Paris.

FRANÇOISE FLAMANT, M.D. Assistant, Department of Pediatric Oncology, Institut Gustave-Roussy, Villejuif, France.

M. FRANCE GAGNADOUX, M.D. Chief of Clinic, Hôpital des Enfants Malades, Paris.

MARIE CLAIRE GUBLER, M.D. Research Associate, Institut National de la Santé et de la Recherche Médicale (INSERM). Hôpital des Enfants Malades, Paris.

RENÉE HABIB, M.D. Professor of Research, Institut National de la Santé et de la Recherche Médicale (INSERM). Hôpital des Enfants Malades, Paris.

CLAIRE KLEINKNECHT, M.D. Research Associate, Institut National de la Santé et de la Recherche Médicale (INSERM). Hôpital des Enfants Malades, Paris.

MICHELINE LEVY, M.D. Research Associate, Institut National de la Santé et de la Recherche Médicale (INSERM). Hôpital des Enfants Malades, Paris.

CHANTAL LOIRAT, M.D. Associate Professor, Faculté de Médecine de Paris. Hôpital des Enfants Malades, Paris.

HENRI MATHIEU, M.D. Professor of Pediatrics, Faculté de Médecine de Paris. Hôpital Bretonneau, Paris.

GINETTE RAIMBAULT, M.D. Master of Research, Institut National de la Santé et de la Recherche Médicale (INSERM). Hôpital des Enfants Malades, Paris.

PIERRE ROYER, M.D. Professor of Pediatrics, Faculté de Médecine de Paris. Hôpital des Enfants Malades, Paris.

ODILE SCHWEISGUTH, M.D. Professor of Pediatric Oncology, Institut Gustave-Roussy, Villejuif, France.

Author's Preface

This book is the work of a team, a devoted team that in 1963 published *Current Problems in Childhood Nephrology* and now presents the fruits of 10 years additional experience. The text expresses the views of a group of doctors who have worked together for more than 15 years. On the credit side this has the advantage that the authors have been in the habit day after day of submitting their ideas to mutual and comprehensive criticism. On the debit side is the difficulty in avoiding bias and perhaps inadequate consideration of certain aspects of the subject, despite the exceptional amount of case material at our disposal. We are offering an account of experience and its interpretation rather than mere knowledge. This will explain the too few references, the errors of omission, and the occasional didactic statements. No doubt the balance will be restored by many well-deserved criticisms.

Each of the four principal authors, in line with his main interests, has taken responsibility for one part of the book, but all have collaborated in the whole work. For many of the chapters we have sought the aid of many other members of our team. We are deeply grateful to these collaborators and friends, especially E. Bois, F. Flamant, M. F. Gagnadoux, M. C. Gubler, C. Kleinknecht, M. Levy, C. Loirat, G. Raimbault, and O. Schweisguth. Our thanks are due also to our designer, our photographer, our secretaries, and our publishers, whose task was often difficult.

However imperfect or incomplete, however justly criticized this new book may be, let no one suggest that we should do better next time: the task has proved so formidable that we have no hesitation in promising never to do it again.

P. ROYER

Foreword

We are proud to present to the pediatric reading public this eleventh volume in the Major Problems in Clinical Pediatrics series. The principal author is Professor Pierre Royer, Chairman of the Department of Pediatrics at the Université Necker and the Hôpital des Enfants Malades of Paris. His name has become almost synonymous with pediatric nephrology. In the task of writing this book he was assisted by three colleagues in his extremely active nephrology clinic, Drs. Renée Habib, Henri Mathieu and Michel Broyer. The translation from the original French was accomplished by Mr. Anthony Walsh of Jervis Street Hospital, Dublin.

This volume is a gold mine of information, most of it based upon the authors' personal observations on their own patients. Everything is included—from embryology and genetics, through pathogenesis, symptomatology, diagnosis, and prognosis, to therapy—of a host of renal disorders to which the newborn, infant, child and adolescent are liable. This book is a must for everyone who aspires to be, or already is, a pediatrician.

ALEXANDER J. SCHAFFER, M.D.

Translator's Preface

In this series devoted to Major Problems in Pediatrics it is very appropriate that the volume on Pediatric Nephrology is translated from the French. The advances in Nephrology in the last two decades have been little short of phenomenal and the great French school of renal medicine has been one of the foremost contributors. Professor Royer heads a team that is known the world over, and the present work is the distillate of their experience blended with a wide-ranging knowledge of the world literature.

As a urologist who believes strongly in the importance of very close collaboration between urology and nephrology, I am happy to have had the opportunity to make Professor Royer's work more easily accessible to English-speaking physicians.

Lastly, I must place on record my very deep appreciation of the superb professionalism of the firm of W. B. Saunders which has made my task very much easier.

ANTHONY WALSH

Contents

PART II. URINARY INFECTION AND THE PATHOLOGY
OF INTERSTITIAL TISSUE
H. Mathieu

Chapter Four

Chapter Five

Chapter Six

PART III. GLOMERULOPATHIES
R. Habib

Chapter One

Chapter Two

Chapter Three

Congenital Disorders of the Kidney

PIERRE ROYER

EMBRYOLOGICAL DEVELOPMENT OF THE KIDNEY AND GENETIC FACTORS

Knowledge of the biology of normal and abnormal kidney development, and of the hereditary nephropathies, is growing rapidly. This area of nephrology is peculiar to the newborn, the infant, and the young child.

THE EMBRYONIC KIDNEY

There are three embryonic renal structures in man: the pronephros, the mesonephros or Wolffian body, and the metanephros. These are all derived from the nephrogenic cord. Development proceeds in a craniocaudal direction, with metamerization being clear-cut at the cranial extremity, where the pronephros develops, slight in the middle part of the metanephros, and nil in the mesonephros.[6]

Pronephros

The human pronephros is a cervical kidney. It differentiates at the end of the third week and disappears at the end of the fourth week. It does not function. The solid nephrotomes transform into vesicles that do not form tubules and which degenerate without forming true nephrons or opening into the collecting duct. At the end of the vesicle a diverticulum develops which evolves into the Wolffian duct. The pronephros disappears and only the Wolffian duct persists.

Mesonephros

Development

The mesonephros is a thoracic kidney. It begins to appear about the twenty-fourth or twenty-fifth day in the 3.7 mm. embryo, and degenerates between the eighth and tenth weeks. It opens into the Wolffian duct. In the female, the mesonephros and Wolffian duct disappear during the third month.

In the male, a few tubules persist in the region of the testis, and the remains of the Wolffian duct form the epididymis and the vas deferens.

Structure

The formation of the nephron structures of the mesonephros resembles that of the definitive kidney, with formation of a vesicle, development of an S-shaped body, elaboration of a tubule, and the appearance of a glomerular tuft. The chief differences from the definitive kidney are: the glomeruli are twice or three times as big; the vessels forming the tuft come directly from the aorta; the proximal tubule is well differentiated, with a brush border, but there is no loop of Henle and no distal tubule, nor is there any juxtaglomerular apparatus. The mesonephros has been shown to function in certain mammals and there is probably some slight function in the human embryo.

Metanephros or Definitive Kidney

Development

Development of the metanephros begins about the fifth week and is complete about the thirty-second week, when some 800,000 nephrons have been formed. The metanephros develops from two sources, the renal blastema and the ureteral bud. The renal blastema gives rise to the nephrons, and the ureteral bud gives rise to the collecting apparatus (ureter, pelvis, calyces, papillary ducts, ducts of Bellini, and collecting tubules). In the course of this development, the definitive kidney undergoes three changes. First is the elongation in a cranial direction of the ureteral bud, which arises from the dorsal aspect of the caudal extremity of the Wolffian duct. This brings the kidney from a pelvic to a lumbar position, but it is not a true migration, being instead an effect of the very rapid growth of the lumbosacral region of the embryo. Second, at the same time, the kidney rotates through 90 degrees, so that the pelvis, which originally faced the ventral surface of the embryo, now faces the midline. Third, the fetal kidney is very lobulated; the lobulation is still obvious at birth but disappears during infancy.

Morphogenesis of the Collecting System

The collecting system derives from the pyriform extremity of the ureteral bud by an alternating process in which there are many successive generations of dichotomous branching and enlargement in several planes. Using a micro-dissection technique, Potter and Osathanondh[6] have shown that this process continues from the end of the sixth week to the thirty-second week and ends only three or four weeks before birth. The pelvis and major calyces derive from the third to fifth generations of branches; the minor calyces arise by formation of multiple short branches in one generation; the papillary ducts are formed from the seventh to eleventh generations of branching; and the medullary and cortical collecting tubules in the final four to seven branchings. In all, there are some 20 to 38 generations, and the first differentiated vesicles appear at the end of the first week.

Between the fourteenth and twentieth weeks, arcades of nephrons are formed; the ampullae or growing ends of branches of the ureteral bud cease to branch but continue to give rise to new vesicles, until four to seven nephrons attached to each other are appended to each ampulla. The glomerulus of the oldest nephron is juxtamedullary; it is large and has a long loop of Henle. The younger glomeruli are smaller and have a short loop of Henle. From the twentieth to the thirty-second weeks the terminal ampullae continue to grow and give rise to independent vesicles in the subcapsular cortex. Some of the large juxtaglomerular glomeruli and some of the small subcapsular glomeruli may regress or degenerate before or just after birth.

The initial part of the ureteral bud develops in several stages. First the cornu of the urogenital sinus is formed from the end of the Wolffian duct. The two horns unite to form the posterior wall of the sinus, to which the ureters and Wolffian ducts are attached separately (seventh week). The trigone of the bladder is then formed between the orifices of these four openings (eighth week), the bladder is established and the Wolffian ducts regress in the female. This development is linked closely with the development of the genital organs. The lower end of the ureter is blocked for a short time by Chwalla's membrane.

Morphogenesis of the Nephron

The terminal ampulla of the collecting system is covered by a cap of cells derived from the renal blastema. Differentiation of the cap cells produces a renal vesicle surrounded by a basal lamina. This vesicle becomes S-shaped and the end close to the ampulla fuses with it. The other, unattached extremity forms the Bowman's capsule from the distal bend of the S. The afferent artery, the glomerular tuft, and the efferent artery are derived from an interlobular arteriovenous shunt and are enfolded in the same bend of the S. The tubule forms at the other bend of the S. Differentiation into distal tubule, loop of Henle, and proximal tubule is complete four to five weeks after the formation of the primitive vesicle. Thus, the initial glomerular epithelium and the first glomerular capillaries have their own basal laminae, which unite to form the definitive glomerular basement membrane with its three layers.[3]

The mesenchymal cells of the nephrogenic zone that are not used in the formation of the nephron form the interstitial tissue of the kidney. These cells follow the capillaries in the formation of the tuft and are the source of the mesangial tissue. Some of the mesenchymal cells form the juxtaglomerular apparatus.[1] The macula densa is recognizable early in the formation of the glomerulus; its cells contain glucose-6-phosphate dehydrogenase, and at an early stage dense granules are visible in the basal part of the cells.[3]

Induction of Nephron Formation

The morphogenesis of the nephron depends on a sequence of stimuli. The first inductor is the ureteral bud; the second is the renal blastema, which has inductive properties even for other organs. These inductions have been studied in cultures of embryonic kidney and have been found to depend on dialyzable chemical substances. It seems that glycogen level and diffusion of an enzyme, phosphomonoesterase, are important factors in these induction phenomena.[8]

Function

At a very early stage, the metanephros elaborates a urine whose composition is very similar to an ultrafiltrate of plasma. Much information about the function of the fetal kidney has been acquired from dye and isotope techniques and from enzyme studies.

GENETIC FACTORS IN KIDNEY DISEASE

At first sight, genetic studies in infant nephrology might seem to be of little more than speculative interest, useful for example in defining nosology, in providing coherent and reproducible models for studying abnormal structure and function, and in defining the role of heredity in adult kidney disease, touching as well on the problem of hereditary predispositions to certain acquired nephropathies or their variants.[7]

But genetic studies of kidney diseases in children are no longer of purely academic interest; they do indeed have many practical applications. The hereditary nephropathies very often follow a similar pattern from one patient to another, especially within one family. The general prognosis, the duration of the disease, and length of survival are often easy to foretell. Knowledge of the mode of transmission of a nephropathy will often indicate the intrafamilial risk. In addition, the extension of kidney transplantation to ever younger children renews interest in genetic studies. In cases of hereditary kidney disease, when a donor is chosen from within the family, it is essential to be certain that the donor himself is not affected. There is little knowledge of the course of events in cases of dominant diseases of variable expression, and we need also to know a good deal more about the behavior of a transplanted kidney from a heterozygous subject.[2, 5, 7, 9, 10]

Hereditary Nephropathies

The incidence of the problem can be summarized by our own experience: of 1450 nephropathies studied in a 10 year period, 201 (13 per cent) were hered-

Table 1. Classification of 201 Cases of Hereditary Nephropathy, Seen from 1960 Through 1970, of a Total of 1450 Cases of Kidney Disease in Children*

Category	*Number of Cases*
I. Hereditary malformations of the kidney	10
II. Hereditary nephropathy progressing to overall renal failure	86
III. Nephrotic syndromes	19
IV. Hereditary primary tubular disease	53
V. Renal disease secondary to hereditary disorders of metabolism	33
Total	201

*From Royer, P., *et al.*: Les néphropathies héréditaires. Arch. Franç. Pédiat. *27*:293, 1970. Masson & Cie, Paris.

itary nephropathies. We have classified these into five groups (see Table 1).[7] These diseases are considered in more detail in the chapters that follow.

Hereditary Malformations of the Urinary Tract

Congenital absence of a kidney has been reported in two brothers, in a boy and his uncle, and in four sisters suffering from one, two, or all of these conditions: renal dysgenesis, malformations of the internal genital apparatus, or anomalies of the middle ear. In certain cases, only male subjects are affected, exhibiting a syndrome that includes renal dysplasia associated with congenital torticollis, multiple keloids, and cryptorchidism.

Intrafamilial *malformations of the urinary tract* have been reported, often of varied type in the same family, such as familial nonobstructive megaureter or unilateral hydronephrosis affecting only the males in one family. It is not certain that these "familial" cases are purely hereditary because the recurrence of congenital malformations within one family might result either from factors other than genetic ones or from an interplay of genetic and other factors. The incidence of malformations induced by some exogenous factor is often much greater in families that have a natural predisposition for this malformation (Table 2).

Table 2. Malformations of the Kidney and Urinary Tract.*

Sex ratio	1.4/1 (≠1)
Birth rank	2.45 (2.36)
Father's age (at birth of child)	31.05 (31.05)
Mother's age (at birth of child)	27.63 (27.64)
Mean birth weight (kg.):	
Boys	3.371 (3.344)
Girls	3.356 (3.220)
Birth month	Identical to national distribution
Mean consanguinity ($\times 10^5$)	84 (23.4)
Incidence in close relatives:	
Father	2.9 per cent
Mother	4 per cent
Siblings	1.5 per cent
Age at time of diagnosis (percentage of cases):	
Birth	4 per cent
0–12 months	30 per cent
1–12 years	66 per cent
Other associated malformations:	
One	9 per cent
More than one	17 per cent
Chromosome aberrations	7 (including 5 with XO)

*Figures taken from a study of 473 patients by J. Feingold and E. Bois. The figures in parentheses are those for the general population of France.

Malformations and Chromosome Aberrations

Malformations of the kidney and urinary tract have been reported in association with aberrations of both the sexual chromosomes and the autosomes. Such defects seem to be common in Turner's syndrome, which is frequently accompanied by malrotation, horseshoe kidney, congenital hydronephrosis, renal agenesis, or duplication of the kidney, pelvis, and ureters. Of the autosomal syndromes, trisomy 18 has produced abnormal urinary apparatus (horseshoe kidney and hydronephrosis) in one case in three. Various malformations — hydronephrosis, megaureter, and hypoplasia or dysplasia of the kidney with cortical cysts — have also been noted in trisomy 13. These conditions can also be found, though rarely, in trisomy 21. Finally, chromosome deletion syndromes affecting chromosome 18, such as deletion of the short arm, deletion of the long arm, or ring chromosome formation, are sometimes also accompanied by kidney malformations.

CONCLUSIONS

Better knowledge of the biology and pathology of prenatal kidney development provides a valuable basis for the study of embryonic kidney disorders of children. Indeed, genetics has become one of the most useful basic disciplines in the analysis and classification of childhood nephropathies. Valuable guides to individual and intrafamilial prognosis, as well as improved understanding and treatment, can be derived from progress in genetic studies. Models of disease can be found in spontaneous mutants among laboratory animals. For example, three hereditary kidney diseases have been identified in mice: the autoimmune nephropathy of NZB/B1 mice, the nephropathy of periarteritis nodosa type in the PN strain, and the nephronophthisis of KD strain mice.[4]

REFERENCES

1. Bouissou, H., Régnier, C., and Fabre, M. T.: Etude du développement embryonnaire du mesangium glomérulaire. J. Urol. Nephrol. *71*:241, 1965.
2. Cook, R.: Genetic aspects of hereditary renal diseases. *In* J. Metcoff, ed.: Hereditary, Developmental and Immunologic Aspects of Kidney Diseases. Chicago, Northwestern University Press, 1961.
3. Kazimierczak, J.: Development of the renal corpuscle and the juxtaglomerular apparatus. Acta Path. Microbiol. Scand. *Suppl. 218,* 1971.
4. Lyon, M. F., and Hulse, E. V.: An inherited kidney disease of mice resembling human nephronophthisis. J. Med. Genet. *8*:41, 1971.
5. Perkoff, G. T.: The hereditary renal diseases. New Eng. J. Med. *177*:79, 129, 1967.
6. Potter, E. I., and Osathanondh, V.: Normal and abnormal development of the kidney. *In* F. K. M. Mostofi and D. E. Smith, The Kidney. Baltimore, Williams and Wilkins, 1966.
7. Royer, P., Frézal, J., Bois, E., and Feingold, J.: Les néphropathies héréditaires. Arch. franç. Pediat. *27*:293, 1970.
8. Turchini, J.: Recherches récentes sur l'induction enzymatique. *In* E. Wolff: De l'embryologie expérimentale à la biologie moleculaire. Dunod, Paris, 1967.
9. Whalen, R. E., and McIntosh, H. D.: The spectrum of hereditary renal diseases. Amer. J. Med. *33*:282, 1962.
10. Zweymüller, E.: Genetically determined diseases of the kidney. Wien. Klin. Wschr. *79*:382, 1967.
For recent additions to the literature, see:
a. Egli, F., and Stalder, G.: Malformations of kidney and urinary tract in common chromosomal aberrations. Human Genet. *18*:1, 1973.

Chapter Two

MALFORMATIONS OF
THE KIDNEY

These are sometimes hereditary or secondary to chromosomal aberrations. Most often they result from some accidental disturbance of development of unknown origin. Such anomalies of the kidneys are sometimes associated with malformations of the urinary tract as well.

ANOMALIES OF POSITION AND NUMBER

Some abnormalities, such as simple malrotation of the kidney, unilateral renal aplasia with compensatory hypertrophy of the contralateral kidney, the very rare true supernumerary kidney, and iliac or pelvic ectopia, usually are well tolerated and have no pathologic significance. Fusion of the two kidneys can take various forms; the most common variety is the horseshoe kidney, in which the two kidneys are joined by an isthmus of renal tissue in front of the vertebrae, with malposition of the kidneys, pelves, and calyces. The horseshoe kidney may give rise to various complications, such as hematuria, pyuria, and calculi. This condition is easily diagnosed by intravenous urography.

RENAL HYPOPLASIA

The renal hypoplasias are not hereditary. They are disorders of development acquired during intrauterine life and the intrafamilial prognosis is good. There are at least five varieties. In *simple hypoplasia* (unilateral or bilateral), the kidney tissue is found to be normal on biopsy. This condition causes no problems and is discovered only by chance. In *cortical hypoplasia*, the renal cortex is very thin, and this condition is sometimes accompanied by various malformations of the urinary tract. *Hypoplasia with dysplasia* is characterized by the presence of fetal tubules, immature glomeruli, undifferentiated mesenchyme, cortical cysts, and islets of cartilage. It may occur unilaterally or bilaterally, and may be diffuse or patchy. This type is often associated with malformation of the urinary tract and persistent urinary infection. In some cases, it is isolated and bilateral, producing chronic renal insufficiency. Multicystic kidney is a particular form of this condition, in which there is renal hypoplasia with intense cystic dysplasia. The two remaining types of renal hypoplasia, *oligomeganephronia* and *segmental hypoplasia*, merit more detailed description.

9

Oligomeganephronia

Oligomeganephronia is a condition we have described in children suffering from chronic uremia of early onset. In this condition, there is bilateral renal hypoplasia with a reduction in the number as well as hypertrophy of the nephrons.[8, 9] The characteristic features of the condition are: it is congenital but not familial; both kidneys are reduced in size; there is considerable hypertrophy of the glomeruli and tubules, and a secondary interstitial fibrosis that is not inflammatory; there is an alarming degree of renal failure in the first two years of life, but this remains stable for many years before going on to terminal uremia. This disorder provides a spontaneous model in man of the effects of reduction in the nephron population with defective conservation of water and sodium. Other authors have confirmed our description[1, 3, 4, 7] and added further information. Glomerulometric studies have shown that the hypoplastic kidneys continue to grow.[2] Microdissection reveals a considerable increase in the length of the nephrons.[5] In addition, electron microscopy has revealed ultrastructural abnormalities.[10] The condition has been recorded in a girl but was absent from her identical twin;[10] also, it has been associated with auditory, ocular, and mental abnormalities[6] and has been recorded in a case of single kidney with aplasia of the contralateral kidney.[11] The following description is derived from our own cases.

Anatomy

Macroscopic Appearance.   Both kidneys weigh less than normal and often one is smaller than the other. The actual weights vary from 12 to 45 g., with a mean of about 20 to 25 g. The kidneys are pale and firm, with an irregularly granular surface. On section, no clear distinction can be found between the cortex and medulla, and there are only five or six kidney segments, much fewer than normal. No abnormalities of the upper urinary tract or of the blood vessels have been found. The bladder is generally large and thick-walled.

Microscopic Appearance.   The *number* of glomeruli per field at equal magnification is on average one fifth of the number found in a normal kidney from a child of the same age. The *diameter* of the glomeruli varies from 250 to 325 micrometers (μm.), compared to a mean diameter of 100 to 150 μm. in normal children of the same age (Figure 1). The glomerular volume is seven to 10 times as great as in normal subjects.[3, 9] Microdissection shows that the nephron is very much longer than normal.[5] In the simplest cases, the only really obvious features are the scant number of glomeruli and their hypertrophy, and also the hypertrophy of the juxtaglomerular apparatus and the increased diameter of the proximal convoluted tubules. However, there is no abnormality of glomerular morphology apart from the hypertrophy of the epithelial cells, whose cytoplasm is abnormally basophilic. The tubular epithelium is also normal. Distinct bands of fibrosis may be seen in the interstitial tissue (Figure 2).

In other cases, in addition to the reduction in number and the increase in volume of the glomeruli, there may be various *modifications* of the renal parenchyma of varying degree. These affect chiefly the interstitial tissue and the tubules and are not necessarily a function of age, but serial studies have shown an unrelenting progression that can be divided into three stages: pure oligo-

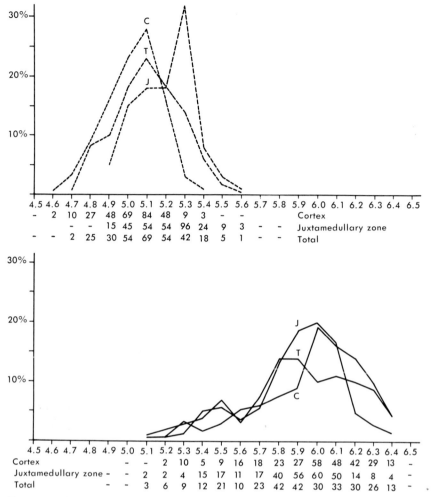

	4.5	4.6	4.7	4.8	4.9	5.0	5.1	5.2	5.3	5.4	5.5	5.6	5.7	5.8	5.9	6.0	6.1	6.2	6.3	6.4	6.5	
	-	2	10	27	48	69	84	48	9	3	-	-										Cortex
		-	-	15	45	54	54	96	24	9	3	-	-									Juxtamedullary zone
	-	-	2	25	30	54	69	54	42	18	5	1	-	-								Total

	4.5	4.6	4.7	4.8	4.9	5.0	5.1	5.2	5.3	5.4	5.5	5.6	5.7	5.8	5.9	6.0	6.1	6.2	6.3	6.4	6.5
Cortex				-	-	2	10	5	9	16	18	23	27	58	48	42	29	13	-		
Juxtamedullary zone	-	-	2	2	4	15	17	11	17	40	56	60	50	14	8	4	-				
Total			-	-	3	6	9	12	21	10	23	42	42	30	33	30	26	13	-		

Figure 1. Glomerulometric curve of the logarithmic values of glomerular volumes: upper graph, in the normal child; lower graph, in oligomeganephronia. Note the greatly increased glomerular volumes in oligomeganephronia. *C*, cortex; *J*, juxtamedullary zone; *T*, total.

meganephronia; the appearance of interstitial and periglomerular fibrosis with some tubular lesions; dense interstitial fibrosis, with some of the glomeruli partially or totally hyalinized; and gross tubular lesions.

Clinical Features

Oligomeganephronia is not hereditary. It occurs in boys three times more often than in girls. It is rarely associated with other congenital malformations. In 33 per cent of cases the birth weight of the infant is less than 2500 g. Also, in one third of the cases, the mother was 35 years or older.

Natural History. In 75 per cent of cases, the disease presents very early, in the first days or months of life, and it progresses in three stages.

INITIAL STAGE. In breast-fed infants, the symptoms tend to appear between 4 and 6 months, but symptoms often date from the neonatal period in infants fed with formulas or cow's milk. The principal clinical features in the first

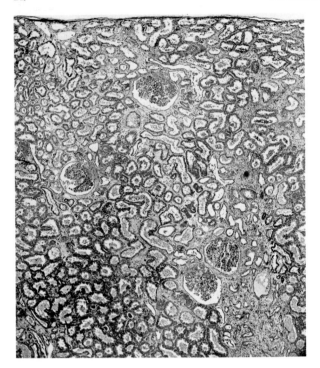

Figure 2. Oligonephronic hypoplasia. The glomeruli are sparse, enlarged, and in places partly hyalinized. There is diffuse interstitial fibrosis and also foci of tubular atrophy. ×25.

two years of life are gastrointestinal disorders, especially vomiting and anorexia, unexplained fever, polyuria with intense thirst, and attacks of acute dehydration. The most significant laboratory findings include a very early lowering of endogenous creatinine clearance to a figure between 10 and 50 ml./min./1.73 m.^{2}, a rise in the blood urea value to between 50 and 200 mg. per 100 ml., and especially loss of concentrating power in the kidney so that the urine has a maximum specific gravity between 1.007 and 1.012. Moderate proteinuria is common but not constant. Neither red nor white blood cells are found in the urine. The blood potassium and sodium levels are normal. The plasma pH is often below 7.30, and there are low bicarbonate and high blood chloride levels. Radiologic studies demonstrate very small kidneys. In this first stage, there is nearly always adequate concentration of contrast medium in the urine to exclude the possibility of malformation of the urinary tract.

Stage of stable uremia. The polyuria-polydipsia syndrome may be moderate or very severe. Retardation of growth, expressed as a standard deviation from the median corresponding to the chronologic age, varies from 1 to 4 standard deviations (S.D.). Abnormalities of bone structure have been noted in 40 per cent of cases. The radiologic picture may be one of rickets or of mixed renal osteopathy combining rickets and fibro-osteolysis. The degree of anemia is variable, generally moderate, relatively late in onset, and well tolerated. Hypertension does not develop. Moderate proteinuria is an almost constant finding, but there is no glycosuria or hypoaminoaciduria, and the red and white blood cell counts in the urine are normal. Water restriction tests reveal a considerable diminution in maximum specific gravity of urine (between 1.004 and 1.012), and with water loading tests the specific gravity may drop below 1.004.

The blood urea level is elevated and stable. Endogenous creatinine clearance is lowered. There is moderate acidosis, with normal blood potassium and sodium levels. Calcium, phosphorus and alkaline phosphatase levels are often within or just outside normal limits, but account must be taken of the fact that these patients may have been treated with calcium or vitamin D, or both. The urinary calcium output is usually below 1 mg./kg./24 hours. There is a renal salt losing syndrome detected by salt restriction in about 50 per cent of cases; this salt loss is usually moderate. Acid loading or ammonium chloride tests give the following results: The urinary pH drops normally, but there is an inadequate rise in titratable acidity and urinary ammonium levels. The ammonium coefficient is low, indicating defective production, but when the urinary ammonium level is corrected for the glomerular filtration rate, it is found to be normal.

Endogenous creatinine clearance corrected for surface area shows progressive deterioration, whereas the uncorrected clearance tends to remain stable for a long time (Figure 3).

STAGE OF PROGRESSIVE UREMIA. This stage presents no unusual features. The blood urea level is very high, there is marked anemia and acidosis, a low blood calcium level, and a high blood phosphorus level. Complications from water overload are common. Even in this stage, the blood pressure is generally normal or subject to increases that are only transient. There is a rapid lowering of clearances, both net and corrected for surface area. The terminal stage is reached in a matter of months and its onset is marked by the appearance of a urinary

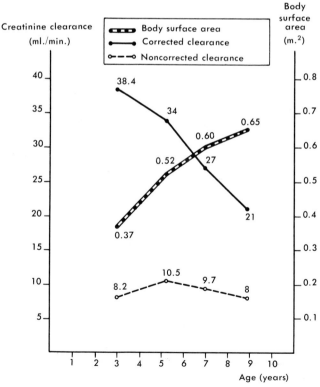

Figure 3. Oligomeganephronia: Comparative changes in body surface area (in m.²) and of endogenous creatinine clearance (in ml./min.) both uncorrected and corrected for surface area.

protein loss of over 2 g./24 hours, a stable acidosis, a deterioration in uncorrected glomerular clearance and severe anemia. Life expectancy is on the average 13 years for those cases beginning in the neonatal period and 12 years for cases presenting between 1 and 24 months.

Cases with Late Onset. In about 25 per cent of cases, the clinical onset occurs after the age of 2 years, with isolated proteinuria, failure to thrive, renal osteodystrophy, or uremic coma.

Treatment

In the first stage of the disease, treatment consists in combating the water loss by a high fluid intake and a diet that is low in osmotically active components. Salt loss and acidosis should also be treated. In the stable stage, protein intake should be limited to 1.5 g./kg./day, with a normal intake of salt and an excess water intake. Vitamin D, calcium, transfusion of packed red cells, and aluminum hydroxide may be indicated. In the terminal stage, placement on a dialysis-transplantation program is indicated when glomerular clearance falls below 5 ml./min./1.73 m.^{2}

Conclusions

Oligomeganephronia is one of the principal causes of chronic uremia of congenital origin in children. Diagnosis is not difficult and depends principally on renal biopsy. Prognosis is poor, especially after the age of 8 to 10 years. There are good indications for maintenance dialysis and kidney transplantation in this disorder. Because the condition is not hereditary, the intrafamilial prognosis is good. Two problems remain to be resolved.

What causes the reduction in number of nephrons and their hypertrophy? This reduction suggests premature interruption of the process of nephrogenesis, probably between the fourteenth and twentieth weeks of intrauterine life, at the stage when the arcades are formed. The causative factors at this "critical time" are unknown. It may be that advanced maternal age and certain (drug) intoxications are predisposing factors, but this is purely hypothetical. The factors that allow hypertrophy of the nephrons are also unknown; such hypertrophy does not occur in simple renal hypoplasia.

What causes the development of secondary interstitial fibrosis? This is a condition that occurs only rarely in the young child. The fibrosis destroys nephrons and is responsible for the transition from the stage of stability to the stage of rapidly progressing uremia. The causes of this interstitial fibrosis are unknown.

Segmental Hypoplasia (Ask-Upmark Kidney)

In 1929, Ask-Upmark[12] described a renal anomaly that he had observed in six patients with malignant nephroangiosclerosis. Five of the six patients were adolescents. The hypoplastic kidney had few pyramids and a furrowed surface, corresponding to pseudocalyceal dilatation. Histologically, beneath the furrowed areas the tubules showed a pseudo-thyroid appearance, vessels were thick-walled, and glomeruli were absent. Ask-Upmark regarded the condition as congenital. His description has been confirmed by many other authors.[13–18, 21, 23, 25]

Since 1963 we have been studying this condition in children, in whom it had not previously been recognized.[18] The following description is based on the 38 cases we have encountered.

Anatomic Description

Gross Appearance. The kidney is small, between 12 and 35 g. Its external surface is marked by one or more transverse furrows, giving the appearance of notches on the outer border. The renal arteries are small and sometimes multiple, but otherwise they are normal in appearance. On section, some segments are seen to be normal while others are atrophied. The normal segments appear identical to those of a normal kidney with the exception that they are often very much smaller than would be seen in a kidney of a normal child of the same age. The abnormal segments seldom occupy the whole kidney but may be found at either pole or between the poles. There may be several abnormal segments in the same kidney. The hypoplasia affects both cortex and medulla and is juxtaposed to the pseudodiverticular dilatation of the calyces.

Histology of the Abnormal Segments. The abnormal segments are clearly demarcated from the healthy tissue. The *medulla* is reduced to a narrow band. In the region of the corticomedullary junction, there are a few small tubular cavities filled with colloid casts. Between these tubules and the pelvic mucosa, the mesenchyme contains scattered collecting tubules arranged at random. There are no loops of Henle. The *cortex* is greatly thinned. Three abnormalities occur, affecting the glomeruli, the tubules, and the intrarenal vessels, respectively (Figure 4). In most cases, routine stains reveal no glomeruli in the abnormal zones, but PAS stains reveal glomerular vestiges in the form of small fibrohyaline masses in which the capillary network of the tuft can still

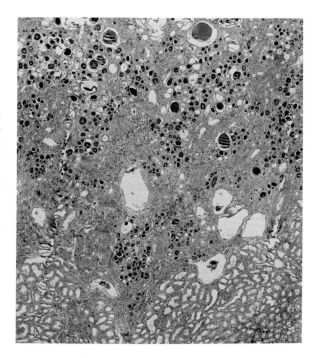

Figure 4. Segmental hypoplasia. Within an atrophic zone clearly delimited from the adjacent normal parenchyma can be noted the absence of glomeruli, the presence of numerous thyroid-like tubules, many arteries with thickened walls, and some vascular lacunae. The inflammatory infiltration of the interstitial tissue is slight. ×25.

be recognized. In some cases, alongside the so-called "aglomerular" zones, there are other areas in which the glomeruli are more easily seen; these glomeruli appear ischemic. The tubules are collapsed, lined with a clear epithelium, and have an almost invisible lumen, or alternatively they may be dilated with cubical epithelium and have a lumen filled with colloid casts, producing a pseudo-thyroid appearance. The arcuate and interlobar arteries show an intense fibroelastic chronic endarteritis that may or may not be obstructive. On section, these arteries appear much more numerous than usual because of their tortuous, corkscrew path, as demonstrated by microangiography.[21] Glomus formations are present in many cases, and doubtless form the "obstructions" in kidneys in which circulation anomalies are the main problem. In places there are vascular lacunae, which are interpreted as empty blood vessels. An important negative finding is the almost constant absence of any inflammatory infiltration of the interstitial tissue in the abnormal segments.

Histology of the Normal Segments. The normal areas may resemble normal renal parenchyma, but in some cases there are lesions secondary to hypertension, endarteritis of the medium sized vessels (never nearly so severe as the endarteritis in the abnormal segments), subendothelial hyalinization and necrosis of the afferent arterioles, and sometimes more or less segmental hyalinization of the glomerular tuft. The main renal artery is normal.

These histologic findings have been observed in kidneys removed at autopsy or at nephrectomy or renal biopsy. In theory, renal biopsy should be a useful method of confirming the diagnosis, but in practice it is difficult, even at open biopsy, to ensure that a specimen of abnormal tissue is being taken, either because, as in many cases, the abnormal tissue lies at the upper pole of the kidney or because it lies at the bottom of a furrow. More often than not, the biopsy specimen will include only "normal" tissue; however, even this has some prognostic value in giving an idea of the degree of nephroangiosclerosis secondary to hypertension and especially the degree of glomerular damage.

Clinical Features

Girls are affected twice as often as boys. The condition is not familial. It presents most often after the age of 10, but cases with severe hypertension have been seen before the age of 2 years.

Diagnosis. Diagnosis is based on clinical and radiologic findings. In the vast majority of cases, the clinical picture is of severe hypertension, with marked retinopathy occurring in half of the cases. Half of the cases also show a definite retardation of growth. Two thirds of the patients have left ventricular hypertrophy, and half present moderate or severe renal insufficiency, as revealed by a high blood urea level, reduction in glomerular clearances, and diminished ability to concentrate urine.

Urography reveals the calyceal abnormalities in the involved segments: The calyces have a swallowtail appearance (Figure 5), with diminution of the corticopapillary distance, and often lie opposite a notch on the outer border of the kidney. The moderate dilatation of the calyces contrasts with the normal size of the renal pelvis. Renal arteriography reveals a regular renal artery with a clear outline, whose caliber is in proportion to the size of the kidney—it becomes very small with severe hypoplasia. In the nephrogram phase, the notches

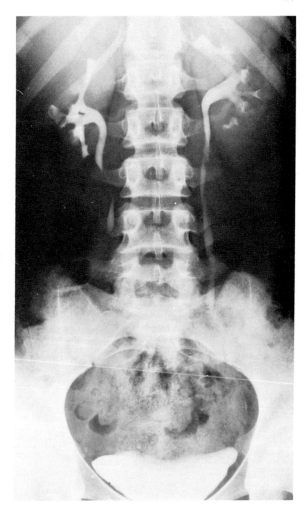

Figure 5. Intravenous urography in bilateral segmental hypoplasia. The swallowtail deformity of the calcyces can be seen in the upper poles.

on the kidney border, and also the nonvascular transverse bands corresponding to involved segments (Figure 6), are easily seen.

Prognosis. In every case, it is important to evaluate the chances of obtaining good results before advising surgery. In our experience, favorable indications are the absence of proteinuria, normal renal function, strictly unilateral disease, and the development of compensatory hypertrophy in the healthy kidney as determined by direct measurement[20] and by fixation of a radioactive isotope of mercury.[24] If part of a "normal" segment has been obtained by renal biopsy, it will give a good idea of the degree of secondary nephroangiosclerosis. The presence of hyalinization in the glomerular tufts suggests a poor prognosis when surgical relief of hypertension is being considered.

Classification

The patients in our series can be classified into five groups (Table 3).

The first group includes patients with *strictly unilateral segmental hypoplasia*. There is nearly always compensatory hypertrophy of the other kidney and

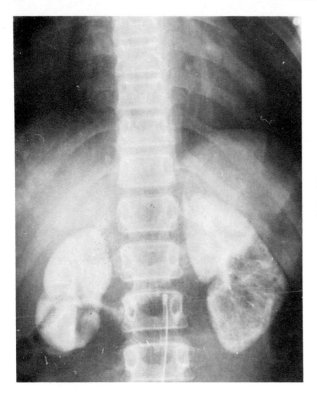

Figure 6. Aortography (nephrogram) in segmental hypoplasia. The right kidney is small and there is a deep notch on the midportion of its outer border.

compensatory hyperfixation of mercury on that side. Renal function is normal, and we have never found proteinuria. Sometimes the involved kidney is extremely small. In other cases, the diseased kidney is not quite so small and only the upper pole seems involved.

The second group includes cases of *bilateral segmental hypoplasia,* with involvement of the two sides being very different. In these cases, one of the kidneys is very small; the other is about normal size, although it has a hypoplastic segment, usually without compensatory hypertrophy. Renal function is slightly if at all diminished, at least in the early stages, but in nine of 11 cases there was proteinuria.

The third group includes *bilateral segmental hypoplasia* with almost equal

Table 3. Segmental Hypoplasia of Kidney: Classification of Author's Series (1970)

Only one kidney affected	9
Both kidneys affected but very unequally	11
Bilateral disease	12
Latent segmental hypoplasia	3
Segmental hypoplasia with malformation of the urinary tract	3
Total	38

involvement of the two sides. Both kidneys are small, with one or more segments involved. Proteinuria is common. Renal insufficiency is the rule, with a blood urea level above 50 mg. per 100 ml. There is no compensatory hypertrophy.

The fourth group includes *latent forms*. These patients are children with segmental hypoplasia of a kidney without hypertension or renal insufficiency. The condition is discovered by chance. The existence of this latent form is not surprising, because sometimes hypertension does not set in until adult life.

The fifth group includes *segmental hypoplasia* with special problems, owing to the association of malformations of the urinary tract or renal dysplasia.

Therapeutic Problems

The plan of treatment is variable. In strictly unilateral cases, with one very small kidney and compensatory hypertrophy on the other side, but with no segmental involvement of the hypertrophied kidney, removal of the small kidney or of the involved pole of that kidney always cures the hypertension.

In the symmetrical bilateral forms with renal insufficiency, the hypertension can generally be controlled satisfactorily by medical treatment with hypotensive drugs if the treatment is carefully maintained. Some patients have been maintained in good health in this way for many years. Others have died of uremia. Those who reach terminal renal failure should be considered for a dialysis-transplantation program.

There is a choice of two approaches for the asymmetrical bilateral forms. The first approach is medical treatment, and this is satisfactory if carefully controlled. The second approach is removal of the smaller kidney and partial nephrectomy of the involved segment in the other kidney.[23]

Monitoring the blood pressure every three months and renal function once a year is all that is necessary for the latent forms.

Conclusions

In children, segmental hypoplasia of the kidney is one of the principal causes of serious hypertension, and when the condition is bilateral it is one of the main causes of chronic uremia.

Classification. The classification into five groups shows that the concept of segmental hypoplasia, initially applied to very small unilateral kidneys, has subsequently been extended to very asymmetrical bilateral forms and then to a disease affecting both kidneys virtually to the same extent. The degree of renal insufficiency depends on the degree of bilateral involvement. The condition may be latent. It may also be associated with dysplasia and malformations of the urinary tract. This classification contrasts the benign nature of the unilateral forms with the seriousness of bilateral forms, especially when these are symmetrical (i.e., when there is no compensatory hypertrophy). It is evident that both the development of chronic uremia and the success or failure of nephrectomy in curing hypertension depend much more on the diffusion of the lesions than on nephroangiosclerosis secondary to hypertension, although the latter factor is not negligible.

Nature of the Embryopathy. There is no evidence of genetic transmission. The presence of segments that are normal although very small, the narrow but otherwise normal renal artery, and the near absence of the medulla are all arguments against inflammatory or ischemically produced postnatal contraction of a kidney that was originally healthy and of normal size. There seems little doubt that the renal hypoplasia is the result of an embryopathy. The special anatomic features of segmental hypoplasia suggest that the accident occurs at a stage at which the kidney already has the structure of an adult organ but is still very small. Because of the severity of the vascular lesions and the possibility of interpreting the other features as secondary to ischemia, it might be suggested that the accident initially affected either the development or the permeability of certain intrarenal arteries. There is however, no direct proof of this hypothesis.

Mechanism of the Hypertension.   It is possible that the hypertension that frequently accompanies segmental hypoplasia, albeit in an inconstant fashion and at very different periods of life, belongs to the category of renovascular hypertension with hyperreninemia. Measurements of the renin in peripheral venous blood, in the inferior vena cava, or in the renal veins themselves have confirmed a high renin level in some cases,[16, 22, 23] but in other cases the results have been normal or contradictory, especially in some of our own patients. More information is needed on this point. If in fact overproduction of renin is confirmed, it still has to be explained how an ischemic segment of kidney, whose removal cures hypertension, elaborates renin when no juxtaglomerular apparatus can be found in this segment. It is possible that undifferentiated cortical arterioles may play some part in the elaboration of hypertensive agents.[19]

CYSTS OF THE KIDNEY*

Renal cysts, which are common, may be closed cavities, or they may open into the urinary tract. Much is still obscure about their classification and morphogenesis, despite study in serial sections and microdissection.[39] Certain aspects of renal cystic disease can be reproduced in adult rats or in the litters of pregnant rats by the administration of a diphenylamine, the impurities of which have been found to be the teratogenic factors.[32]

Cystic diseases may be divided into hereditary and nonhereditary types.

Hereditary Cystic Diseases

The Hereditary Polycystic Diseases

These are diffuse polycystic diseases affecting both kidneys. It is usual to distinguish three varieties—infantile, juvenile, and adult.

Infantile Polycystic Disease.[30, 32-34, 38]   This condition is transmitted as an autosomal recessive trait. There may be several subvarieties.[31]

Infantile polycystic disease often proves fatal in the *perinatal period.* The kidneys are enormous. The facies are often abnormal (Potter syndrome). There may be associated malformations in the nervous, gastrointestinal, skeletal, muscular, genitourinary, cardiovascular, and pulmonary systems. Death in the neonatal period often occurs from respiratory failure owing to atelectasis or pneumomediastinum.

---

*This section has been written in collaboration with Dr. Micheline Levy.

It is certain that a significant number of cases may run a *prolonged course.*
In one sibship both perinatal death and prolonged survival may be observed,[34, 35]
The early manifestations include large kidneys, hypertension, uremia, anemia,
a salt-losing syndrome, defective concentration of urine, and, more rarely,
hematuria and persistent urinary infection. Intravenous urography reveals the
large bosselated kidneys, elongation and curvilinear deformity of the calyceal
stems, and sometimes persistence of dye in the medulla with the nephrogram
still present after 24 hours. Some children die in the first year, but most survive
much longer, perhaps 10 years or more,[38] during which time the kidneys reduce in size, the uremia is stabilized, and the hypertension disappears. In some
children there is a large palpable liver and portal hypertension ensues, hence the
necessity in all cases to look for esophageal varices and to perform a liver
biopsy.[35, 38]

The anatomic lesions in the kidney are diffuse cystic dilatations lined by
flat or cuboidal epithelium (honeycomb or sponge kidney). There are zones of
normal renal parenchyma, especially in the subcapsular region. These zones are
very limited in patients who die early but may be quite extensive in children
who survive for many years. In the latter patients, repeated biopsy has revealed
the development of progressive interstitial fibrosis. Microdissection shows that
the abnormality is localized to the collecting tubules (Group 1 of Osathanondh
and Potter). In the liver there is always interstitial fibrosis, with dilatation of the
biliary ducts and the canals of Hering. Cysts may also be found in the pancreas,
thymus, lungs, and seminal vesicles.

Juvenile Polycystic Disease.[26, 30, 32, 37]   This type is transmitted as an autosomal recessive trait and generally appears in children between the ages of 5
and 10 years. The condition is commonly called "congenital hepatic fibrosis"
or "biliary fibroadenomatosis." In fact, in the great majority of cases, the clinical
features depend on the hepatic involvement—a large, firm liver, portal hypertension, and sometimes cholangitis. Generally the serum alkaline phosphatase
levels are raised, with bromsulphalein retention and esophageal varices. The
renal involvement, which is sometimes latent, is most commonly manifested
by proteinuria, uremia, hypertension, defective concentration of urine and large
kidneys with deformed pelvis and calyces on intravenous urography. Renal
insufficiency may develop after treatment of the portal hypertension.

The liver lesions are more severe and the kidney lesions less diffuse, but
otherwise the condition resembles that seen in the newborn. An abnormality
that is sometimes associated is *intracranial aneurysm,* and the incidence of this
complication is much higher than in other renal diseases.

Adult Polycystic Disease.   This is a common condition, transmitted as
an autosomal dominant trait. Little is known about the course of the condition in childhood, but some cases may present clinically and radiologically
at an early age.

The three types of polycystic disease are not yet clearly defined. It is
possible, though rare, to find the "adult type" of polycystic disease in children,
and from genetic and histologic viewpoints this type is well defined; there are
no hepatic lesions or only very localized ones, and the liver is not enlarged.
It is possible, on the other hand, that the juvenile and infantile types are not
truly distinct, and that they form but one group of polycystic hepatorenal
disease transmitted as an autosomal recessive, which, because of variation in the

renal lesions, presents as four *subgroups* with different prognoses in the prenatal, neonatal, infantile, and juvenile periods.[31]

Other Hereditary Cysts

The Meckel syndrome is an infantile polycystic disease of the kidneys associated with encephalocele or anencephaly. In another syndrome the cerebral malformation of Dandy-Walker is associated with polycystic disease. In the *hepato-cerebro-renal syndrome* of Zellweger, transmitted as an autosomal recessive, a peculiar craniofacial deformity occurs, associated with severe hypotonia, cortical cysts of the kidney, hepatomegaly, and a Sudanophil leukodystrophy; the condition proves fatal within a few weeks.

Cortical *cysts* have been noted in the phakomatoses: tuberous sclerosis and von Hippel-Lindau disease,[33] in the oral-facial-digital syndrome, and in asphyxiating thoracic dystrophy. Cysts of the renal cortex have also been found in trisomies E and D, which are nonhereditary chromosomal aberrations.

Two hereditary varieties of renal cysts pose special problems: *microcystic disease of the kidney*, which is considered with the congenital nephrotic syndrome (see page 47), and *medullary cystic disease*, which seems to be closely related to nephronophthisis (see page 42).

Nonhereditary Cystic Diseases

Cysts Without Dysplasia[34, 37]

Parapelvic Cyst. This is rare in children. It is a cyst that develops beside the pelvis or in the hilum, which may limit its expansion. It produces a filling defect on intravenous urography. The origin of parapelvic cyst is disputed.

Pyelogenic Cyst (Calyceal Diverticulum or Cystic Diverticulum of the Calyces). This results from an abnormality of the junction of parenchyma and calyx and is characterized by a cystic cavity of varying size communicating with the calyces close to the fornix by a narrow channel, which is rarely obvious on intravenous urography. Most commonly it is a chance radiologic discovery. In some cases it may give rise to abdominal pain, urinary infection, or lithiasis.

Serous Cysts. These cysts are unilateral, and most often they occur singly, although there may be two or three cysts in one kidney. Their site in the cortex is variable—they may occur within the parenchyma or in the subcapsular region. They vary greatly in size from small cysts that are discovered only radiologically to very large cysts that present as an abdominal mass. On intravenous urography there is a regular homogenous shadow that deforms the pelvis and calyces but rarely obstructs them. Selective renal angiography associated with nephrotomography will distinguish this condition from Wilms' tumor: in the arterial phase the vessels are seen to be displaced and curved around the cyst, and the nephrogram shows an avascular zone with regular outlines.

Multilocular Cyst (Cystadenoma). The cyst is composed of multiple juxtaposed cavities separated by strands of connective and vascular tissue. It often occupies one pole of the kidney, with the normal renal parenchyma stretched out as a narrow band. It presents clinically as an abdominal mass and must be distinguished from malignant tumor, but in many cases the true diagnosis is evident only at operation.

Renal Dysplasia with Cysts

Histologically, renal dysplasia is characterized by primitive tubules surrounded by fibromuscular rings in association with islets of cartilage in the renal cortex. There may also be primitive glomeruli and cysts.

Cystic dysplasia may be unilateral or bilateral, segmental or diffuse, and there may or may not be associated abnormalities of the urinary tract. Four types can be distinguished.

Cystic Dysplasia Associated with Lower Urinary Tract Obstruction.[27] This is doubtless due to the effects of hydroureter and hydronephrosis on renal development. The inner cortex appears normal, whereas the cysts and the dysplasia are found at the periphery; the medulla shows a few sparse tubules scattered throughout a dense tissue. Microdissection studies reveal dilatations at the extremity of the collecting tubules. Bilateral cystic dysplasia is most frequently associated with persistent urethral valves, urethral atresia, and sometimes with megaureter-megacystis. Unilateral obstruction is associated with dysplasia on the same side; a dysplastic renal segment may represent obstruction of one ureter compressed by a ureterocele in cases of ureteral duplication.

Segmental Cystic Dysplasia.[28, 29] The patient presents with abdominal pain or stone, and intravenous urography demonstrates a small kidney with deformed pelvis and calyces, the deformity often being restricted to the upper pole of the kidney. The kidney has fewer lobes than normal, but the general architecture is preserved. The cysts are mainly subcapsular.

Bilateral involvement is possible, in which case the condition presents with gastrointestinal disturbances, retardation of growth, and rapidly progressive renal failure.

Multicystic Dysplasia. The dysplasia and cystic degeneration may be more severe in *multicystic kidney.* The major form is aglomerular multicystic aplasia.[28, 29, 34, 37] The most common presenting sign is an abdominal mass in a newborn or older child. Ring calcification of the cysts may be visible on plain x-ray films. On intravenous urography, the involved kidney is not visualized. At cystoscopy, the ureteral orifice is nearly always absent, but it is sometimes possible to catheterize the ureter for a few centimeters. On examination, the kidney is unrecognizable as such. It may be small, but it is often very large and deformed by masses of cysts joined by dense connective tissue, containing primitive glomeruli, primitive tubules, and dysplastic elements (Figure 7). The cysts do not communicate with the urinary tract. The renal vessels are very small and the "kidney" has a poor blood supply. Microangiography shows a defect in corticomedullary differentiation. Microdissection of this lesion (Group II of Osathanondh and Potter) shows that nephrons are almost nonexistent, that there is a reduction in the number of divisions of the collecting tubules, and that most of the tubules terminate in cysts.

The prognosis for unilateral multicystic kidney is excellent after nephrectomy. However, frequently there are abnormalities in the urinary tract on the contralateral side and these must be sought and treated.

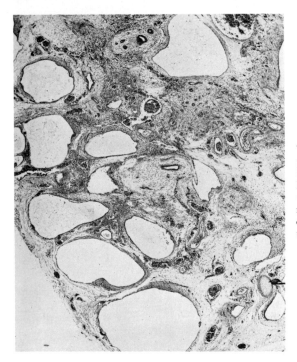

Figure 7. Multicystic kidney. There is no trace of recognizable renal parenchyma, which is replaced by connective and vascular tissue containing large cystic formations and some primitive tubules surrounded by a cuff of mesenchymal tissue. Note also the presence in the center of an island of cartilage. ×24.

Bilateral multicystic disease may be found in the newborn. It is probably the most common form of cystic disease in this age group (see page 119).

Pluricystic Hypoplasia. In six cases we have found a peculiar variety called *"pluricystic hypoplasia with dysplasia."* Within a few days of birth, these children present with renal failure and rapidly progressive acidosis. The kidneys are small and there are no malformations of the urinary tract. There are regular dilatations of all the tubules in the cortex and dysplastic elements are constantly found (Habib [unpublished data]) (Figure 8).

Although the dysplasia is usually sporadic, *familial cases* have recently been reported.[27, 38] Cystic dysplasia is sometimes associated with cerebral malformations and disease in the pancreas and liver (dilatation of the pancreatic ducts and proliferation of the biliary ducts) (Ivemark syndrome).

Medullary Sponge Kidney (Cacchi-Ricci Disease, Medullary Tubulectasis)

Some authors regard this condition as hereditary,[30, 32] others disagree.[40] It is the result of a failure of development of the collecting tubules in the medulla. The cysts communicate with the calyces. Medullary sponge kidney has been found at autopsy in infants but is very rarely diagnosed in children.[34, 36, 37] The clinical picture is the same in children as in adults—lumbar pain, renal colic, hematuria, pyuria, and proteinuria. Renal function is normal. The clinical features are due to infection and lithiasis. A plain x-ray film will often show nephrocalcinosis in the form of tiny stones in the papillary part of the pyramids. The cysts are apparent on the earliest films in intravenous urography, and they remain opaque for a long time. The cysts can take various shapes, such as rounded or triangular or opaque parallel streaks. Various

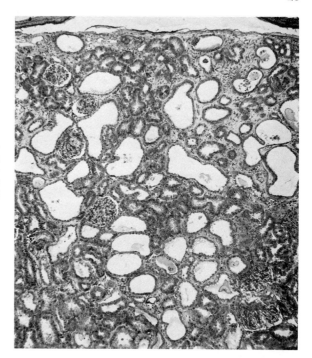

Figure 8. Pluricystic hypoplasia. Note the presence, within otherwise normal renal parenchyma, of numerous cystic cavities whose tubular nature is indicated by the epithelial border. ×60.

descriptive terms (such as mottled, flame-shaped, and bouquet of flowers) have been applied to the appearance of the cysts. The pelvi-calyceal system is generally normal, but associated deformities of the ureters have been described.

Conclusions

Kidney cysts are common in childhood. Their morphogenesis, classification, and diagnosis need to be clarified in the future, and genetic studies will obviously be important. It is already possible to distinguish clearly between hereditary hepatorenal polycystic disease with its various evolutionary potentials and nonhereditary cysts with or without renal dysplasia. The individual and intrafamilial prognosis and treatment vary enormously in the different varieties of cysts.

REFERENCES

OLIGOMEGANEPHRONIA

1. Bueno, M., Hermida, F., Vasquez, J., Ferragut, J., Guerendiain, J. M., and Garcia-Fuentes, M.: Hipoplasia renal oligonefronica. Bol. Soc. Vasco-Navarra Pediat. *4*:273, 1969.
2. Callis, L., Castello, F., Vidal, M. T., and De Fortuny, G.: Hypoplasie rénale avec oligonéphronie. Arch. franç. Pédiat. *27*:267, 1970.
3. Carter, J. E., and Lirenman, D.: Bilateral renal hypoplasia with oligomeganephronia. Amer. J. Dis. Child. *120*:537, 1970.
4. Cruveilier, J., Boquet, L., and Dun, N. M.: Etude clinique, biologique et anatomique d'un cas d'oligonéphronie. Sem. Hôp. Paris *42*:3306, 1966.
5. Fetterman, G. H., and Habib, R.: Congenital bilateral oligonephronic renal hypoplasia with hypertrophy of nephrons (oligomeganephronia). Amer. J. Clin. Path. *52*:199, 1969.
6. Hirooka, M., Kubota, N., and Ohno, T.: Congenital nephropathy associated with hearing

loss, ocular abnormalities, mental retardation, convulsions, and abnormal EEG. Tohoku J. Exp. Med. *98*:329, 1969.

7. Roget, J., Beaudoing, A., Couderc, P., and Lagier, A.: Un cas d'insuffisance rénale chronique à début précoce avec rachitisme sévère: hypoplasie rénale bilatérale oligonéphronique. Pédiatrie *20*:969, 1965.

8. Royer, P., Habib, R., Mathieu, H., and Courtecuisse, V.: L'hypophasie rénale bilatérale congénitale avec réduction du nombre et hypertrophie des néphrons chez l'enfant. Ann. Pédiat. *38*:753, 1962.

9. Royer, P., Habib, R., Courtecuisse, V., and Leclerc, F.: L'hypoplasie rénale bilatérale avec oligonéphronie. Arch. franç. Pédiat. *24*:249, 1967.

10. Scheinman, J. I., and Abelson, H. T.: Bilateral renal hypoplasia with oligonephronia. J. Pediat. *76*:369, 1970.

11. Van Acker, K. J., Vincke, H., Quatacker, J., Senesael, L., and Van Den Brande, J.: Congenital oligonephronic renal hypoplasia with hypertrophy of nephrons (oligonephronia). Arch. Dis. Child. *46*:321, 1971.

SEGMENTAL HYPOPLASIA

12. Ask-Upmark, E.: Über juvenile maligne Nephrosclerose und ihr Verhältnis zu Störungen in der Nierenentwicklung. Acta Path. Microb. Scand. 7:383, 1929.

13. Batzenschlager, A., Blum, E., and Weill-Bousson, M.: Le petit rein unilatéral (étude anatomo-clinique). Ann. Anat. Pathol. 7:427, 539, 1962.

14. Chaptal, K., Jean, R., Bonnet, H., Pages, A., Dumas, R., and Baldet, P.: Hypertension artérielle secondaire à une hypoplasie rénale segmentaire. J. Méd. Montpellier, *3*:325, 1968.

15. Fahr, T.: Uber Pyelonephritische Schrumfniere und hypogenetische Nephritis. Virchow. Arch. Path. Anat. *301*:140, 1938.

16. Favre, R.: Hypertension artérielle rénale et son traitement chirurgical. Helv. Paediat. Acta *22*:54, 1967.

17. Guedon, J., Cormier, J. M., and Wascher, G.: Les hypertensions artérielles avec petit rein unilatéral. Problèmes diagnostiques et thérapeutiques. Presse méd. *74*:1805, 1966.

18. Habib, R., Courtecuisse, V., Ehrensperger, J., and Royer, P.: Hypoplasie segmentaire du rein avec hypertension artérielle chez l'enfant. Ann. Pédiat. *12*:262, 1965.

19. Hatt, P. Y., Duojakovic, M., and Cornet, P.: Contribution de la microscopie électronique à l'étude du mécanisme de l'hypertension artérielle expérimentale d'origine rénale. Path. Biol. *10*:23, 1962.

20. Jodson, C. J., Drewe, J. A., Karn, M. N., and King, A.: Renal size in normal children. Arch. Dis. Child. *37*:616, 1962.

21. Ljungqvist, A., and Lagergren, C.: The Ask-Upmark kidney. Acta Path. Microbiol. Scand. *56*:277, 1962.

22. Meyer, P., Ecoiffier, J., Guize, L., Alexandre, J. M., Devaux, C., and Milliez, P.: Valeur de la détermination de l'activité rénine plasmatique dans la prévision de la curabilité chirurgicale d'une hypertension d'origine rénale. In Actualités Néphrologiques Hôpital Necker. Paris, Flammarion, 1967.

23. Mozziconacci, P., Attal, G., Boisse, J., Pham-Huu-Trung, M. T.: Guy-Grand, D., and Durand, C.: Hypoplasie segmentaire du rein avec hypertension artérielle. Ann. Pédiat. *15*:337, 1968.

24. Raynaud, C., Schoutens, A., and Royer, P.: Intérêt de la mesure du taux de la fixation rénale du Hg dans l'étude de l'hypertrophie rénale compensatrice chez l'homme. Nephron 5:300, 1968.

25. Spach, M. O., Imbs, J. L., and Schwartz, J.: Hypertension artérielle de l'adulte par hypoplasie segmentaire aglomérulaire. Presse méd. *78*:1879, 1970.

KIDNEY CYSTS

26. Benhamou, J. P., Antoine, B., Debray, C., Nézelof, C., Roux, M., Watchi, J. M., and Pequignot, H.: La fibrose hépatique congénitale. Presse méd. *77*:167, 1969.

27. Bernstein, J., and Meyer, R.: Parenchymal maldevelopment of the kidney. In Brennemann and Kelley: Practice of Pediatrics. Vol. III. New York, Harper and Row, 1967.

28. Bernstein, J.: Developmental abnormalities of the renal parenchyma. Renal hypoplasia and dysplasia. In S. C. Sommers: Pathology Annual 1968. New York, Appleton-Century-Crofts. 1968.

29. Bernstein, J.: The morphogenesis of renal parenchymal maldevelopment (renal dysplasia). Ped. Clin. N. Amer. *18*:395, 1971.

30. Bernstein, J.: Heritable cystic disorders of the kidney. The mythology of polycystic disease. Ped. Clin. N. Amer. *18*:435, 1971.

31. Blyth, H., and Ockenden, B. G.: Polycystic disease of kidneys and liver presenting in child-hood. J. Med. Genet. *8*:257, 1971.
32. Crocker, F. S., Brown, D. M., Borch, R. F., and Vernier, R. L.: Renal cystic disease induced in newborn rats by diphenylamine derivates. Amer. J. Pathol. *66*:343, 1972.
33. Elkin, M., and Bernstein, J.: Cystic diseases of the kidney. Radiological and pathological con-siderations. Clin. Radiol. *20*:65, 1968.
34. Fauré, C.: Les maladies kystiques des reins chez l'enfant. J. Can. Ass. Radiol. *18*:356, 1967.
35. Gaisford, W., and Bloor, K.: Congenital polycystic disease of kidneys and liver. Portal hyper-tension. Portacaval anastomosis. Proc. Roy. Soc. Med. *61*:304, 1968.
36. Habib, R., Mouzet-Mazza, M. T., Courtecuisse, V., and Royer, P.: L'ectasie canaliculaire pré-calcielle. Ann. Pédiat. *12*:288, 1965.
37. Lemaître, G. W., Michel, J., and Tavernier, J.: Kystes du rein. *In* Traité de radiodiagnostic. Paris, Masson, 1970.
38. Lieberman, E., Salinas-Madrigal, L., Gwinn, J., Brennan, P., Fine, R., and Landing, B.: In-fantile polycystic disease of the kidneys and liver. Clinical, pathological, and radiological correlations and comparison with congenital hepatic fibrosis. Medicine *50*:277, 1971.
39. Osathanondh, V., and Potter, E.: Pathogenesis of polycystic kidneys. Arch. Path. *77*:459, 1964.
40. Torti, G., D'Amico, E., and Radice, G.: Malattia di Cacchi e Ricci. Min. Pediat. *22*:1883, 1970.

For recent additions to the literature, see:
a. Lyons, E. A., Murphy, A. V., and Arneil, G. C.: Sonar and its use in kidney disease in children. Arch. Dis. Child. *47*:777, 1972.
b. Naffah, J., Ghosn, G., and Gharios, N.: A propos de trois nouveaux cas dans une même fratrie de syndrome de Meckel. Arch. franç. Pédiat. *29*:1069, 1972.
c. Vuthibhadgee, A., and Singleton, E. B.: Infantile polycystic disease of the kidney. Amer. J. Dis. Child. *125*:167, 1973.

Chapter Three

EMBRYONAL TUMORS*

TUMOR OF THE RENAL BLASTEMA
(NEPHROBLASTOMA OR WILMS' TUMOR)

Incidence

These tumors, called nephroblastomas or tumors of the renal blastema, were described by Wilms in 1899. Wilms' tumor occurs in approximately two in every 100,000 children between the ages of 1 and 4 years. Eighty per cent of cases present between the ages of 1 and 5; certain forms are congenital. The sexes are affected equally, and cases have been described in adolescents and even in adults. There seems to be a slightly higher incidence on the left side than on the right; approximately 5 per cent are bilateral. These tumors account for about one fifth of all malignant tumors in childhood.[7, 8, 15]

There is a particular association between these tumors and certain congenital malformations, and children with such malformations constitute a high-risk population. The malformations include hemihypertrophy of the body, sometimes limited to one limb or to the face[3]; aniridia, often associated with microcephaly (aniridia is found in one in 80 cases of nephroblastoma, in contrast to an incidence of one in 50,000 births in the general population)[19]; and urogenital malformations.[2] Some familial cases have been reported, and it has been established that certain nephroblastomas are hereditary, in which case the clinical presentation is often early and bilateral.

Pathologic Anatomy

These are very large tumors that may weigh over 1 kg. They develop in the parenchyma and are separated from the healthy kidney by a pseudocapsule. They may invade the renal vessels or the calyces, and they may extend through the capsule and rupture into the peritoneal cavity.

Histologically, these tumors resemble the mesonephros, and consist of two parts. The blastemic part comprises small undifferentiated cells interspersed with zones of epithelium showing varying degrees of differentiation into tubules and glomeruli. The sarcomatous, fibroblastic part very commonly contains cells differentiating into muscle tissue and sometimes even chondroblasts or osteoblasts. Small blastemic islets have been found at autopsy in apparently normal kidneys in newborn children, and these islets may be the source of Wilms' tumors.

---

*This chapter was written in collaboration with Odile Schweisguth and Françoise Flamant.

28

Clinical Features

In the great majority of cases, the initial symptom is a swelling, which is palpable in 95 per cent of cases. The tumor may be found by chance at routine examination or during examination for some commonplace problem, such as gastrointestinal disorder or abdominal pain. The tumor fills the lumbar fossa and rapidly extends forward. It may extend beyond the umbilicus and down into the iliac fossa as far as the pubis. The tumor is firm, smooth or nodular, and not well defined, and because of its size it is not mobile.

Episodes of painless hematuria occur in 25 per cent of cases. However, hematuria is the first symptom in only 10 per cent of patients, and then it may precede the discovery of the tumor by weeks or even months. Such hematuria is always an indication for intravenous urography. One case in 10 presents as an acute surgical problem, in rare instances as a result of hemorrhage and intraperitoneal rupture, most often because of acute abdominal pain, often of a type suggesting the diagnosis of appendicitis. Apart from the swelling, the clinical examination is generally negative; a varicocele has been noted on the left side on rare occasions. The blood pressure is normal or slightly raised, and overall renal function is normal. The general condition usually is good, although there may be fever, dysuria, and digestive upsets. Severe hypertension[6] and polycythemia[12] have been reported. Renal failure never occurs. An associated nephrotic syndrome is also possible; we have seen one such case.[10]

The most important examination is intravenous urography without compression, including lateral views. The principal finding is distortion of the calyces. Tumors of the upper pole push down the entire kidney, and it may be difficult to distinguish this type of tumor from a suprarenal tumor, especially neuroblastoma. Tumors of the lower pole may elevate the calyces and pelvis and displace the ureter medially. In lateral views, the calyces are usually seen to be pushed forward. The picture is sufficiently typical for diagnosis in the majority of cases, although a similar picture can be produced by multilocular cysts of the kidney.

In 10 per cent of cases, the kidney is silent, even on very late films. In such cases, the best additional evidence can be had through renal arteriography, which will reveal very accurately the disordered vasculature of the tumor and the normal nephrographic appearance of the remaining healthy parenchyma.

Other laboratory studies are of little value, but it is important to look for pulmonary metastases (by far the most frequent type) by obtaining good chest x-rays, including lateral views, and for liver metastases, by palpation and by a liver scintiscan.

Treatment

Treatment consists of a combination of surgery, radiotherapy, and chemotherapy.[8]

Surgery. The required surgery is an extended transabdominal nephrectomy by a transperitoneal approach, including the perirenal fat and the ureter down as far as the bladder. The renal vessels should be tied as early as possible in the course of the operation, and in upper pole tumors the adrenal gland should be removed. Any suspect renal lymph glands and para-aortic glands should be removed. It is important to palpate the opposite kidney and the liver and also to look for any malignant seedlings on the peritoneum.

Radiotherapy. The aim of radiotherapy is to complete the work of the surgery by local sterilization of the tumor field. The radiation should include the whole of the tumor field up to the diaphragm above, and medially to include the vertebral column and great vessels. The total tumor dose is usually 3000 to 3500 rads, given at a rate of 1000 rads per week. The dose is increased to 4000 rads in any particularly suspect zone. The radiation may be given immediately after surgery or as combined preoperative and postoperative radiation, 2000 rads being given before surgery to reduce the tumor volume and make the surgery easier, with the treatment being completed by giving 1500 rads postoperatively.

Chemotherapy. The drugs used are actinomycin D and vincristine. Actinomycin D is given strictly intravenously, generally in a series of five doses of 15 mg./kg. body weight each, in association with the postoperative radiation. Vincristine has been used both instead of preoperative radiotherapy, in order to diminish the tumor size, and after surgery, as a supplement to the radiotherapy.

Therapeutic Indications

In the majority of *nephroblastomas in childhood*, except in very young infants, two views of treatment hold sway: (1) perform immediate surgery, or (2) delay operation while giving preoperative radiation. Our preference has been for the latter technique, which serves to facilitate surgery of these large and very necrotic tumors, except in cases in which uncertainty of diagnosis or a small size of tumor indicates the desirability of immediate operation.

In the *neonate and young infant*, it seems that nephrectomy alone, without chemotherapy or radiotherapy, will produce a considerable number of definitive cures. For this reason the complementary methods of treatment are reserved for situations in which they are obviously indicated, such as discovery at operation or on histology of extension of the tumor beyond the kidney, or of numerous vascular emboli, or of the presence of metastases.

In *very large tumors*, whatever the age of the child, it is preferable to reduce the tumor size, either by chemotherapy or by radiotherapy, to make surgery easier.

If *metastases* are present at the time of diagnosis, they pose a special problem, and, depending on the degree of tumor extension, a choice may be made to treat the pulmonary metastases first or to begin with surgery of the primary tumor and then treat the metastases.

Tumors ruptured into the abdomen present a difficult problem. They require emergency surgery and irradiation of the entire abdominal cavity. In such cases, the remaining kidney must be masked after 1200 rads to avoid subsequent radiation nephritis. In these cases, the addition of actinomycin D to the treatment plan after extensive radiation may not be well tolerated by the very small child, and it is often preferable to reserve the chemotherapy to a later date.

Bilateral tumors[11] can be treated with a distinct chance of success. The treatment must be very carefully planned, and arteriography is essential in order to determine what parts of the renal parenchyma are not involved. To reduce tumor volume as much as possible, a choice can be made between a moderate dose of radiation—not more than 1200 to 1300 rads, in order to avoid damage to the healthy kidney parenchyma—or, preferably, treatment by vincristine sulfate in doses of 1.5 mg./m.^{2} per injection, giving two or three injections at intervals of one week, a regime that offers less risk to the healthy kidney tissue. In some cases, the remaining kidney is found to be involved months or years after the first kidney has been removed. In such situations, this preoperative treatment must be followed by a carefully planned partial nephrectomy. Total nephrectomy followed by kidney transplantation is a counsel of despair. Bilateral involvement is sometimes discovered at the outset. In these cases, abdominal exploration will make it possible to decide which kidney is likely to be more suitable for partial nephrectomy. The partial nephrectomy should be done first, and operation should not be carried out on the second kidney until it is certain that there is adequate function in the remnant of the first kidney.

Treatment of Metastases[16, 17]

Distinction must be made between pulmonary metastases, which are often successfully treated, and abdominal metastases, which are much more difficult to manage.

Pulmonary metastases are often multiple and bilateral. The entire lung field on both sides can be irradiated without undue risk to respiratory function with a dose of up to 2000 rads, given over a period of 16 to 18 days. This treatment is supplemented by a series of injections of actinomycin D, and usually results in complete clearance of the pulmonary lesions. Subsequent courses of chemotherapy may be given to consolidate the results. Thoracotomy is justified for a solitary metastasis. The metastasis is removed by wedge resection, or sometimes by segmental resection or lobectomy. The remainder of the lung is examined carefully; if there are no other metastases, radiation need not be given and courses of chemotherapy should suffice. If, on the other hand, there are microscopic metastases, the lungs are irradiated as for cases of multiple metastases. There may be other indications for thoracic surgery—for example, when new, relatively localized metastases appear after irradiation of multiple metastases.

Abdominal metastases may occur at various sites. Small *liver metastases* discovered at the time of surgery may be removed without particular trouble. More often the metastases appear at a later stage; these can be localized in the liver by arteriography, and partial hepatectomy is sometimes possible. If liver surgery does not seem possible, the entire liver can be irradiated, with supplemental actinomycin D being given, but the results are not nearly so good as in the treatment of pulmonary metastases. Other *abdominal metastases* may occur on the peritoneum or in intra-abdominal or retroperitoneal lymph nodes. Their treatment is always very difficult because it is impossible to judge the extent of the disease without further exploratory laparotomy. At such a laparotomy, any lesions that can be resected are removed, and the entire abdomen is then irradiated. If possible, actinomycin D is given as well, but the difficulties with this form of management have already been indicated.

Other metastases are much rarer. They may occur in mediastinal or supraclavicular lymph nodes or in the bones, and often they are multiple. In such cases there is little chance of cure, and only palliative treatment for pain and functional disorders is possible.

Follow-up

A regular and meticulous follow-up of every patient with nephroblastoma is essential in order to detect any metastases as soon as possible and to institute the necessary treatment. Follow-up supervision should include full clinical examination, especially palpation of the remaining kidney, and also chest radiography. These examinations should be carried out every six to eight weeks during the first year, every three months for the second year, every six months for the third year, and then once yearly. It is a good idea to repeat the intravenous urogram one year after the initial treatment or at any time when there is any doubt about the remaining kidney.

Results

Success of treatment can be judged at the end of two years. Ninety-five per cent of patients who show no recurrence or metastases in the first two years will prove to be permanently cured. In our own series of 248 cases examined or treated in whole or in part at the Institut Gustave-Roussy between 1952 and 1967, 124 (50 per cent) are living at two years or longer. Of these patients, 205 had received their entire treatment at the Institut Gustave-Roussy, and of these, 114 are living (56 per cent). The presence of metastases is not necessarily fatal; when there was only a single pulmonary metastasis, 57 per cent were cured. Even with bilateral pulmonary metastases, the definitive cure rate was as high as 29 per cent. Abdominal and bone metastases, on the other hand, are far more serious, and are nearly always fatal.

The results obtained with bilateral tumors are encouraging. Of six children seen before 1960, who were treated only palliatively, all are dead. Since 1960, 14 children with bilateral tumors have been treated in an attempt at cure and have been followed up for more than two years. Of these 14, six died, in most cases in less than one year. However, eight of the 14 are alive with no evidence of tumor and with normal renal function after nine and 10 years, respectively, in two cases, and after two to four years in the other six.

It is still difficult to define the prognostic factors. The prognosis is better in infants under the age of one year and especially in the first three or four months of life. Limitation of the tumor within the kidney capsule is an important favorable factor. Rupture of the tumor, invasion of neighboring organs, thrombosis of the renal vein, and metastases in lymph nodes, on the other hand, indicate a poor prognosis. Definite differentiation of the tumor tissue into glomeruli or tubules seems to be a good prognostic factor.

Other Kidney Tumors

Congenital Mesoblastic Nephroma.[1] This is a rare embryonic tumor, variously described as fibroma, fibrosarcoma, leiomyoma, and rhabdomyoma. It resembles nephroblastoma but is composed of fibroblastic tissue with no malignant epithelial component, and there are also foci of renal dysplasia. The prognosis is apparently good after simple nephrectomy.

Benign Renal or Para-Renal Tumors. These tumors are very rare; they include adenoma, subcapsular fibroma, and fibrolipoma.[7]

Clear Cell Tubulopapillary Carcinoma of the Kidney. Such carcinomas are rare; they are found in older children and adolescents. The presenting signs are hematuria and tumor. Radiological evidence of peripheral calcification is very suggestive. The tumor usually invades the urinary tract and the lymphatics, and bone metastases are common. The prognosis is often favorable after nephrectomy supplemented by postoperative radiation or chemotherapy.[4]

The Leukemic Kidney.[13] This condition has become much more common now that leukemic children survive so much longer with chemotherapy or steroid treatment. Such patients present with bilateral renal tumors, often very large, which are produced by massive invasion of the kidneys by leukoblastic tissue. The effect on renal function is very variable. Most often renal function is normal, but there may be hematuria owing to the leukemic hemorrhagic syndrome, and the blood urea and uric acid levels may be raised because of cell destruction caused by the chemotherapy. However, sometimes a rapidly fatal renal failure sets in, with albuminuria, hematuria, oliguria, hypertension, a rising blood urea level, and diminishing renal clearances. Exceptionally, leukosarcomatosis may begin with signs of renal involvement—proteinuria, raised blood urea levels, hematuria, and enlarged kidneys—and in such cases the hematologic diagnosis of leukemia may not be made for many weeks.

Renal lithiasis is a common complication of leukemia in children, varying with the pattern of the particular disease and the degree of skeletal involvement. Stone formation may also be related to treatment. The calculi may be calcium or urate. During steroid therapy, the administration of potassium chloride should be avoided, because this salt acidifies the urine and encourages precipitation of urates.

Radiation Nephritis

Radiation nephritis is the result of irradiation of one or both kidneys by x-rays. Glomerular filtration and renal plasma flow are depressed when the radiation dose exceeds 400 rads, but the real risk of radiation nephritis comes with doses higher than 1200 rads in children. In this age group, such radiation is most likely to have been given for the treatment of Wilms' tumor, but even in patients with this disease radiation nephritis has become much less common with modern methods of calculating dosages and accurate localization of radiation fields.

Histologically, there are always severe lesions in the small vessels, with fibrinoid necrosis and hyalinization. In the acute stage, there is interstitial edema, glomerular ischemia, and "endocrine" involution of the renal tissue. In the chronic stage, there is glomerular fibrosis, interstitial fibrosis, and tubular atrophy.

When the condition develops some months after irradiation, the clinical presentation is usually malignant hypertension and uremia, and the condition is then often fatal. The child should undergo bilateral nephrectomy if both kidneys have been irradiated, and he should then be placed on a dialysis-transplantation program. In other cases, radiation nephritis is chronic and appears a long time after the radiotherapy. In these cases, it presents with proteinuria and particularly hypertension, which may be benign or malignant.

A newborn infant whose mother had been irradiated during pregnancy presented, in addition to other disorders, a chronic radiation nephritis, which proved fatal at the age of 8 years.[14]

Conclusion

Great improvements have been made in recent years in the treatment of embryonal tumors of the kidney. However, some questions remain to be answered.

1. Should surgery be performed immediately, whatever the size of the tumor, or is it preferable to use preoperative irradiation? 2. What is the exact value of the chemotherapy currently associated with radiotherapy and surgery in the treatment of these tumors? Should the child be given repeated courses of chemotherapy or only one course at the time of the definitive treatment? 3. Should the radiotherapy and chemotherapy be altered in particular cases or in various categories of cases? If the last question is answered in the affirmative, there must be precise criteria for classification.

The answers to all these questions can come only from carefully designed controlled therapeutic trials. Some trials are already in progress, but because of the relatively small number of cases, only a few trials are possible, and even these require the collaboration of many centers in one country. Perhaps even international collaboration may prove necessary. One can only hope that answers will be found in the not too distant future.

SARCOMA OF BLADDER AND PROSTATE

Embryonic sarcoma, arising in muscle (rhabdomyosarcoma) is in practice the only malignant tumor of the lower urinary tract in children.[5, 9, 18]

Pathologic Anatomy

Macroscopically, these tumors present in two forms: (1) a botryoid sarcoma formed of bunches of translucent cysts, developing in the natural cavities, and (2) a dense tumor developing in the connective tissue of bladder and prostate. Histologically, the tumor is composed of small, highly undifferentiated, stellate or ovoid cells, sometimes loosely dispersed in a loose mucoid stroma, sometimes arranged in dense masses. Only in some cases is myoblastic differentiation revealed, either by the presence of larger cells with an eosinophilic cytoplasm, or by the presence of elongated cells with abundant cytoplasm in which transverse striation can be shown by special stains.

Symptomatology

Although these tumors may occur at any age, the majority occur in children under the age of 5 years. In most cases, urinary symptoms predominate, such

Table 4. Sarcoma of Bladder and Prostate*

Sex of Patient	Age (years)	Initial Symptom	Initial Treatment	Secondary Treatment	Interval Until Death (in months)	Survival (follow-up in years)
M	8/12	Acute retention of urine	DXT† (3000 r)	Surgery	2	
M	2	Tumor	Surgery	DXT (2000 r)	5	
M	8	Acute retention of urine	DXT (4000 r)		3	
F	10	Acute retention of urine	Surgery	DXT (4300 r) + actinomycin	3	
M	3	Acute retention of urine	Surgery	DXT (5000 r) + actinomycin	6	
M	9	Tumor	DXT (4000 r)		9	
M	5	Pyuria	Surgery	Surgery + DXT (5000 r)	24	
M	10	Tumor	DXT (3000 r)		11	
M	7	Acute retention of urine	Surgery	DXT (4500 r) + actinomycin		4
F	1/12	Tumor	DXT (5000 r) + actinomycin	Surgery + actinomycin		3
F	4	Tumor	Surgery	DXT (5000 r) + actinomycin		2
M	3	Acute retention of urine	Surgery	DXT (5000 r) + actinomycin		3
F	2	Hematuria	Surgery	DXT (5000 r) + actinomycin		7/12
M	3	Acute retention of urine	Surgery	DXT (4500 r)		4/12

*Data of O. Schweisguth and F. Flamant.
†DXT, Radiotherapy.

as persistent urinary infection with fever and dysuria, or the rapid onset of acute retention of urine. Much more rarely, the tumor may appear at the urethral meatus as a botryoid protrusion. In some cases, the only clinical finding may be the discovery of a pelvic tumor (Table 4).

On examination, abdominal palpation reveals a midline suprapubic tumor, but this may be mistaken for a distended bladder. Rectal examination provides the essential information that the pelvic tumor is anteriorly and medially situated. Some small intravesical tumors are not palpable.

Urography, with anteroposterior and lateral cystograms, is essential. In the intravesical forms, the polypoid tumor shows as a "parachute" type filling defect. In the parietal tumors, the bladder is deformed and compressed, and the urethra is deviated by the tumor. Where the bladder is obstructed, the upper urinary tract is often greatly dilated. The tumor extends principally by local infiltration, but a search should also be made for metastases in the lungs and sometimes in bones and lymph nodes.

Treatment

In boys, surgical ablation involves at least a total cystoprostatectomy; in girls, anterior exenteration is necessary. Sometimes total exenteration of the pelvis is necessary. Usually the ureters are implanted into the sigmoid colon. Extensive and mutilating as this surgery is, it is often inadequate for complete local removal of tumor, and pelvic recurrence is common. Postoperative radiation may be given to the pelvis, and for this at least 4500 rads are necessary. Recent trials suggest that chemotherapy (actinomycin D, vincristine, Endoxan) may be helpful, but the correct use of these drugs has yet to be established.

The results are still bad. No patient has been cured by surgery alone. In the most recent cases, routine radiation has been given postoperatively, in association with chemotherapy. Although follow-up is as yet inadequate, there are grounds for hope. Four patients are alive two years after starting treatment, with no signs of local recurrence or metastases, but unfortunately three of these developed serious intestinal and urethral complications of radiotherapy.

REFERENCES

1. Bolande, R. P., Brough, A. J., and Izant, R. J.: Congenital mesoblastic nephroma of infancy. Pediatrics *40*:272, 1967.
2. Denys, P., Malvaux, P., Van Den Berghe, H., Tanghe, W., and Proesmans, W.: Pseudo-hermaphrodisme masculin, tumeur de Wilms, néphropathie parenchymateuse et mosaïcisme XX/XY. Arch. franç. Pédiat. *24*:729, 1967.
3. Fraumeni, J. F., Geiser, C. F., and Manning, M. D.: Wilms' tumor and congenital hemihypertrophy. Pediatrics *40*:886, 1967.
4. Imbert, M. C., Gerard-Marchant, R., Schweisguth, O., and Nezelof, C.: Le carcinome tubulopapillaire du rein de l'enfant. Ann. Pédiat. (Paris) *15*:302, 1968.
5. Jarman, W. D., and Renealy, J. C.: Polypoid rhabdomyosarcoma of the bladder in children. J. Urol. *103*:227, 1970.
6. Joseph, R., Job, J. C., and Courtecuisse, V.: Nephroblastome et hypertension artérielle chez l'enfant. Arch. franç. Pédiat. *17*:593, 1960.
7. Koop, C. E.: Abdominal tumors in infants and children. Arch. Dis. Child. *35*:1, 1960.
8. Ledlie, E. M., Mynors, L. S., Draper, G. J., and Gorbach, P. D.: Natural history and treatment of Wilms' tumor: an analysis of 335 cases occurring in England and Wales 1962–66. Brit. Med. J. *4*:195, 1970.
9. Legier, J. F.: Botryoid sarcoma and rhabdomyosarcoma of the bladder. Review of the literature and report of 3 cases. J. Urol. *86*:583, 1961.
10. Lines, D. R.: Nephrotic syndrome and nephroblastoma. J. Pediat. *72*:274, 1968.
11. Martin, L. W., and Kloecker, R. J.: Bilateral nephroblastoma (Wilms' tumor). Pediatrics *28*: 101, 1961.
12. Marie, J., Levèque, B., Auvert, J., Perelman, R., Boivin, P., Corvin, J. L., Watchi, J. M., and Roy, C.: Le syndrome "polyglobulie-tumeur rénale" chez l'enfant. Ann. Pédiat. (Paris) *39*:118, 1963.
13. Mikulowski, V.: Urämische Syndrome im Verlauf von Leukämien bei Kindern. Ann. paediat. (Basel) *192*:360, 1959.
14. Schärer, K., Mühlethaler, J. P., Stettler, M., and Bosch, H.: Chronic radiation nephritis after exposure in utero. Helv. Paediat. Acta *23*:489, 1968.
15. Schweisguth, O., and Bamberger, J.: Le néphroblastome de l'enfant. Ann. Chir. Infant. *4*:335, 1963.
16. Schweisguth, O., and Bamberger, J.: Les métastases dans le néphroblastome de l'enfant. Arch. franç. Pédiat. *22*:939, 1965.
17. Tan, C. T.: Long-term survival with metastatic Wilms' tumor in children. Proc. Amer. Ass. Cancer Res. *5*:63, 1964.
18. Williams, J. D.: Rhabdomyosarcoma of the genitourinary tract. Proc. Roy. Soc. Med. *59*:413, 1966.
19. Woodard, J. R., and Levine, M. K.: Nephroblastoma (Wilms' tumor) and congenital aniridia. J. Urol. *101*:140, 1969.

Chapter Four

HEREDITARY NEPHROPATHIES CAUSING CHRONIC RENAL FAILURE*

This group of diseases includes hereditary polycystic disease (see page 20) and certain nephropathies secondary to hereditary disorders of metabolism, such as cystinosis, oxalosis, and Fabry's disease (see page 99). We shall consider here Alport's syndrome, nephronophthisis, and the congenital nephrotic syndrome.

ALPORT'S SYNDROME

Introduction

Described by Alport in 1927,[1] this disease is found in the three major racial groups (Oriental, Negroid, and Caucasian).[8] Apparently it is a common disorder. The disease is hereditary and transmitted as an autosomal dominant trait. In most families, it is less serious in girls than in boys. It presents as a nephropathy with hematuria or proteinuria or both that progresses to chronic renal failure, and there are also extrarenal manifestations which include, in order of frequency, loss of hearing, ocular involvement, and sometimes macrothrombocytopathy. This syndrome is often described as "familial hematuria with deafness." The presenting symptom is usually hematuria, but rarely it is deafness, occurring between the ages of 6 months and 13 years.[3, 11, 12, 14] We have studied 10 families comprising 59 patients (Table 5).

Renal Involvement

Hematuria is the dominant symptom in 80 per cent of cases. It was present in all our patients. There is continuous microscopic hematuria with episodes of macroscopic hematuria that may be provoked by infection, by severe exercise, or by eating certain foods. The degree of microscopic hematuria varies from one patient to another and from time to time in the same patient. It has been

---

*This chapter was written in collaboration with Dr. Etienne Bois.

Table 5.   Alport's Syndrome*

	Boys		Girls	
	Affected	Healthy	Affected	Healthy
Mother affected	26 (15)	14	17 (1)	15
Father affected	0	0	2 (1)	0
Affected parent unknown	6 (2)	3	8	8
TOTAL	32 (17)	17	27 (2)	23
TOTAL with probands excluded	15	17	25	23

*In the analysis of the 10 families of these patients, we have noted that, excluding the probands (figures in parentheses), the ratio of healthy and affected in the two sexes is close to one, a finding that suggests dominant transmission of the disease. The greater proportion of girls is the same as that in the population at large. (Prepared by J. Feingold and E. Bois.)

noted, in the sibships affected, from the first days or weeks of life. Proteinuria is almost as common and may precede the hematuria, but most often it appears after some years. The degree of proteinuria is moderate. In three of our patients, the proteinuria was sufficient to produce a nephrotic syndrome at an early stage of the disease. Progressive increase in proteinuria is a sign of aggravation of the nephropathy. In women, there may be a transient increase in proteinuria during pregnancy. In some reported series, there is a high incidence of leukocyturia and pyuria, but we have never seen isolated leukocyturia, and in only three cases have we seen transient pyuria.

The kidneys are not enlarged. Blood pressure is normal until the terminal stage. In one of our cases, there was early and relentlessly progressive hypertension. Renal function remains normal for many years and then the first defect is in concentration power. Once uremia develops, it is progressive.

Extrarenal Disease

Leaving aside certain probable coincidences, Alport's syndrome may involve three extrarenal areas.

Auditory Involvement

Deafness is more common in males. It is not a constant manifestation. It may skip one generation, only to appear in the next. It may be found in patients who do not exhibit nephropathy but who are carriers of the kidney disease. The age at which the deafness appears is variable, but it is most often found at the stage at which the renal condition becomes aggravated. Two years is the earliest age at which the deafness has been discovered. It is recognized between the ages of 6 and 10 in 50 per cent of cases and before the age of 15 years in 75 per cent.

The deafness is neurogenic, due to involvement of the nerve itself or of the organ of Corti. Hence, the deafness is a perception defect and hearing aids are of no value. The auditory deficit is bilateral but often asymmetrical. The audiometric curve generally shows a lesser ability to hear the high pitch sounds. In the lower range (250 to 500 cycles per second), the hearing loss is of the order of 20 to 40 decibels, and in the higher range (2048 to 4096 cycles per second), the loss is of the order of 40 to 64 decibels. Hence, there is selective involvement of the higher frequencies, at least in the early stages, and this explains why the deafness may be missed if audiometry is not performed. The patient begins to complain of the deafness when the conversational range (from 1024 cycles per second) is involved. In some patients, especially in females, the condition remains latent throughout life and is detectable only by audiometry. According to some authors, the deafness may increase in men during attacks of gross hematuria, leading progressively to total deafness. In one of our patients, the deafness took an unusual pattern. At the age of 13 his deficit was of the order of 10 decibels in all frequencies. At 15 years 6 months, the deficit was 40 decibels at 128 cycles per second, 20 decibels at 512 cycles per second, and only 15 decibels at frequencies above 1024 cycles per second. The increased incidence of ear infection that occurs with this disease is well known, and this may at times complicate the interpretation of hearing disorders.

The deafness is not accompanied by any signs of vestibular disorder.

Ocular Involvement

The occurrence of ocular manifestations in Alport's syndrome is now recognized.[2, 7, 16] However, these are not common and were not present in any of our cases. It may be that eye involvement will be recognized more often by the practice of routine ophthalmological examination. The essential feature is a congenital lesion of the lens that may affect either its shape or its transparency. In the former instance, it may produce anterior lenticonus (usually bilateral, with progressive loss of sight) or a spherophakia that causes myopia. Changes in transparency may produce cataracts that may be cortical, posterior, coronal, or nuclear.

Macrothrombocytopathy

Two families have been recorded which, in addition to having renal and auditory disease, exhibited thrombocytopenia, marked by giant platelets with an abnormal ultrastructure, prolonged bleeding time, and defective platelet adherence. There was an abnormal aggregation in response to epinephrine and defective liberation of platelet factor 3. The involved women had severe renal disease.[5]

Clinical Course

The course of the Alport syndrome varies both with the sex of the patient and from one family to another. The dominant feature is chronic renal insufficiency which, from the time of its onset, progresses in a few years to death. The renal disorder appears earlier and is more serious in boys, of whom some 40 per cent die, generally between the ages of 15 and 25 years. In the female, the disease in both renal and auditory manifestations is often latent, and the mortality rate is no more than 10 per cent, with no peak age of death. Mild cases have, however, been seen in males and severe cases in females.

The association of renal and auditory symptoms also has a bearing on the prognosis of the disease. Deafness is associated with the nephropathy in 56 per cent of men and 24 per cent of women. It is associated with the serious forms and, in both sexes, mortality rates are higher in deaf patients. However, death, when it occurs, takes place at about the same age whether or not the patient is deaf. Hence, the presence of deafness has considerable prognostic significance in both sexes in predicting more severe renal involvement.

Pathologic Anatomy

Kidney

The material on which our study is based derives from 12 biopsies, one autopsy, and one kidney removed surgically. The age range of patients from which this material was taken varies from 2 years 5 months to 16 years 8 months. The histopathologic findings are variable, but two groups can be clearly distinguished. In one group, comprising eight cases, the renal changes were slight (Figure 9). The glomerular lesions were minimal, often characterized by hypertrophy of the epithelial cells or discrete intercapillary hyalinization. The tubular lesions were also discrete. There were very occasional atrophic tubules within minimal bands of fibrosis. Red cell casts were commonly found in the tubular lumen, indicating the renal origin of the disease. In the second group, consisting of four cases, the glomerular lesions varied in degree and extent, but all were of the same type, with irregular intercapillary hyalinization producing adhesions of several capillary loops and sometimes adhesions to Bowman's capsule. This hyalinization was accompanied by minimal endocapillary hypercellularity and thickening of some of the capillary walls. These glomerular lesions were focal or diffuse. All degrees of glomerular involvement could be seen in the same preparation, and the tubular lesions were proportional to

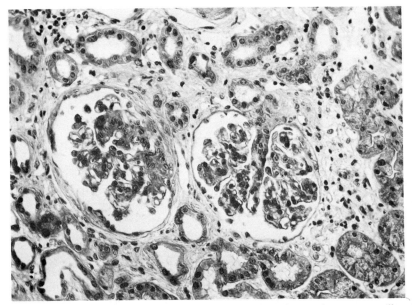

Figure 9. Alport's syndrome. Segmental and focal hyalinization sparing many capillary loops, whose walls are simply and irregularly thickened in places. There is slight interstitial fibrosis infiltrated by occasional round cells and studded with groups of lipophages. ×220.

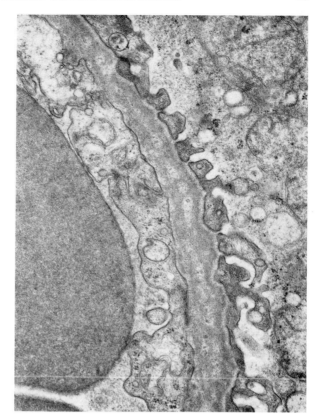

Figure 10. Electron micrograph in Alport's syndrome. Note, in the basement membrane, the numerous clear zones containing a finely granular material. ×21,000.

the glomerular lesions. The lesions might be minimal (with only a few dilated tubules containing red cell casts) or severe, with, in addition to the atrophic lesions, lipoid infiltration of the tubular epithelium. In all four cases, the tubular lesions were associated with varying degrees of severe interstitial fibrosis, and with collections of lipophages (foam cells) disseminated in the fibrous tissue. There was also a thickening of the arteriolar walls and, in one case, endarteritis involving the medium-sized arteries.

These histologic findings, varying from case to case in the same family, could be classified either as interstitial nephritis or pyelonephritis, or as glomerulonephritis, depending on the predominance of one or the other lesion. In a recent study of nine autopsies, seven biopsies, and two nephrectomy specimens, Krickstein and his colleagues[10] described these lesions as a combination of different glomerular, tubular, and interstitial lesions.

It is probably wise, for the present, to admit that there is no characteristic histologic picture in Alport's syndrome. Foam cells containing cholesterol and phospholipids may be found in the interstitial tissue in other nephropathies, particularly acquired chronic glomerulonephritis, and they cannot be regarded as specific for Alport's syndrome. Two facts, however, are important. The absence of abnormal deposits on immunofluorescence in a case of chronic hematuric nephropathy is a negative finding of diagnostic significance on renal biopsy.[17] Ultrastructural studies seem to show early glomerular changes with duplication of the basement membrane and the presence of granular inclusions[9] (Figure 10). It may be, then, that Alport's syndrome begins as a focal and segmental glomerular nephropathy that evolves progressively into global involvement of the kidney.

The Ear

The lesions are found in the organ of Corti, more specifically in the ciliated cells and their supporting cells. They are similar to the lesions produced experimentally by noise, x-rays, and ototoxic antibiotics.

Genetics

The familial and hereditary character of Alport's syndrome was suggested in the earliest reports, but it was not until 1951 that Perkoff[12] demonstrated the dominant autosomal mode of transmission.[4, 6] Some disproportion of sex distribution in this condition has been reported, including a preponderance of daughters who either display or transmit the disease, a dearth of affected sons in the progeny of both male and female patients, or a high proportion of affected persons in a kindred.[13, 15] Many hypotheses have been put forward to explain these observations, including transmission partly linked to sex, higher mortality rate for the male fetus, and preferential segregation during meiosis of the gene at fault. We have found no abnormal distribution in any of our 10 families.[6]

Attention must also be paid to the manner of transmission of the association of renal and auditory involvements. From studies of the genealogical trees of involved families, it is possible to eliminate the idea of two independent genes or two linked genes carried on the same chromosome. It is probable that only a single gene, one with a pleiotrophic action, is involved. Certain factors favor this hypothesis: hematuric patients without deafness can transmit deafness to their descendants, while deaf patients without kidney disease can have children who present all the features of Alport's syndrome. The ocular manifestations may also be a supplemental pleiotrophic facet of the defective gene.

Treatment

The only treatment is symptomatic. Renal insufficiency is treated in the usual manner, and kidney transplantation may be contemplated and indeed has been practiced in some cases with success. We have experience of transplantation in two cases. The principal problem is of course the choice of donor, and obviously the best solution is to use a cadaver kidney. Certainly the mother or sisters of the patient must not be used as a donor because, although they may be healthy, they may be carriers of the hereditary lesion.

The deafness cannot be helped either by surgery or by use of a hearing aid.

NEPHRONOPHTHISIS

In 1951, Fanconi and his colleagues[21] described a hereditary nephropathy, the characteristics of which have been elaborated in subsequent reports. We have observed 21 families with this condition.

Clinical Features[21, 22, 24, 26, 29, 35]

Symptoms most commonly appear between the ages of 2 and 5 years, rarely earlier, and sometimes as late as 8 to 10 years. There is gradual deterioration with death from renal failure from 10 to 15 years after the onset.

This slowly progressive nephropathy has important characteristics that are of diagnostic significance. The first is the fairly long interval between birth and the onset of symptoms. The second is the initial predominance of three manifestations: proteinuria that is moderate and variable at the outset; marked thirst and polyuria owing to a serious defect in the concentrating power of the kidney (the maximal osmolarity of urine after restricting water intake is between 150 to 300 mOsm./kg. water); and anemia, which is present in 75 per cent of cases at an early stage. The blood pressure is normal until the terminal uremic stage. Growth is defective in only 50 per cent of cases, and when present it appears late, is of moderate degree, and is accompanied by abnormalities of skeletal maturation and structure, as with any case of renal failure. Glomerular filtration remains normal for a long time, then drops, and the blood urea level rises with the other usual manifestations of chronic renal failure. There have been reports of transient glycosuria, of an early lowering of the TmPAH, of the possibility of early hypokalemia, and of a high incidence of hyponatremic complications with the salt-losing syndrome.

The urine contains neither red nor white cells. Intravenous pyelography shows a normal urinary tract, and the kidney may be normal or decreased in size.

The disease evolves slowly and progressively. Death occurs from renal failure after several years, most often about the age of 10 years. In our cases, the average survival time, dating from the age of clinical onset, has been 6 years 3 months. In some cases, however, even though the symptoms start at the same age, the evolution may be slower so that it is possible to find the disease in a young adult.

Pathology

We have been fortunate enough to obtain histologic material from all our patients, either by renal biopsy, or, in some cases, at autopsy (Figure 11).

Macroscopically, the kidneys are pale and they may be normal in size, or slightly or greatly reduced. They are sometimes grossly atrophied. The disease is bilateral. The kidney surface is covered with granules resembling semolina, and sometimes there is bosselation. Section reveals diffuse atrophy, with particular involvement of the cortex, and in six of our cases there were varying numbers of cysts, which sometimes were very large, in both medulla and cortex.

Histologic study shows diffuse tubulo-interstitial disease. The tubular changes are very marked, and there are zones in which the dilated tubules are grouped to form adenoma-like structures alternating with zones in which the tubules are greatly atrophied, with remarkable thickening of the basement membrane. These changes affect both the proximal and the distal tubules. Ivemark emphasizes the hypertrophy of the descending limb of the loop of Henle and the thickening of the basement membrane in the ascending limb of the loop. There is sometimes cystic dilatation of the bend of the loop. There may be dilatation of the collecting tubules, and this can progress to cyst formation.[23]

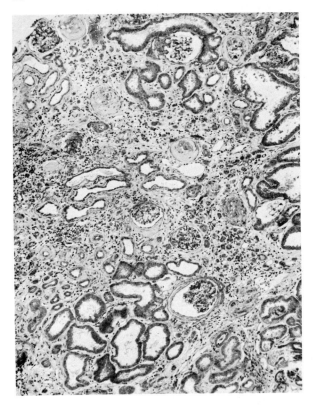

Figure 11. Nephronophthisis. The appearance is that of a diffuse tubulo-interstitial nephropathy with periglomerular and intraglomerular fibrosis, numerous islets of atrophic tubules with markedly thickened basement membranes and interstitial fibrosis infiltrated by occasional round cells. ×65.

In the interstitial tissue, there is considerable inflammatory infiltration of round cells, lymphocytes, and plasmocytes. Most authors regard these findings as resulting from the pathologic process and not as evidence of infection. There is progressive invasion of the interstitial tissue by generalized fibrosis.

At an early stage of the disease, the glomeruli are normal, apart from slight thickening of Bowman's capsule. At a later stage, after they have become entrapped in interstitial fibrosis, they undergo hyalinization. More rarely, they may in places undergo cystic dilatation. The arteries are normal except when hypertension occurs. By microangiography, Ivemark has shown that the interlobular arteries and the afferent arterioles run irregular and tortuous courses.[23]

In conclusion, this is essentially a tubulo-interstitial nephropathy, with the glomeruli becoming involved only at a late stage of the disease. Microdissection studies have shown diverticula throughout the nephron; the cysts develop only from the distal and collecting tubules.[34]

Genetics

The horizontal distribution of cases, the normal sex ratio, and the high degree of consanguinity in parents of affected patients are all evidence that the disease is transmitted as an autosomal recessive trait.

We have studied 21 families, and the following observations are compatible with this mode of transmission: (1) With regard to the established criteria, we have found no significant difference between the familial and the isolated forms of the disease; (2) the sex distribution was normal, with a sex ratio of 1.14 for all patients; (3) we found two cases of consanguinity, and in six families the parents had both come from the same small village; (4) in the parents of the patients, we found a history of renal disease ("pyelonephritis," proteinuria, uremia, renal failure) on four occasions, but water concentration tests in the parents did not show disturbances similar to those in the patients; (5) the 21 families studied included a total of 71 children, and of these, the 21 probands and 10 other children were affected. The proportion of affected subjects, analyzed by the proband method, was 0.200, a figure that does not differ significantly from the 0.25 incidence expected for an autosomal recessive trait. There are, however, many facts that make it clear that the problem of the mode of transmission of nephronophthisis is not so simple as it might seem: the very high proportion of cases in certain families, the vertical distribution of cases in other families, and the unusually early or late appearance of symptoms in still other patients. These facts have been interpreted in two ways. Some postulate the existence of an infantile recessive type appearing early and developing rapidly, and a dominant "adult" type that appears later and is less serious. According to other authors, the transmission in all cases can be explained by the hypothesis of "dominance with variable expression."[35]

In fact, it is difficult to come to a clear conclusion from genetic studies because of varying interpretations of the nosologic limits of the condition.

Nosologic Problems

Idiopathic Chronic Interstitial Nephropathies[29]

The only difference between these and the disease described by Fanconi lies in the absence of a familial element, and this poses a nosologic problem. Hereditary diseases commonly include "sporadic forms." It is legitimate to include with nephronophthisis certain chronic idiopathic tubulo-interstitial nephropathies that are clinically, biochemically, and histologically indistinguishable, but the possibility must not be excluded that certain nonfamilial cases may in fact be other morbid entities and not genetic. In this context, a particularly acute problem is posed by the "Balkan nephropathy," which clinically and histologically is very similar to nephronophthisis but has a special geographic distribution. It is true that this disease affects adults more frequently than children, but there are cases of nephronophthisis that appear during adolescence or adult life.

Medullary Cystic Disease

In 1945, Smith and Graham described a disease characterized by familial incidence, dominant transmission, and occurrence in children (but also in adults), the pathology of which included a tubulo-interstitial nephropathy and cysts in the medulla.[33] In adults, this condition progresses very slowly. It is generally thought that this condition and nephronophthisis are one and the same disease.[19, 22, 27, 28] Certainly any differences between the two may be only apparent. The presence of cysts in the medulla was not recorded in earlier reports but has been noted in many pathologic studies of nephronophthisis, and we have found cysts in six of our patients. The development of cysts may in fact be a secondary process. There are, however, a certain number of cases of nephronophthisis in adults in which no cysts occur. Nephronophthisis and cystic disease of the pyramid have been reported within the same family.[33]

Senior's Syndrome

Another nosologic problem concerns the association of nephronophthisis and tapetoretinal degeneration. This association was described first by Contreras[19] and later by Senior and associates[31] in six members of a sibship of 13 children. Since then, there have been some 30 reports of the presence of these two hereditary diseases in many members of the same sibship. We have studied two related sibships (Figure 12), and in each we found both the full syndrome and the nephropathy or the retinal disease alone. In addition to these two sibships, we have picked out six other families, and these eight families make up a relatively homogenous group with regard to both renal and ocular manifestations.[18] In all the cases, tapetoretinal degeneration was confirmed on ophthalmoscopy and electroretinography. The kidney condition in every case fulfilled all the criteria for a diagnosis of nephronophthisis. Genetic studies indicate that both diseases are apparently transmitted as autosomal recessive traits. The ratio of healthy to affected subjects makes it improbable that the two diseases are transmitted independently, but search for a linkage between the two genes involved has not been conclusive. It is thus very prob-

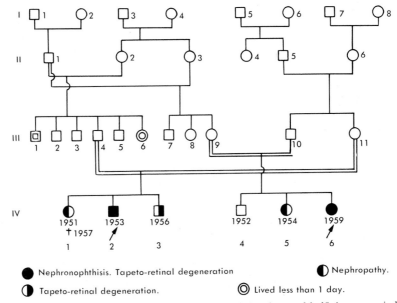

● Nephronophthisis. Tapeto-retinal degeneration   ◐ Nephropathy.

◐ Tapeto-retinal degeneration.   ◎ Lived less than 1 day.

Figure 12. Senior's syndrome. Note in III that a half-brother and half-sister married a sister and brother. In IV, 5 of 6 children are diseased; *2* and *6* have Senior's syndrome; *1* and *5* have nephronophthisis and *3* has tapetoretinal degeneration.

able that Senior's syndrome is induced by a single gene that is pleiotrophic and of variable expression. Systematic study of the families leads us to conclude that changes in the electroretinogram in nephronophthisis, like changes in the audiogram in Alport's syndrome, are very common, and that Senior's syndrome is probably not a separate condition.

Nervous Disorders

The association of nephronophthisis with tapetoretinal degeneration and neurologic disorders has been the subject of recent studies. Among these are a report by Saldino and Mainzer,[30] who found nephronophthisis, retinitis pigmentosa, cerebral ataxia, and cone-shaped epiphyses in a brother and sister, and a report by Durand and his colleagues[20] of the association of chronic tubulointerstitial nephropathy with tapetoretinal degeneration, deafness, mental deficiency, and generalized visceral lipidosis.

Animal Model

An important factor in the study of this disease is the discovery by Lyon of a spontaneous mutation in mice producing an inherited kidney disease with characteristics identical to nephronophthisis associated with tapetoretinal degeneration. This mutant strain has been named KD.[25]

Treatment

In the absence of any etiologic treatment the only possibility is symptomatic management of the renal insufficiency to prolong the life of these children with nephronophthisis.

Renal transplantation can be considered. The genetic situation makes it unwise to choose a donor from the family, and a cadaver graft should be preferred. In one of our cases, there has been apparent cure and good long-term survival after removal of both diseased kidneys and transplantation.

THE CONGENITAL NEPHROTIC SYNDROME

The congenital nephrotic syndrome is a hereditary condition transmitted as an autosomal recessive trait. It appears in the first few weeks of life and is lethal. The first detailed observation was reported by Gautier and Miville in Geneva.[41] More than 200 cases have been studied, and about half of these were from Finland. The reason for this geographic distribution is not clear: it may be real, or it may be a result of failure to recognize the condition in other countries. Most of the work on the disease has been carried out by the school of Hallman in Helsinki, and Hallman and his colleagues made a very complete review of the subject in 1970.[42] Our own observations and the French cases were reviewed in 1968.[37, 44]

The "Finnish" Type of Congenital Nephrotic Syndrome

The "Finnish" type of congenital nephrotic syndrome is a hereditary disease transmitted as an autosomal recessive trait. Parents of the affected children do not themselves have the disease. Cousins may be involved. Neither sex predominates, in contrast to the finding in the idiopathic nephrotic syndrome of older children, in which boys are more often affected. Parental consanguinity is a possibility to be considered. The condition can affect identical twins, and three pairs of nonidentical twins have been seen — in one case, both members were affected, and in the other two cases only one twin was involved. Of 204 cases, more than one member of a family was involved in 44 kindreds.[45]

Clinical Features

The pregnancy is usually normal. Proteinuria, edema, hypertension, and toxemia have been noted, but with no greater frequency than in the general population.

Premature birth was recorded in 20 per cent of the involved children. The birth weight was low, even when the infant was not premature. The placenta is nearly always very large, weighing more than 25 per cent of the weight of the infant.

The affected infants have a small nose, wide-set eyes, and low ears. The cartilage of the nose and ears is soft and poorly developed. There is often bilateral flexion of the foot. Respiratory distress in the postnatal period has been noted in a few cases. Edema may be present at birth or may manifest itself in the weeks that follow, usually appearing in the first four weeks, with an outer limit of 4 to 5 months. Abdominal distention owing to meteorism and ascites is very common, and this is accompanied by dilatation of the veins of the abdominal wall. Intense and persistent diarrhea may produce severe malnutrition and endanger survival. Routine examination of the urine of newborn children in affected sibships sometimes reveals proteinuria at a very early stage, even though edema may appear relatively late. The blood pressure is nearly always normal. Height and weight are below normal. Ossification is retarded, and the cranial sutures are very wide. At a later stage, the teeth are poorly developed and of poor quality.

The proteinuria may be moderate or severe. There is microscopic hematuria, not always seen at the outset, but appearing later. This may be associated with a moderate degree of leukocyturia.

Hypoproteinemia is marked, with very low albumin and gamma globulin levels, and a considerable elevation in the α2-lipoprotein levels. Immunoelectrophoresis shows the albumin level to be low, the gamma globulins nearly impossible to quantitate, and the β2-M globulin level increased. The cholesterol level rises, and that of the complement fractions drops as the disease progresses. In most cases, the blood urea and creatinine levels rise relatively late. In the beginning, the renal plasma flow and glomerular filtration rate are normal, but these decline progressively. Hypocalcemia is common, and there may be attacks of tetany.

Clinical Course

There may be tubular signs, such as glycosuria and hyperaminoaciduria. The greatest dangers are sudden electrolyte disorders, serious deficiency in growth, muscular atrophy with hernia, and, in particular, extreme sensitivity to infection.

Death usually occurs from one or another of these complications between the ages of 6 months and 1 year, most often before the development of renal failure.

Treatment

Steroid therapy is useless and may be poorly tolerated. Antimitotic and immunosuppressive drugs do not appear to be of any value. The only treatment is symptomatic: spironolactone for the edema; antibiotics for infection; correction of secondary electrolyte disturbances. Many attempts have been made at very early renal transplantation, but these have not met with success.[42] Diarrhea and malnutrition may be indications for prolonged, exclusively parenteral feeding.

Pathology

It is quite common to find a very peculiar, rosary chain *pseudocystic dilatation* in the proximal tubules. This has been noted both on light microscopy and by microdissection.[46] In most cases, the tubular cells are hyperplastic at the site of dilatations; only very rarely are they atrophic. There is good evidence that this appearance develops only at a later stage in the evolution of the disease.

Immunofluorescence studies have revealed intense glomerular deposits of IgG, IgM, and beta-1-C, most marked after the disease has been progressing for some months.

The progressive character of the lesions and the fact that they begin in the deep zone of the cortex, as well as the chance nature of renal biopsy, explain why biopsy may show either a normal kidney or a microcystic appearance, with normal or abnormal glomeruli.

Etiology

The condition is the result of a gene abnormality, but the mechanism of its expression remains obscure.

Immunologic Features.[42] There is definite evidence of immunologic incompatibility between fetus and mother in cases of congenital nephrotic syndrome. A substance that precipitates human kidney and placenta has been found in affected infants and in their mothers before and after delivery. Skin grafts from the infants to their mother are rejected very early, whereas when such grafts are transplanted to other persons they are tolerated normally. IgG, IgM, and beta-1-C are precipitated in the glomeruli and the beta-1-C

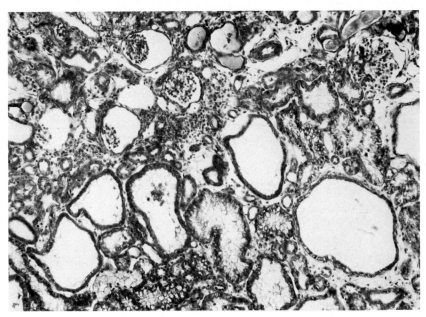

Figure 13. Microcystic kidney in infantile nephrotic syndrome. The glomeruli are normal though slightly hypercellular in places. The only abnormality is the gross dilatation of the proximal tubules in the deeper part of the cortex. ×100.

fraction of the complement decreases progressively in the serum of these patients. It has been demonstrated in rats that antikidney sera labeled with ^{131}I cross the placenta and can be found in the spleen, kidney, liver, and stomach, and that antikidney sera labeled with fluorescein are deposited in the juxtamedullary glomeruli.

Experimental Features. Attempts have been made to reproduce the disease experimentally by injecting pregnant females with nephrotoxic serum, amino-nucleoside, and indium sulfate, with little success.[37] Nevertheless, amino-nucleoside produces kidney lesions in newborn rats, notably tubular dilatation, but it has not been possible to reproduce the progressive characteristics of the nephropathy.[42]

In conclusion, the mechanism of the condition remains unknown, and there are two hypotheses to be considered: (1) either the abnormal gene in the homozygous state alters the synthesis of the basement membrane and is responsible for changes in the structure and permeability, with secondary immunologic reactions, or (2) the gene induces an immunologic disorder, toxic or enzymatic, that secondarily produces the changes in the kidneys, placenta, cartilage, and other tissues.

The Infantile Nephrotic Syndromes and the Hereditary Late Nephrotic Syndromes

The Finnish type of congenital nephrotic syndrome appears to be a well-defined hereditary disease. There are, however three diagnostic or nosologic problems.

Nephrotic Syndromes of Specific Origin in the Newborn

Nephrotic syndromes in the newborn have been described as resulting from mercury poisoning, from the toxins of *Escherichia coli* and from renal tuberculosis. There is no doubt that early congenital syphilis can produce a nephrotic syndrome with hypergammaglobulinemia which is easily cured by penicillin.[47] Many cases of cytomegalic inclusion disease with congenital nephrotic syndrome have been reported. Most authors consider that the association is coincidental and that there is no link between the inclusion disease and the congenital nephrotic syndrome.[36] Many cases of nephrotic syndrome with thrombosis of the renal veins have been noted in the newborn. The vein thrombosis may possibly be secondary, a hypothesis that is supported by the possibility of association of renal vein thrombosis with microcystic lesions of the proximal tubules.

Idiopathic Infantile Nephrotic Syndromes (INS)

The concept of INS is more factual than that of the congenital nephrotic syndrome. It includes all idiopathic nephrotic syndromes that appear during the first year of life.

We have studied the pathology in 37 cases of INS. These cases can be classified into four groups (Table 6). The first group includes 11 cases of nephrotic syndrome with microcystic lesions. In these, the placenta was always very large and the clinical onset was early, before the fifth month; the disease was familial in two cases; and the condition terminated fatally before the age of 1 year from infection, electrolyte disorders, and renal vein thrombosis. A second group can be described as *"diffuse mesangial sclerosis of infants"*; it was familial in three of six cases. In most of these cases, the onset was later than in the first group (9 to 11 months); death resulted from renal failure and occurred between 14 and 36 months (Figure 14). The third group includes 17 patients; in these the kidney exhibits minimal glomerular lesions or segmental and focal hyalinization as in the nephrotic syndrome of the older child. The clinical onset was

Table 6. Infantile Nephrotic Syndrome (Onset Before the Age of One Year) (37 Cases)

Histologic Type	Number of Cases	Number of Boys	Familial Cases	Age at Onset	Age at Death
Microcystic kidney	11	7	2	1 day to 5 months	1 to 12 months
Diffuse mesangial sclerosis	6	4	3	1 month to 11 months	14 to 36 months
Segmental and focal hyalinization	17	11	4	1 day to 11 months	7 deaths between one month and 17 years
Glomerulonephritis with extramembranous deposits	3	3	0	6 months to 11 months	1 death at 8 years

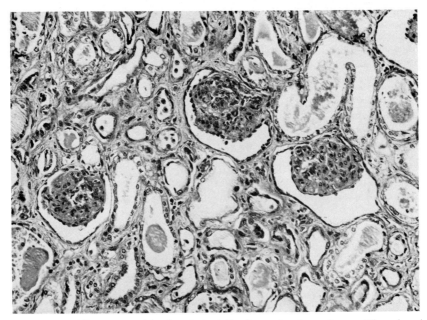

Figure 14. Diffuse mesangial sclerosis in infantile nephrotic syndrome. The sclerosis has invaded the mesangium of all the glomeruli, causing retraction of the tuft, which is surrounded by a wreath of epithelial cells. ×185.

between one day and 11 months. Thirteen patients did not respond to steroid therapy; seven of the children died, in most cases after several years; in four cases the disease was familial. The fourth group included three nonfamilial cases of glomerulonephritis with extramembranous deposits that set in between the ages of 6 and 11 months.

Hereditary Late Nephrotic Syndromes

The association in four sisters of *congenital heart disease* (narrowing of the pulmonary infundibulum) with congenital nephrotic syndrome, which appeared in the first weeks of life and proved fatal about the age of five years, was reported by Fournier and his colleagues.[40] The parents were first cousins, and had one child who was normal. The pathologic condition was a chronic glomerulonephritis. There is perhaps a correlation with our observation of INS with cardiac malformation.

Zunin and his colleagues have reported the association of *nephroblastoma* and *INS* in two children of the same sibship. In one case removal of the tumor was followed by amelioration of the nephrotic syndrome.[49]

One very special etiologic type of familial nephrotic syndrome is that linked to *Mediterranean periodic disease*. It occurs in certain groups of Israelites and in Armenians. This syndrome is definitely familial. Children in certain families exhibit renal amyloidosis with gross proteinuria, a nephrotic syndrome, and renal failure, most often between the ages of 8 and 15 years. There is no known treatment.

The *syndrome of Muckle and Wells*, described in 1962, is a condition transmitted as an autosomal dominant trait. It includes attacks of arthralgia and urticaria that appear in childhood or adolescence, late and progressive deafness, and renal amyloidosis with a nephrotic syndrome and uremia.

Conclusions

Congenital nephrotic syndrome of the Finnish type should be suspected in any newborn infant when the weight of the placenta is more than 25 per cent of the weight of the infant; or when, from the very beginning, the urine contains large amounts of protein; or when a typical nephrotic syndrome develops in the first 4 months of life. From a practical viewpoint, at the present time, this signifies: (1) a fatal outcome, almost always before the age of 1 year, although some children have survived for several years; (2) ineffectiveness of steroids and immunodepressive drugs in treatment; (3) a high intrafamilial risk, with one chance in four that every child will be affected by congenital nephrotic syndrome.

There is still much that is obscure. The following questions require answers particularly urgently. Is the predominance in Finland only apparent or real, and what are the reasons for it? How can an error in the genetic code cause the kidney disease by immunologic means? What are the chances of detecting the risk of disease before birth? Can we develop any active preventive or curative treatment?

REFERENCES

ALPORT'S SYNDROME

1. Alport, A. C.: Hereditary familial congenital hemorrhagic nephritis. Brit. Med. J. *1*:504, 1927.
2. Arnott, E. J., Crawfurd, M., and Toghill, P. J.: Anterior lenticonus and Alport's syndrome. Brit. J. Ophthal. *50*:390, 1966.
3. Cassady, G., Brown, K., Cohen, M., *et al.*: Hereditary renal dysfunction and deafness. Pediatrics *35*:967, 1965.
4. Chazan, J. A., Zacks, J., Cohen, J. J., and Garella, S.: Hereditary nephritis: clinical spectrum and mode of inheritance in five new kindreds. Amer. J. Med. *50*:764, 1971.
5. Epstein, C. J., Shaud, M. A., Piel, C. F., Goodman, J. R., Bernfield, M. R., Kushner, M. R., Kushner, J. H., and Ablin, A. R.: Hereditary macrothrombocytopathia, nephritis and deafness. Amer. J. Med. *52*:299, 1972.
6. Feingold, J., and Bois, E.: Génétique du syndrome d'Alport. Human Genetik *12*:29, 1971.
7. Goldbloom, R. B., Fraser, F. C., Waugh, D., Aronovitch, M., and Wiglesworth, F. C.: Hereditary renal disease associated with nerve deafness and ocular lesions. Pediatrics *20*:240, 1957.
8. Grace, S. G., Suki, W. N., Spjut, M. J., Eknoyan, G., and Martinez-Maldonado, M.: Hereditary nephritis in the Negro. Report of a kindred. Arch. Intern. Med. *125*:451, 1970.
9. Gribetz, D., Churg, J., Cohen, S., Kasen, I., Mathaway, L., and Griskman, E.: Hereditary nephropathy: pathology and genetics. *In* Second International Symposium of Pediatric Nephrology. Paris, Sandoz, 1971, p. 167.
10. Krickstein, H. I., Gloor, F. J., and Balogh, K.: Renal pathology in hereditary nephritis with nerve deafness. Arch. Path. *82*:506, 1966.
11. Marie, J., Royer, P., Habib, R., Mathieu, H., and Reveillaud, R. J.: La néphropathie hématurique héréditaire avec surdité. Sem. Hôp. Paris *36*:84, 1960.
12. Perkoff, G. T.: Hereditary chronic nephritis. *In* M. Strauss and L. Welt: Diseases of the Kidney. Boston, Little, Brown Co., 1963, p. 1033.
13. Preus, M., and Fraser, F. C.: Genetics of hereditary nephropathy with deafness (Alport's disease). Clin. Genet. *2*:331, 1971.
14. Purriel, P., Drets, M., Pascale, E., Cestau, R. S., Borras, A., Delucca, A., and Fernandez, L.: Familial hereditary nephropathy (Alport's syndrome). Amer. J. Med. *49*:753, 1970.
15. Shaw, R. F., and Glover, R. A.: Abnormal segregation in hereditary renal disease with deafness. Amer. J. Hum. Genet. *13*:89, 1961.
16. Sohar, E.: Renal disease, inner ear deafness and ocular changes. Arch. Intern. Med. *97*:627, 1956.

17. Spear, G. S., Whitworth, J. M., and Konigsmark, B. W.: Hereditary nephritis with nerve deafness. Immunofluorescent studies on the kidney, with a consideration of discordant immunoglobulin-complement immunofluorescent reactions. Amer. J. Med. *49*:52, 1970.

NEPHRONOPHTHISIS

18. Bois, E., and Royer, P.: Association de néphropathie interstitielle chronique et de dégénérescence tapéto-rétinienne. Etude génétique. Arch. franç. Pédiat. *27*:471, 1970.
19. Contreras, B. C., and Espinoza, S. J.: Discussion clinica y anatomopatologica de enfermos que presentaron un problema diagnostico. Pediat. (Santiago) *3*:271, 1960.
20. Durand, P., Bugiani, O., Pallidini, G., Borrone, C., Della Sella, G., and Siliato, F.: Néphropathie tubulo-interstitielle chronique, dégénérescence tapéto-rétinienne et lipidose généralisée. Arch. Franç. Pédiat. *28*:915, 1971.
21. Franconi, G., Hanhart, E., Albertini, A., Uhlinger, E., Dolivo, G., and Prader, A.: Die familiäre juvenile Nephronophtise. Helv. paediat. Acta *6*:1, 1951.
22. Giselson, N., Heinegard, D., Holmberg, C. G., Lindberg, L. G., Lindstedt, E., Lindstedt, G., and Schersten, B.: Renal medullary cystic disease or familial juvenile nephronophthisis: a renal tubular disease. Amer. J. Med. *48*:174, 1970.
23. Ivemark, B. I., Ljungquist, A., and Barry, A.: Juvenile nephronophthisis. Part II. A histologic and microangiographic study. Acta Paediat. Scand. *49*:480, 1960.
24. Koyayashi, A., Masashi, I., Murata, H., and Sato, H.: Familial juvenile nephronophthisis. Report of cases in two siblings. Acta Paediat. Jap. *9*:1, 1967.
25. Lyon, M. F., and Hulse, E. V.: An inherited kidney disease of mice resembling human nephronophthisis. J. Med. Genet. *8*:41, 1971.
26. Mangos, J. A., Optiz, J. M., Lobeck, C. C., Cookson, D. V.: Familial juvenile nephronophthisis. Pediatrics *34*:337, 1964.
27. Mongeau, J. G., Worthen, H. G.: Nephronophthisis and medullary cystic disease. Amer. J. Med. *43*:345, 1967.
28. Pedreira, F. A., Marmer, E. L., and Bergstrom, W. H.: Familial juvenile nephronophthisis and medullary cystic disease. J. Pediat. *73*:77, 1968.
29. Royer, P., Habib, R., Mathieu, H., and Courtecuisse, V.: Les néphropathies tubulo-interstitielles chroniques idiopathiques de l'enfant. Sem. Hôp. Paris *39*:2636, 1963.
30. Saldino, R. M., and Mainzer, F.: Cone-shaped epiphysis (CSE) in siblings with hereditary renal disease and retinitis pigmentosa. Radiology *98*:39, 1971.
31. Senior, B., Friedmann, A. I., and Braudo, J. L.: Juvenile familial nephropathy with tapetoretinal degeneration. Amer. J. Ophthal. *52*:625, 1961.
32. Sherman, F. E., Studnicki, F. M., and Fetterman, G. H.: Renal lesions of familial juvenile nephronophthisis examined by microdissection. Amer. J. Clin. Path. *55*:591, 1971.
33. Smith, C. H., and Graham, J. B.: Congenital medullary cysts of kidney with severe refractory anemia. Amer. J. Dis. Child. *69*:369, 1945.
34. Sworn, M. J., and Eisenger, A. J.: Medullary cystic disease and juvenile nephronophthisis in separate members of the same family. Arch. Dis. Child. *47*:278, 1972.
35. Victorin, L., Ljungquist, A., Winberg, J., and Akesson, H. O.: Nephronophthisis. Acta. Med. Scand. *188*:145, 1970.

CONGENITAL NEPHROTIC SYNDROME

36. De Luca, G., Delendi, N., and D'Andrea, S.: Un raro caso di nefrosi congenita e malattia de inclusioni citomegaliche. Min. Pediat. *16*:1164, 1964.
37. Durroux, R., Mayzou, J., Régnier, C., and Bouissou, H.: Le syndrome néphrotique congénital. Rev. Méd. Toulouse *4*:25, 1968.
38. Fanconi, G., Kousmine, C., and Frischknecht, W.: Die knostitutionnelle Bereitschaft zum Nephrosesyndrom. Helv. Paediat. Acta *6*:199, 1951.
39. Feinerman, B., Burke, E. C., and Bahn, R. C.: The nephrotic syndrome associated with renal vein thrombosis. J. Pediat. *51*:385, 1957.
40. Fournier, A., Paget, M., Pauli, A., and Devin, P.: Syndromes néphrotiques familiaux. Syndrome néphrotique associé à une cardiopathie congénitale chez quatre soeurs. Pédiatrie *18*:677, 1963.
41. Gautier, P., and Miville, D.: Syndrome de néphrose lipoïdique congénitale. Rev. Méd. Suisse Rom. *68*:740, 1942.
42. Hallman, N., Norio, R., Kouvalainen, K., Vilska, J., and Kojo, N.: Das kongenitale nephrotische Syndrom. Erg. inn. Med. Kinderheilk. *30*:1, 1970.

43. Marie, J., Rouer, P., and Lévèque, B.: Le syndrome néphrotique familial de l'enfant. Ann. Pédiat. 7:76, 1960.
44. Mathieu, H., and Habib, R.: Syndromes néphrotiques congénitaux. *In* Journées parisiennes de Pédiatrie. Paris, Flammarion, 1968, p. 287.
45. Norio, R.: Heredity in the congenital nephrotic syndrome. A genetic study of 57 Finnish families with a review of reported cases. Ann. Paediat. Fenn. *12* (Suppl. 27):1, 1966.
46. Paatela, M.: Renal microdissection in infants with special reference to the congenital nephrotic syndrome. Ann. Paediat. Fenn. *9* (Suppl. 21):1, 1963.
47. Papaioannou, A. C., Asrow, G. G., and Schuckmell, N. H.: Nephrotic syndrome in early infancy as a manifestation of congenital syphilis. Pediatrics *27*:636, 1961.
48. Worthen, H. G., Vernier, R. L., and Good, R. A.: The syndrome of infantile nephrosis. Amer. J. Dis. Child. *96*:585, 1958.
49. Zunin, C., and Soave, F.: Association of nephrotic syndrome and nephroblastoma in siblings. Ann. Paediat. (Basle) *203*:29, 1964.

For recent additions to the literature, see:

a. Habib, R., and Bois, E.: Hétérogénéité des syndromes néphrotiques à début précoce du nourisson (syndrome néphrotique infantile). Helv. Paediat. Acta *28*:91, 1973.
b. Hinglais, N., Grünfeld, J. P., and Bois, E.: Chracteristic ultrastructural lesion of glomerular basement membrane in progressive hereditary nephritis (Alport's syndrome). Lab. Invest. *27*: 473, 1972.
c. Senior, B.: Familial renal-retinal dystrophy. Amer. J. Dis. Child. *125*:442, 1973.

Chapter Five

THE HEREDITARY
TUBULAR DISEASES

Hereditary disorders of tubular function, which may be simple or complex, are rare. In some of these there have been significant therapeutic advances. For convenience they can be divided into four groups: simple transfer disorders, tubular acidoses, pseudoendocrinopathies, and complex tubulopathies.

SIMPLE ANOMALIES OF TUBULAR TRANSFER

Various abnormalities of amino acid transport are summarized in Table 7. Cystinuria is discussed with urinary lithiasis. Renal glycosuria, chronic hypokalemia, idiopathic resistant rickets, and idiopathic hypercalciuria have an apparent renal expression, but there are doubts about the primary tubular character of the last three named.

Hereditary Normoglycemic Glycosuria (Renal Glucose Diabetes)

Clinical Features

The symptoms consist simply of glycosuria without hyperglycemia. The glycosuria may be intermittent and may appear only after meals. Most often, however, it is continuous and can be noted even in fasting morning urine. The degree of glycosuria is often moderate—between 5 and 30 g. per 24 hours. Sometimes the glucose output is greater and may even be more than 100 g. in 24 hours. In any given patient, the urinary glucose output is fairly stable and is little affected by diet. Polyuria, ketosis, and hypoglycemia are rare.

Laboratory Studies

The laboratory investigation of renal glucose diabetes includes measurement of the renal threshold for glucose, establishing the maximal tubular reabsorption of glucose (TmG) and titration tests.[6, 7] The purpose of these tests is to distinguish two varieties of renal diabetes.[6] The first variety, or type A, is characterized by lowering of both the renal threshold for glucose and the TmG, and by a normal "nephron dispersion." It is the result of an abnormality in the tubular glucose transport systems. The second variety, or type B, is characterized by a lowering of the renal threshold for glucose, a normal TmG, and a greatly

Table 7. Abnormalities of Amino Acid Transport

Condition	Amino Acids	Organs Involved	Mode of Transmission*	Clinical Features
Blue diaper syndrome	Tryptophan	Intestine	R	Hypercalcemia
Methionine malabsorption	Methionine	Intestine	R	Mental retardation Diarrhea
Hypercystinuria	Cystine	Kidneys	R	Urinary lithiasis
Glycinuria	Glycine	Kidneys	D	Urinary lithiasis
Hartnup disease	Tryptophan and others	Kidneys Intestine	R	Pseudopellagra
Classic cystinuria	Cystine Lysine Arginine Ornithine	Kidneys Intestine	R, D	Urinary lithiasis
Dibasic hyperaminoaciduria	Lysine Arginine Ornithine	Kidneys Intestine	R, D	Dwarfism, sometimes mental retardation
Iminoglycinuria	Proline Hydroxyproline Glycine	Kidneys Intestine	R, D	Variable
Glycoglycinuria	Glycine Glucose	Kidneys	D	None
Protein intolerance with dibasic aminoaciduria	Lysine Arginine Ornithine	Kidneys Intestine	R	Vomiting and diarrhea with high blood ammonium level, dwarfism, and hepatomegaly

*R, autosomal recessive; D, autosomal dominant.

increased "nephron dispersion." It has been suggested that this dispersion results from a difference in the length of the nephrons. The distinction between the two types is not yet completely clear. Taggart[7] has correlated the various published reports, and he has shown that there is a continuous spectrum of Tm values from very low to very high. In other words, there is no true distinction between the two groups.

Evolution

Renal glucose diabetes is more an anomaly than a disease. It is a tubular disorder that is not progressive and remains unchanged throughout life, without causing secondary complications.

The only point that has given rise to controversy is the appearance of true diabetes mellitus in later life. The incidence of true diabetes in patients with renal glycosuria is the same as in the general population.

Pathology

Most renal biopsy specimens from patients with renal glycosuria have proved to be normal on light microscopy.[4] However, Monasterio and his colleagues[5] have made somewhat different observations. They have found the configuration of the nephron to be normal on microdissection, but there are changes in the cells of the proximal tubules, including vacuolization, annulation of PAS-positive material, and abnormalities of the brush border and mitochondria.

Pathogenesis

The pathogenesis of renal glycosuria may depend on a global abnormality of the tubular transfer mechanisms, which lowers the TmG; on changes in the kinetics of the transport reaction, augmenting the "dispersion" of the titration curve; or on a functional heterogeneity of the nephrons.[1-3, 6] It is certain, however, that the condition is not the result of a defect in the phosphorylation of glucose by hexokinase or of a defect in alkaline phosphatase or glucose-6-phosphatase.

Bartter's Syndrome
(Familial Chronic Hypokalemia with Hyperkaluria)

The features of this condition are chronic hypokalemia, elevation of the circulating renin, an inadequate pressor response to the injection of angiotensin, excessive secretion of aldosterone, and hypertrophy of the juxtaglomerular apparatus. There is often dwarfism, polyuria, globulinuria, hyponatremia, hypomagnesemia, and hypercalciuria. The disease may be sporadic or familial. It is easy to distinguish between this and other causes (renal, adrenal, and cerebral) of chronic hypokalemia in children. The pathophysiology has not yet been clarified.[15] We have studied six cases (Table 8).

Familial Distribution

The disease often manifests itself very early, in the first year of life. In more than 50 per cent of cases, two or more children in the same sibship are involved. The sexes are affected equally. The parents are free of the disease, but sometimes they are blood relatives. The whole picture suggests a hereditary condition transmitted as an autosomal recessive trait.

Clinical Features

Polyuria and polydipsia are common and early manifestations, and these may be accompanied by the complications of dehydration. Gastrointestinal disorders, including anorexia, vomiting, and constipation, and sometimes a chronic fetid diarrhea, are also present. Defective growth is noted in 75 per cent of cases: the children are small and thin, with poor muscular development, are easily tired, and appear sad but intelligent. In some cases, the dwarfism is marked. Recurrent tetany has been reported in many cases. Hypokalemic paralysis is very rare, a suprising observation in view of the very low blood potassium level. The skeleton is sometimes abnormal, with retardation of bone maturation and osteoporosis or discrete metaphyseal lesions. An important negative finding is the normal blood pressure. Nephrocalcinosis has been reported in some cases.[14]

Table 8. Bartter's Syndrome (Personal Series)

Case	Age at Onset (years)	Sex	Familial	Height, cm. (S.D.)	Urinary Output (liters/24 hours)	Serum Potassium (mEq./liter)	Urinary Calcium (mg./kg./24 hours)	Proteinuria	G.F.R. (ml./min./1.73 m.²)	Blood Urea (mg./100 ml.)	Urinary Aldosterone (mcg./24 hours)	Aldosterone Secretion (mcg./24h)	Plasma Renin (ng./ml./M.²)	Angiotensin test	Renal biopsy	Treatment	Follow-up Interval (years)	Follow-up Present Condition
1	9/12	M	0	84 (−4)	2	2.5	3	+	27	57	8.6	?	?	?	I.N.	Potassium citrate	5	Dead
2	6/12	F	+	79 (−3)	3	1.8	4–9	0	130	28	4	?	?	?	J.G.A., I.N.	Potassium chloride, spironolactone	3	Dead
3	6/12	F	+	94 (−6)	2	1.5	4–10	0	120	30	8–110	?	61	No response	J.G.A., I.N.	Potassium chloride, triamterene	19	H = −3.5 S.D. Urea, 80 mg. per 100 ml.
4	4/12	F	+	69 (−1)	0.8	2	0.4	±	41	50	8–189	45	?	No response	J.G.A., I.N.	Potassium chloride, triamterene	9	H = −3 S.D. Renal failure
5	6/12	M	+	70 (−1)	0.3	1.9	?	±	74	42	?	?	?	?	?	Potassium chloride	4/12	H = −2 S.D. G.F.R. = 74 ml./min./ 1.73 m.²
6	2	M	C	78 (−4)	1.5	2	7	0	135	18	40	?	80	No response	J.G.A.	Potassium chloride, spironolactone	2	H = −4.5 S.D. G.F.R. = 124 ml./min./ 1.73 m.²

C, Consanguinity; H, height; J.G.A., hypertrophy of juxtaglomerular apparatus; I.N., diffuse interstitial nephritis; G.F.R., glomerular filtration rate; S.D., standard deviations.

Biochemical Abnormalities

A marked and very stable hypokalemia, usually in the region of 2 mEq./liter, is a constant feature. The urinary potassium level is normal or raised. Spironolactones raise the blood potassium level and sometimes diminish urinary potassium output. Exchangeable potassium and muscle potassium are low. Hyponatremia is nearly always present and may be considerable, below 125 mEq./liter. The urinary sodium is normal. The exchangeable sodium and tissue sodium values are slightly raised. Hypochloremic alkalosis is found in nearly 50 per cent of cases. The urinary pH is generally close to 7.0. The blood calcium level is over 11.0 mg. per 100 ml. in one third of cases. Urinary calcium output has rarely been studied; on two occasions it was normal, and in two familial cases it was elevated. In two cases, we have studied the calcium balance and found it negative, owing to the rise in fecal and urinary calcium outputs. The serum magnesium level is normal or low. The plasma lipid, cholesterol, triglyceride, and fatty acid levels may sometimes be elevated, but this is not a constant finding. A high platelet count has been reported.

Renal function studies constantly show a serious defect in the concentrating ability of the kidney that cannot be corrected by pitressin. The dilution power is normal. There is no glycosuria, and the amino acid output in the urine is normal. The urine contains neither red nor white cells. The urogram, when obtainable, is normal. In some cases there is proteinuria of the tubular type, diminution of glomerular clearance rates, and a renal salt-losing syndrome.

Adrenal function studies show a normal urinary output of 17-ketosteroids and 17-hydroxycorticosteroids. With a normal sodium intake, there is an abnormally high urinary excretion of tetrahydroaldosterone and true secretion of aldosterone. Plasma renin and angiotensin levels are raised. A pressor response to intravenous injections of angiostensin is obtained only with doses at least 10 times as great as are required in the normal child.[9] There is sometimes a considerable rise in the urinary corticosterone level, with a normal 11-desoxycorticosterone level.

Pathology

Lesions are found in two organs, the adrenals and the kidneys.

In the *adrenals*, there is considerable lipoid infiltration of the cortex. This may involve the whole cortex or may affect principally the zona glomerulosa and the zona fasciculata.

In the *kidney*, there is considerable hypertrophy of the juxtaglomerular apparatus. Electron microscopy reveals a relative paucity of secretory granules and a large number of protogranules.[17] The remainder of the kidney is normal apart from apical vacuolization of the cells of the proximal tubule, owing to the hypokalemia. In late stages of the disease, biopsy may show a distinct interstitial fibrosis, tubular atrophy, and intercapillary hyalinization in the glomeruli. In one of our patients, the first renal biopsy showed a normal kidney with hypertrophy of the juxtaglomerular apparatus, and a second biopsy three years later showed a glomerulotubular nephropathy.

Course and Treatment

The disease progresses in a chronic fashion. Some forms may be complicated by tubulo-interstitial renal lesions and uremia after some time. Death may occur during acute intercurrent infection or bacterial diarrhea owing to violent disturbances of the water and electrolyte balance.

Spironolactone given in doses of 10 to 15 mg./kg./day raises the blood potassium level, but the sodium intake must be adjusted to avoid aggravating the hyponatremia. We have found triamterene in doses of 10 mg./kg./day to be equally effective. The best treatment, nevertheless, is the continuous administration of high doses of potassium chloride. Dosages need to be considerable to maintain the serum potassium level above 3.5 mEq./liter. With doses of potassium chloride approaching 1 g./kg./day, we have found improvements in the general condition, in growth, and in strength, as well as reduction of the polyuria. A trial of total adrenalectomy failed to correct the potassium loss.[16]

Pathophysiology

Many hypotheses have been put forward. The most common hypothesis is of a *functional tubular nephropathy* with selective renal potassium loss. Some authors claim that atrophy or dilatation of the distal tubules is a primary factor and that this can be confirmed by microdissection of the nephron. Many cases progress to glomerular hyalinization and renal failure.

Another explanation has been proposed by Bartter and his associates,[9] who made the discovery that intravenous perfusion of angiotensin, even in very high doses, does not raise the blood pressure. The primary factor is the *insensitivity of the vessels to the action of angiotensin.* The secondary chain of reactions includes hypertrophy of the juxtaglomerular apparatus, hypersecretion of renin, and the abundant formation of angiotensin. This increased angiotensin formation causes increased synthesis of aldosterone and possibly also of corticosterone.

Gall and his colleagues[11] report the interesting finding of excessive *permeability of the red cell membrane to sodium,* with an increased sodium concentration within the erythrocyte. This would explain the finding of a high level of rapidly exchangeable sodium. This exaggerated cell permeability to sodium could produce chronic hypovolemia, giving rise in turn to the high blood renin levels, and the increased secretion of aldosterone and would account for the increased reabsorption in the tubule of sodium at the expense of potassium.

Morphologic abnormalities of the *macula densa* have been described, including hypercellularity, pyknosis of the nucleus, and sometimes the presence of an abnormal, PAS-positive membrane between the macula densa and the afferent arteriole. The macula densa is the sensory structure responsible for inhibiting renin secretion when the sodium concentration or output rises in the distal tubular urine. Disorder of this receptor apparatus would raise the the blood renin level and consequently stimulate the secretion of aldosterone.[10]

In conclusion, the pathophysiology of this syndrome is far from clear, but there is certainly a disordered regulation of fluid volumes and chronic hypovolemia. Bartter's syndrome may possibly include several entities with different mechanisms.[14]

Variants: Liddle's Syndrome

In 1964, Liddle and his colleagues[13] described eight patients in one family who suffered from hypertension, hypokalemic alkalosis, inability of the kidney to retain potassium, and a low rate of both actual secretion and urinary excretion of aldosterone. The disease is apparently transmitted as an autosomal dominant trait and is the result of abnormal transmembrane sodium transport.[12] Many other cases have been reported in children.[8] According to most reports, the condition can be treated effectively by triamterene in doses of 10 mg./kg./day.

We have seen one other variant, in a boy who presented with hypokalemia, hypercalciuria, and a salt-losing syndrome, and the histologic picture included dilatation of the tubules without hypertrophy of the juxtaglomerular apparatus.

Hereditary Idiopathic Vitamin-Resistant Rickets

Vitamin D is extremely effective in the prevention and treatment of ordinary rickets, and this has made it possible to identify a series of hereditary idiopathic vitamin-resistant osteopathies. These were originally regarded as a "renal phosphate diabetes." Two varieties are clearly defined.

Familial Hypophosphatemia

It is probable, as suggested by Winters and his colleagues,[27] that this condition is transmitted as a hereditary dominant linked to the X chromosome (Figure 15). The primary abnormality, and one that can be used as an indicator of the condition in involved families, is hypophosphatemia, which becomes marked between the ages of 3 and 6 months.

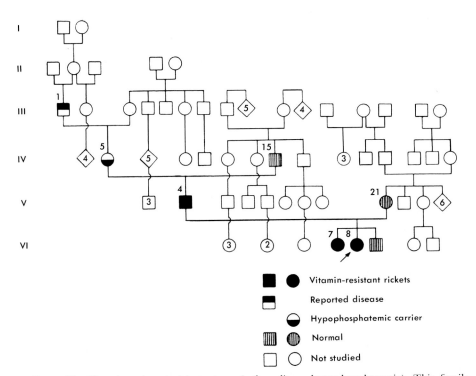

Figure 15. Vitamin-resistant rickets, type 1 (hereditary hypophosphatemia). This family tree is compatible with a dominant transmission linked to the X chromosome.

Clinical Features. The clinical features usually appear during the second year of life, when the children begin to stand upright and learn to walk. The first deformities are noted at this stage, and the initial diagnosis is rickets from defective nutrition. However, there is no improvement on treatment with physiologic doses of vitamin D. The deformities increase, and retardation of growth becomes obvious. The hands and feet are square and thick. The bone deformities affect the lower limbs (coxa vara, genu valgum, bowlegs), spine, and pelvis. Epiphyseal thickenings, a rachitic rosary, a protuberant forehead, and an enlarged bridge of the nose are common findings. The teeth erupt normally, but the first teeth may be lost prematurely. The dentin is defective, but the enamel is normal. There may also be alopecia, albinism, fibrous dysplasia of the bones, or early craniostenosis. The condition evolves chronically; active until adolescence, the disease then enters a quiescent phase. The height of adults is 140 to 155 cm. When fatigability is a dominant symptom, it persists into adult life. Pregnancy and lactation may reactivate the disease. In some cases, after the age of 40 years, varying degrees of osteomalacia occur.

Radiology. *Radiology* shows two types of lesions. The first type is found in the region of the epiphysis and nearby metaphysis, and is identical to that of normal rickets. The second type is more typical, a loose retiform pattern of the bone trabeculae, giving a latticed appearance, which may be generalized or may be seen only in the pelvis, femur, tibia, humerus, and small bones of the wrist. Looser-Milkman striae are rarely found.

Biochemical Disorders. The principal disorder is the severe diminution of plasma phosphorus, usually to a level of 1.0 to 2.5 mg. per 100 ml. Serum calcium level is normal or very slightly lowered. The alkaline phosphatase level usually is elevated but may occasionally be normal. The urinary calcium output is very often low, but this too may be normal. Phosphorus clearance is very markedly elevated, with a lowering of the percentage of tubular reabsorption of phosphorus (TRP). Renal function is normal. There have been some reports of hyperaminoaciduria. In balance studies, a considerable increase in calcium and phosphorus outputs in the stools is a constant finding. On a normal diet, calcium and phosphorus balance are negative or inadequately positive. Intestinal absorption of vitamin D is normal, as is the absorption of 25-hydroxycholecalciferol.

Pathology. Bone biopsy reveals the presence of large osteoid seams. The irregular deposition of tetracyclines along the zones of apposition is an index of the abnormal mineral fixation. Microradiography shows enlarged osteocyte lacunae surrounded by a hazy zone deficient in calcium, characteristic of this condition.[28]

Mechanism. Many simple explanations have been proposed, including primary intestinal calcium malabsorption,[18] a primary disorder of the tubular transfer of phosphorus,[22] and a primary defect of mineralization of bone tissue,[23] but none of these explanations is satisfactory.[26] It has also been shown that a disorder of activation of cholecalciferol, especially its 25-hydroxylation, is not the cause[19] (Figure 16). We are left with the hypothesis that a primary and generalized abnormality of cell transfer of phosphorus is responsible. We have found in the red blood cells an increased glycolytic activity, a rise in ATP levels, a lowering of inorganic phosphorus levels, and enhanced kinetics of phosphorus entry.[21] This makes it difficult to regard the condition as a simple, isolated,

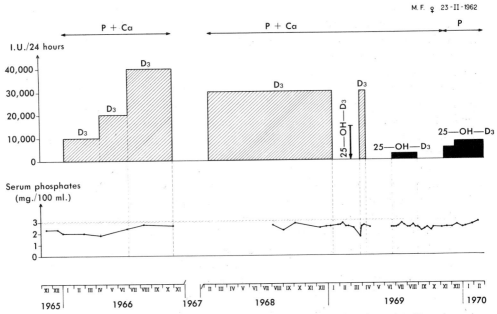

Figure 16. Vitamin-resistant rickets, type 1 (hereditary hypophosphatemia). Note the resistance to vitamin D_3, which does not achieve complete correction of the hypophosphatemia even with a dose of 40,000 I.U. per day. The phosphatemia is corrected by 25-hydroxycholecalciferol (25-OH-D_3) in doses of 10,000 I.U. per day. Hence, there is resistance to 25-hydroxycholecalciferol as well, but it is less than the resistance to cholecalciferol.

and primary disorder of phosphorus transfer in the renal tubule, although an argument has been presented recently in favor of this thesis: the loss of a tubular factor for phosphate transport, a factor responsive to parathormone.[24]

Treatment. The most effective treatment at the present time is the daily oral administration of high doses of phosphorus (1 to 2 g. per day) and of 25-hydroxycholecalciferol in doses of 2500 to 15,000 units per day. The administration of the latter substance is stopped if the urinary calcium output increases beyond 6 mg./kg./day or when an osteotomy is performed. Treatment is continued until growth is completed.[19]

Familial Hypocalcemic Pseudo-Vitamin D-Deficiency Rickets[20, 25]

The familial distribution of this condition is that of a hereditary disease transmitted as an autosomal recessive trait; heterozygous parents are therefore normal. All involved children are seriously diseased; the sexes are affected equally.

The first abnormality to appear—between 4 and 12 weeks after birth—is a progressive lowering of blood calcium level. Clinical signs begin to appear between the second and fourth months of life, including metaphyseal thickening, rachitic rosary, and curvature of diaphyses. Failure to grow and gain weight soon becomes very marked. Muscular weakness is the rule. Attacks of diarrhea and anemia are common. Radiologic study of the skeleton shows severe osteomalacic rickets, with Looser-Milkman striae and multiple fractures. Serum calcium is low, with a normal or low phosphorus level and an elevated alkaline phosphatase level. Urinary calcium is low or normal. There is sometimes hyperaminoaciduria. Prophylactic doses of vitamin D do not prevent the onset of the disease, and normal therapeutic doses have no effect. Attacks of tetany and laryngospasm are common, and the child is in danger of dying from convulsions, pulmonary hypoventilation, and glottal spasm. When high doses of vitamin D (0.5 to 1 mg. per day) and of calcium (500 mg. per day) are given, all these complications are relieved, the skeleton undergoes repair, and the growth defect is corrected. Lower doses are equally effective if 25-hydroxycholecal-ciferol is given as well. If treatment is stopped, relapse follows in 4 to 6 weeks, the first sign being a fall in the serum calcium level. Hence, this hereditary rickets is a pseudo-vitamin D-deficiency condition, and because of its response to treatment, it has been labeled "vitamin-dependent." The exact mechanism remains unknown, although there is some indirect evidence of abnormal 1-hydroxylation of 25-hydroxycholecalciferol.

Idiopathic Hypercalciuria

This was described in adults by Albright and his colleagues in 1953.[29] The clinical presentation is nearly always with calcium oxalate or calcium phosphate stones in the urine. In children, two clinical types have been noted. The first, which is relatively benign, resembles the adult disease, and is the lithogenous hypercalciuria described by Zetterstrom[46] and Rosenkranz.[40] The other, more serious, was described in 1962 by Royer and his colleagues,[41] and includes hypercalciuria with dwarfism, osteoporosis, nephrocalcinosis or lithiasis, defective concentration of urine, and proteinuria of the tubular type.[30-33, 35, 39, 42] We have studied 10 cases (Table 9).

Familial Distribution

No coherent study of the familial distribution has been made. There is a strong predilection for males to be affected, but girls may also be involved. In one family,[30] the father and a brother of the patient had hypercalciuria. In another family,[31] four brothers in the same sibship were affected, but the parents had not been studied. In one of our cases, the father and a brother of the patient had hypercalciuria, and in another family, two brothers were affected, one with rickets, the other with osteoporosis.

Clinical Features[42]

The age at the time of diagnosis varies from 3 months to 18 years. Dwarfism is a significant feature in nearly every case. The height is some 4 to 5 standard deviations less than the mean height for the age. Bone maturation is always delayed in comparison with the chronologic age. The bone age often corresponds to the height or may be a little greater. Maturation of the teeth is normal in relation to chronologic age. The dwarfing is uniform.

In addition to delayed bone maturation, radiology of the skeleton reveals in most cases an intense osteoporosis, with lowering of the corticodiaphyseal ratio in the long bones and decreased density of the skeleton. Some authors have reported a normal skeleton or have found rickets. The rickets may be responsive or resistant to vitamin D.

Table 9.   Idiopathic Hypercalciuria (Personal Series)

Case	Age at Onset (years)	Sex	Familial	Height, cm. (S.D.)	Urinary Output (liters/24 hours)	Proteinuria	Bone Disease	Nephrocalcinosis (on X-ray)	Lithiasis	Urinary Calcium (mg./kg./24 hours)	G.F.R. (ml./min./1.73 m.^{2})	Serum Calcium (mg. per 100 ml.)
1	2	F	C	77 (−3)	2	0	Ost.	0	0	15–24	80	9.9–10.7
2	7/12	F	0	58 (−4)	0.2	0	0	0	0	18–20	51	10.0
3	5	M	0	88 (−5)	1	+	R, Ost.	0	0	9	95	9.6
4	1	M	0	66 (−5)	2	0	Ost.	0	0	11–20	63	9.9
5	4	M	0	80 (−5)	1	+	R	0	0	7–13	80	8.4–10.5
6	10	F	0	112 (−4.5)	0.7	+	0	0	0	8.5	34–74	9.0
7	7 years 10 months	M	C	104 (−4)	2	0	0	0	0	10–25	95	10.0
8	4 years 7 months	M	0	90 (−4)	0.6	+	Ost.	0	0	10–18	67	9.9
9	2	M	0	76 (−3)	2	+	0	+	0	10	76	9.9
10	4	M	0	82 (−5)	2.5	0	Ost.	0	0	15–20	136	9.6

C, Consanguinity; R, rickets; Ost., osteoporosis; I.N., focal interstitial nephritis; H, height; G.F.R., glomerular filtration rate; S.D., standard deviations; T.R.P., tubular reabsorption of phosphorus.

In all cases, there is polyuria, varying from 600 to 2500 ml. per 24 hours. In our patients, the maximal osmolar concentration was between 170 and 178 mOsm./kg. of water. This defect in concentration is resistant to pitressin therapy. It may disappear or persist when the urinary calcium output becomes normal.

Proteinuria is found in two cases of five, in amounts ranging from 0.4 g. to 3.0 g. per day. The proteinuria is of tubular type, with a predominant globulinuria.

Table 9. Idiopathic Hypercalciuria (Personal Series) — *Continued*

Serum Phosphorus (mg. per 100 mL.) and T.R.P.	Acid Loading Test	Renal Biopsy	Treatment	Follow-up	
				Interval (years)	Present Condition
4.7 61 per cent	Normal	I.N.	Low-salt diet	6	H = −2.5 S.D. G.F.R. = 150 ml./min./1.73 m.²
4.2 73 per cent	Normal (pH 5)	I.N. + calcium	Low-salt diet, phosphorus	1 year 6 months	H = −3 S.D. G.F.R. = 30 ml./min./1.73 m.²
3.8	Normal	I.N.	Chlorothiazide, low-salt diet	12	H = −5 S.D. G.F.R. = 67 ml./min./1.73 m.² Nephrocalcinosis
5.9 86 per cent	Normal (pH 5.2)	I.N.	Low-salt diet	8	H = −2 S.D. G.F.R. = 85 ml./min./1.73 m.² Lithiasis
3.0	Normal (pH 5)	Calcium	Low-salt diet	13	H = −6 S.D. G.F.R. = 56 ml./min./1.73 m.²
3.7	Normal (pH 5.2)	Normal	Low-salt diet (not followed)	5	H = −6 S.D. G.F.R. = 47 ml./min./1.73 m.²
4.2	Normal	Normal	Vitamin D	2	H = −3.5 S.D.
3.0 65 per cent	Normal	I.N.	Low-salt diet	0	—
4.0	Normal	0	Low-salt diet	4	H = −3 S.D.
5.0 79 per cent	Normal	I.N.	Vitamin D, low-salt diet	1 year 6 months	H = −4 S.D. G.F.R. = 60 ml./min./1.73 m.²

Renal function is otherwise satisfactory, with a normal blood urea level and normal endogenous creatinine clearance, no glycosuria or hyperaminoaciduria, no salt-losing syndrome, normal blood and urinary potassium levels, and a normal ammonium chloride test in all the cases. The coefficient of tubular reabsorption of phosphorus is decreased and rises inadequately with intravenous infusion of calcium.

Renal biopsy has been carried out in five cases. In two the histology was normal, and in the other three there was focal interstitial nephritis.

The urine is always cell-free and sterile, and urograms are normal. Nephrocalcinosis can appear in the course of the disease and indeed was evident in the first year of life in one of our patients. It may be accompanied by stone formation.

Hypercalciuria

Hypercalciuria may be regarded as pathologic when the urinary calcium output is more than 8 mg./kg./24 hours. In our cases, the mean urinary calcium output was between 5.8 and 20 mg./kg./24 hours, and the maximal urinary calcium output between 11 and 38 mg./kg./24 hours. The hypercalciuria may be stable or may vary with a seasonal rhythm, rising in spring and summer but being less marked during fall and winter. The serum calcium and alkaline phosphatase levels and the blood and urinary citrate levels are normal. Serum phosphorus is normal or low. On occasion, the serum calcium level may be low, with tetany.

There are many important features of this condition. There is no significant rise in urinary calcium output with daily doses of vitamin D of the order of 10,000 units. The urinary calcium output does not fall with the administration of sodium bicarbonate, unlike the finding in idiopathic chronic tubular acidosis. The urinary calcium output can be decreased by a low-calcium diet, by sodium phytate, by hydrochlorothiazide, or by a low-salt diet with increased phosphorus. The calciuria is not affected by injecting calcitonin.

Pure Lithogenous Hypercalciuria of Children

In this variety, calcium oxalate or calcium phosphate stones in the urinary tract represent the only clinical expression of the disease.[40, 46] We have seen four patients with this variety of lithiasis. The relationship to the preceding syndrome, a much more serious condition, is not clear.

Pathophysiology

Hypercalciuria is probably the central phenomenon that explains the defective concentration of urine, the tubular proteinuria, the lithiasis and nephrocalcinosis, and the consequent focal interstitial nephritis. It probably also explains the inadequately positive calcium balance, with resulting dwarfism, defective maturation of bone, and osteoporosis. This hypothesis, however, remains to be proved.

The mechanism of the hypercalciuria is not clear. Intestinal absorption of calcium is normal or increased, and the calcium balance is negative or inadequately positive. In our patients, isotope studies of accretion and osteolysis rates gave normal results, but increased rates of accretion, osteolysis, and turnover of calcium, have been found in adults.[38] A primary abnormality of renal calcium transfer is sometimes suggested, but in one case of kidney transplantation from a hypercalciuric father to a normocalciuric son, the urinary calcium level remained normal after transplantation.[34] Recent studies suggest that the condition may be due to *equilibrated overproduction* of parathormone and calcitonin and that partial parathyroidectomy may be helpful.[44]

Treatment

Hydrochlorothiazide[33] and sodium phytate may be useful. The most encouraging results in the short run are with a diet relatively low in calcium (300 mg./day) and very low in sodium chloride (10 mEq./day). We have shown that this diet is effective[43] following physiologic studies demonstrating the correlation between the clearances of calcium and sodium[36, 37, 45] (Figure 17). In the long run, a low-sodium diet causes secondary hyperaldosteronism, and hence it must be maintained for only two months in three, and potassium gluconate must be given in addition. An oral dose of 350 to 750 mg./day of phosphorus also reduces urinary calcium but the long-term effects are not known.

PRIMARY TUBULAR ACIDOSIS

There are two types of primary tubular acidosis. The first, described by Albright and his colleagues[47] in a patient previously studied by Butler and

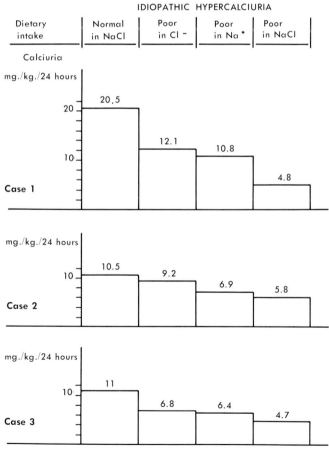

Figure 17.   Effect of intake of sodium and chloride on the urinary calcium level in idiopathic hypercalciuria. The urinary calcium level drops with diminished dietary intake of chloride. With decreased sodium intake, the phenomenon is even more marked. The lowering of urinary calcium output is maximal with a diet containing very little sodium chloride (0.3 mM/kg/24 hours).

associates,[48] results from a defect in the exchange of H^+ ions between the distal tubules and the urine, hence the terms "distal acidosis" or "gradient type acidosis."[54] The second, described by Rodriguez-Soriano and his colleagues,[56] stems from an abnormality of bicarbonate reabsorption, hence the terms "proximal acidosis" or "rate type acidosis." Secondary tubular acidosis and acidosis due to complex tubular disease are primarily of the proximal type.[58]

Primary Distal Tubular Acidosis (DTA)

Clinical Features[54, 58, 62]

Girls are affected twice as often as boys. The onset is usually in the first month of life, with vomiting and failure to thrive.

The clinical features are generalized dwarfism; severe thirst, with polyuria, complications of dehydration, vomiting, and constipation; anorexia; and variable fatigability. The growth defect becomes more evident with the years, and in some cases may long remain the only clinical sign. Skeletal disorders are usual. In young children, there is osteoporosis and delay in bone maturation, but there is little or only slight evidence of rickets in the metaphyses. Often at a later stage there is bowing of the long bones and coxa vara. Extensive osteo-malacia and Looser-Milkman striae are generally found in late childhood and adolescence.

Radiologic disorders of the kidneys are obvious on a straight film. Nephro-calcinosis may be slight, moderate, or gross, the picture varying from that of grains of shot scattered through the medulla to complete petrification of the pyr-amids. Stone formation is common and produces the various clinical compli-cations of lithiasis.

Periodic paralysis with hypokalemia is not uncommon, and in some cases this is the dominant feature. Hypocalcemic tetany is rare. The progress of the disease may be marked by a sudden crisis of acute dehydration, sometimes with collapse, arrhythmia, vomiting, flaccid paralysis, difficult respiration, and some-times coma.

We found a nerve deafness in three of our patients, although this compli-cation had not been previously reported; in addition, two of these developed precocious myopia that was detected in the second year of life, and one de-veloped glaucoma (Table 10).

Biochemical Features

Plasma bicarbonate levels and pH are low. The urinary pH lies between 6.5 and 7.5, with a low titratable acidity and urinary ammonium and, of course, a low net urinary excretion of H^+ ions. Proteinuria is inconstant and in our own patients proved to be a triple globulinuria of tubular type. It is normal to find a low urinary citrate level with a normal blood citrate value. In our cases, we have verified that the very low urinary citrate level contrasts with a normal level of α-ketoglutarate.[57] The hypercalciuria normally reaches a figure of 10 to 20 mg./kg./day, compared to the normal figure of 1 to 8 mg./kg./day. It is accompanied by a normal or low serum calcium level, and a variable but sometimes marked elevation of the alkaline phosphatase. The calciuria is proportional to the acidosis and returns to normal when the acidosis is corrected by administration of bicarbonate or may be aggravated by acid loading with ammonium chloride. The urinary calcium level drops with the onset of uremia.

Hypophosphatemia, with lowering of the coefficient of tubular reabsorption of phosphorus, is inconstant. In one third of our cases there was a high urinary potassium level with low blood potassium level associated with potassium depletion, as measured by isotope techniques. The defective urine concentration and polyuria are resistant to vasopressin. There may be hyperaminoaciduria that disappears when the acidosis is corrected by bicarbonate.

Evolution

The condition develops chronically. Treatment may have remarkable results: growth is restored and any growth deficit is corrected; rickets and osteoporosis are healed, and the general condition is transformed, provided that the acidosis, the hypercalciuria, and the potassium depletion are corrected (Figure 18). Nephrocalcinosis does not regress. Complications caused by urinary calculi may persist during treatment. This very remarkable response persists only as long as treatment continues. Any interruption of treatment is marked by chemical and clinical relapse. In the absence of treatment, after a long interval, chronic renal failure and hypertension may set in, probably due to chronic interstitial nephritis secondary to the nephrocalcinosis.

Pathology

In older patients, the main feature is chronic tubulo-interstitial nephritis, but in our young patients, renal biopsy showed, in addition to nephrocalcinosis, either a normal kidney or striate interstitial nephritis, which varied from minimal to severe, characterized by round-cell infiltration of the interstitial tissue, tubular atrophy, and a varying degree of glomerular sclerosis.

These observations do little to resolve the argument over whether interstitial nephritis is the primary condition, with chronic acidosis as one of its manifestations, or whether interstitial nephritis is secondary to the nephrocalcinosis. The fact that in one of our patients, aged 2 years 6 months, the kidney was normal on light microscopy suggests that the second opinion is probably more reasonable.[58]

Pathophysiology of Symptoms

Patients with DTA are in persistently positive hydrogen ion balance. This leads to metabolic acidosis and the utilization of bone buffers. The defect in renal excretion of hydrogen ions means that the distal reabsorption of sodium is mainly an exchange with potassium, and this explains the potassium loss and hypokalemia. The mechanism of calcium and phosphorus disorders is equally clear. Intestinal absorption of calcium and phosphorus is normal in these patients so long as there is no defect in glomerular function, as we have been able to verify in two patients—although other authors take a different view.[51] The urinary excretion of calcium is very high, probably owing to the effect of the positive hydrogen ion balance on the bones, either directly or

Table 10.   Idiopathic Distal Tubular Acidosis (Personal Data)

Case	Age at Onset (years)	Sex	Familial	Urine pH on Acid Loading	Urinary Calcium (mg./kg./24 hours)	Serum Potassium (mEq./liter)	Serum Immunoglobulins	Height, cm. (S.D.)	Bone Disease	Lithiasis	Nephrocalcinosis (on X-ray)
1	1/12	M	0	6.6	8	2.5	Normal	82 (−3)	0	0	+
2	3/12	F	0	7	7	3.5	?	92 (−4)	Ost., R	+	+
3	5/12	F	0	6.1	7.2	4	?	114 (−3)	Ost., R	0	+
4	3/12	F	0	6.9	13	3.8	?	105 (−3)	Ost., R	+	+
5	2	F	0	6.9	5	4	?	81 (−2)	0	+	+
6	3/12	M	0	6.2	3	6	?	135 (−2)	Ost.	0	+
7	1	M	C	7.5	13	3.7	IgA↗ IgM↗	69 (−2)	Ost., R	0	0
8	2/12	F	C	6.6	7	5.2	?	55 (−3)	Ost.	+	+
9	3/12	F	0	6.5	7	4.8	?	101 (−4)	Ost., R	0	+
10	2/12	M	0	6.4	7	3.2	IgA↗	72 (−1)	0	0	+
11	3/12	F	0	7	4	3.2	Normal	58 (−2)	0	0	0
12	1/12	M	0	7	6	3.6	IgA IgM IgG↗	55 (−2)	Ost.	0	+

N, Nephrocalcinosis; G.F.R., glomerular filtration rate; H, height; R, rickets; Ost., osteoporosis; IN., focal interstitial nephritis; S.D., standard deviations. ↗, increasing amounts.

Table 10.   Idiopathic Distal Tubular Acidosis (Personal Data)—*Continued*

Renal Biopsy	*Treatment*	Interval (years)	Present Condition
Normal	Sodium and potassium citrate and bicarbonate	14	H = −1.5 S.D. G.F.R. = normal; N
N	Sodium and potassium bicarbonate	18	H = −1 S.D. Urea normal; N and lithiasis
I.N.	Sodium bicarbonate	11	H = −1 S.D. Urea normal
N	Sodium bicarbonate	6	H = −3 S.D.
Normal	Sodium and potassium bicarbonate	10	H = −1 S.D. G.F.R. = normal; N
?	0	14	Hemodialysis and transplantation (8 years ago)
Normal	Sodium and potassium bicarbonate	10	H = −2 S.D. G.F.R. = normal; N
N	0	5/12	Death at 7 months
?	Sodium and potassium bicarbonate	19	H = −3 S.D. N.; G.F.R. = 27 ml./min./1.73 m.^{2}
?	Sodium and potassium bicarbonate	10	H = −1.5 S.D. Urea normal; N
Normal	Sodium and potassium	8	H = −0.5 S.D. G.F.R. = normal
N	Sodium and potassium bicarbonate	1 year 6 months	H = −3 S.D. Urea normal

The Follow-up heading spans the Interval (years) and Present Condition columns.

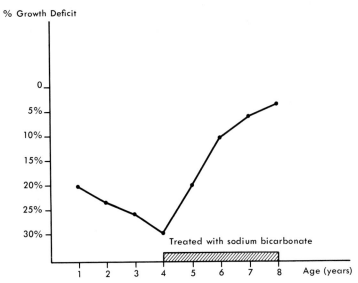

Figure 18. Idiopathic distal tubular acidosis. Correction of growth deficit on treatment with sodium bicarbonate in a case of distal tubular acidosis.

through stimulation of the parathyroids. Calcium balance is either negative or inadequately positive, and this probably explains the defect in growth and the osteoporosis. The combination of hypercalciuria and a high urinary pH leads to nephrocalcinosis and lithiasis, which in turn causes secondary chronic interstitial nephritis. The low urinary citrate level also encourages deposition of calcium salts. The reason for this low citrate level is not clear, but the most probable explanation is the presence of acidosis in the tubular cells. The hypophosphatemia with a low tubular reabsorption of phosphate (TRP) is generally regarded as secondary to hyperparathyroidism, which in turn is secondary to the disordered calcium metabolism. This hypothesis is subject to considerable doubt. We have shown that in rats an acid load has much the same effect on the TRP as parathormone. It is probable that the positive hydrogen ion balance is in fact directly responsible for the hypophosphatemia, which is corrected very rapidly under treatment. The defective concentration of urine is probably related to the hypercalciuria and to the potassium depletion.

Correction of the acidosis by the administration of sodium bicarbonate also corrects the low urinary citrate level, the hypokalemia, the hypophosphatemia, the hypercalciuria, and the defective urine concentration. We have confirmed this in many of our patients. At times, however, some of these disorders may persist, especially the defect in the concentrating power; rightly or wrongly, this is ascribed to the secondary interstitial nephritis.

Mechanism of the Fundamental Disorder

The fundamental disorder in distal tubular acidosis is the total inability to lower urinary pH below 6.0 — in other words, an inability to establish a concentration gradient of hydrogen ions between the tubular cells and the urine.

With acid loading for short or long periods, using either arginine chlorhydrate or ammonium chloride, the urinary pH does not fall below 5.8 or 6.0. Neither can the pH be lowered by the procedures that cause the greatest lowering of urinary pH in normal individuals, such as the administration of sodium sulfate and 9α-fluorohydrocortisone with a low-salt diet. With an acid load, the titratable acidity and urinary ammonium level rise very little. However, the defect in ammoniogenesis is significant only as a function of the inability to lower the urinary pH, because Elkinton's ammoniacal coefficient is normal, and glutaminase activity in renal biopsy material is normal. Bicarbonates are present in the urine because of the high urinary pH, not because of poor proximal tubular reabsorption of bicarbonate. The Tm and bicarbonate threshold are in fact normal.[58] The titratable acidity of the urine can be elevated by perfusion of sodium phosphate, which raises the amount of hydrogen ion acceptors in the urine. This makes it clear that the defect lies not in the elaboration of hydrogen ions but in the establishment of a difference in pH between the tubular cell and the urine. Furthermore, carbonic anhydrase activity, as measured indirectly by the acetazolamide test, or directly on renal biopsy material, is always found to be normal.

It is not known why these patients are incapable of establishing a significant pH difference between the tubular cell and the urine. Two hypotheses have been put forward. The first is that the energy necessary for the excretion of hydrogen ions against a concentration gradient is not available. The second hypothesis is that the excretion of hydrogen ions in the urine is normal, but that these ions are reabsorbed very rapidly and abnormally in the distal tubule, possibly owing to some abnormality of the cell membrane. This theory of excessive retrodiffusion of hydrogen ions may be a better explanation of the fact that the Tm for bicarbonate is normal and the curious finding that mercurial diuretics enable the urinary pH to be lowered in these patients in the normal fashion.

The causative disorder is renal and not the tubular expression of a prerenal abnormality. One of our patients has undergone two kidney transplantations and is alive and well eight years after the first. Neither of the two transplanted kidneys has ever presented any of the functional characteristics of DTA.[58] Enzyme studies on renal biopsy material have provided no evidence to explain the disease on the basis of a metabolic block caused by defective enzyme activity.[53, 57, 66] It may be that there is an electrophysiologic disorder of the cell membranes, the H^+ ion being an elemental particle — a proton.

Etiology

There are two interesting features, concerning genetics and the role of immunoglobulins.

Genetics

Although the majority of cases are sporadic, there is a good deal of evidence in favor of a hereditary origin of the condition. More than 15 families with multiple cases of DTA are known, with up to six members being involved.[62] The sexes are affected equally. Transmission is of the autosomal dominant type.

Table 11.   Classification of Tubular Acidosis

I. Isolated primary tubular acidosis
   A. *Distal tubular acidosis* (D.T.A.)
   B. *Proximal tubular acidosis* (P.T.A.)

II. Associated or secondary tubular acidosis
   A. *Distal tubular acidosis*
       1. Active chronic hepatitis.
       2. Fibrosing alveolitis.
       3. Sjögren's syndrome.
   B. *Proximal tubular acidosis*
       1. Deficiency or toxic.
       2. Secondary to ureterocolic anastomosis.
       3. Associated with complex tubular disorders.
          (Fanconi syndrome, Lowe's syndrome, cystinosis, tyrosinosis, Wilson's disease, galacto-
          semia, and others)

In affected families, some individuals present isolated nephrocalcinosis or isolated nephrolithiasis. A definite abnormality may be revealed in these individuals by an acid loading test (the incomplete type of Wrong and Davies).[65]

Immunoglobulins and DTA

In the serum of patients and of some of their healthy forebears, increased amounts of IgG are commonly found, and sometimes increases in IgA and IgM as well.[51, 64] There is also some evidence of the possibility of distal tubular acidosis associated with autoimmune diseases, such as chronic active hepatitis, Sjögren's syndrome, fibrous alveolitis of the lungs, and Hashimoto's thyroiditis.[51] Research is under way to find the source of the nonspecific organ antibodies found in the serum and their role in DTA. There may indeed be an immunologic explanation for the foci of interstitial nephritis with lymphoid and plasma cells that we have found in renal biopsy material in our patients.[58]

Treatment

The object of treatment is to prevent a positive hydrogen ion balance. This can be done by decreasing the dietary intake of substances such as sulfur containing amino acids and phosphoproteins. A much easier approach is to give sodium bicarbonate to enhance the respiratory elimination of hydrogen ions. The dose required can theoretically be calculated from the dietary intake and urinary excretion of hydrogen ions. It is usually fixed empirically at 2 to 6 g. per day of sodium bicarbonate. The correct dose is that which restores the pH and the plasma bicarbonate and urinary calcium levels to normal. Treatment must be continuous and for the life of the patient. When the serum potassium level is significantly lowered, some of the bicarbonate is given as the potassium salt. This treatment is highly effective. We see no point in adding vitamin D to treat the bone lesions.[58] Some authors have treated DTA successfully with tromethamine.[59]

Chronic Proximal Tubular Acidosis (PTA)

Rodriguez-Soriano and his associates isolated this condition as a distinct syndrome.[56] They studied five infants, all boys, two of whom were first cousins. All showed retardation of growth. Their skeletons were normal. Neither nephrocalcinosis nor lithiasis was present. Biochemical studies revealed hyperchloremia, a low plasma pH and plasma bicarbonate level, a high urinary pH with high bicarbonate output in the urine, an almost normal urinary calcium level, and no hypokalemia. There was no other renal disorder, and renal biopsy was normal. Ammonium chloride loading produced a drop in urinary pH to between 4.9 and 5.2 and a normal or even abnormally high excretion of hydrogen ions in the urine, both as titratable acidity and as the ammonium ion. If sodium citrate was given in addition, the acid loading produced no change. The bicarbonate titration curves were somewhat different in each of two subjects studied. In one, the Tm and threshold for bicarbonate were both lowered, in the other the Tm was normal but the threshold was lowered.

Donckerwolcke and his colleagues[50] studied a girl aged 20 months with dwarfism and bilateral band keratopathy. The acetazolamide test was negative, and the authors suggested that there was defective activity of renal carbonic anhydrase. The treatment with bicarbonate was effective. Hydrochlorothiazide also corrected the disorder,[49] whereas frusemide was ineffective.

The pathogenesis of PTA remains obscure. Three mechanisms are involved in bicarbonate reabsorption: the carbonic anhydrase dependent hydration of CO_2, the non-catalyst dependent hydration of CO_2, and the direct reabsorption of HCO_3^-.[60, 61]

The disease is chronic. It may be compensated for by giving bicarbonate or sodium citrate. The dosage needed is high — 10 to 15 g. per day. With this treatment, growth in height and weight returns to normal.

Nash and his colleagues have recently compared the courses of PTA and of DTA.[55]

More curious findings are the association of PTA with osteopetrosis in two siblings,[52] and the association of proximal and distal acidosis with osteopetrosis.[63]

Conclusions

The primary tubular acidoses are rare, probably hereditary, diseases. They should be sought in every infant who fails to grow normally. When the presence of acidosis has been established by measurement of plasma pH and bicarbonate levels, complex tubular diseases and global nephropathies, such as renal hypoplasia, polycystic disease, or pyelonephritis secondary to urinary tract malformation, should be excluded.

Isolated primary tubular acidoses, in which there is no reduction in glomerular filtration rate, present as two types: distal tubular acidosis, in which the urinary pH will not fall even with an acid load, and proximal tubular acidosis, in which the bicarbonate titration test reveals lowering of the threshold and sometimes of the Tm of bicarbonate. In both types, treatment restores normal growth, and in the distal type it also corrects the bone and kidney complications.

RENAL PSEUDOENDOCRINOPATHIES

Many hereditary conditions present as defects in the renal response to a normal hormonal message. They simulate hormone deficiency and represent hereditary pathology of the cell receptors.

Hereditary Nephrogenic Diabetes Insipidus Resistant to Vasopressin (NDI)

The condition was first defined by Williams[75] and by Waring and his colleagues.[74] We have studied 12 cases of this disorder.

Clinical Features

Nephrogenic diabetes insipidus presents in the first days of life. There is rapid development of a serious clinical disorder dominated by the consequences of the chronic hyperelectrolytemia. Sometimes the major clinical change occurs when breast feeding is abandoned, as a result of the consequent abrupt increase in the osmotic load of the diet. Unexplained and variable fever, anorexia, vomiting, constipation, failure to thrive, and complications of hypernatremic dehydration are common. There is sometimes delay in bone maturation and osteoporosis. Psychomotor retardation very soon becomes apparent; this has been ascribed to cerebral lesions caused by the hypernatremia and also to the fact that normal play activities and adaptation to persons around them is impossible for these infants, because nearly all of their time is devoted to taking liquids and sleeping. Excessive thirst, sometimes selective for water only, is a valuable diagnostic sign, but it is absent in approximately 50 per cent of cases in the first months of life; these constitute the occult cases, in which hypernatremia is often dangerous. The major sign is the severe polyuria, which in a neonate may be 500, 1000, or 2000 ml./24 hours. In order to detect the polyuria at this age, it is necessary to carry out a simple but often forgotten maneuver, the fitting of an apparatus to collect the urine.

After the age of 2 to 4 years, the clinical manifestations of NDI are reduced to thirst, polyuria, and some slowing of growth. Little by little, the spontaneous intake of water becomes adapted to the disorder, which becomes compatible with good physical health, even though it will last throughout life. It should be noted that the precarious equilibrium may at times be compromised by intercurrent infection, surgery, or accidents. The polyuric, polydipsic children, perpetually dogged by their need for water, often find it difficult to adapt to school, and this problem may be aggravated by mental retardation. Adaptation is better in adults. An important feature of the disease is the development of a large bladder (and more rarely of megaureters) as a consequence of the massive polyuria.

Laboratory Studies

The specific gravity of the urine varies from 1.001 to 1.008, being usually about 1.005. With severe acute dehydration, it may rise as far as 1.020. The osmolar concentration generally varies from 80 to 160 mOsm./kg. Neither the polyuria nor the urinary osmolarity is affected by water restriction, by injection of hypertonic sodium chloride, or by vasopressin. Osmolar clearance is normal, but there is a very high clearance of free water, between 6 and 10 ml./min./ 1.73 m.^{2} This free water clearance is not altered by restricting fluid intake or by pitressin. The urine/plasma osmolar ratio is always much less than 1.

Evolution

In the neonate, the evolution of nephrogenic diabetes insipidus is dominated by (1) the complications of acute dehydration that prove fatal in 5 to 10 per cent of cases, (2) by functional disorders, (3) by subdural or intracerebral hematoma, or (4) as we have seen, by bilateral adrenal hemorrhage. Failure to thrive may be extreme. Mental retardation is sometimes regressive, but unfortunately it may persist even with early treatment. In the older child and in adults, the situation is better tolerated. The chief problems, in themselves sufficient to justify treatment, are the discomforts of existence and the inability to adapt to school or work. An apparent late complication is hyperuricemia with a low clearance rate of uric acid and attacks of gout.[71]

In practice patients with this condition can be classified into two main groups. There are serious cases, presenting major problems in the first weeks or months of life, with prodigious polyuria in childhood and adult life. The clearance of free water is positive and very high, and it is unaffected by pitressin. There are, on the other hand, more moderate cases in which the clinical manifestations appear later and are less severe. The clearance of free water is positive but only moderately elevated. It has been said that boys always belong to the first group, whereas girls may be found in either category.

Diagnosis

The pitressin tannate test, with a daily injection for three days of 1 unit for each year of age up to a maximum of 10 units, or the intravenous vasopressin perfusion test, shows the absence or inadequacy of changes in urinary output, urinary osmolarity, clearance of free water, and urine/plasma osmolar ratio. These tests will exclude the possibility of diabetes insipidus that is sensitive to vasopressin, a condition that is sometimes hereditary. The next step is to exclude other causes of pitressin-resistant polyuria. In children, many conditions must be considered, including obstructive uropathy, nephronophthisis, chronic idiopathic hypokalemia, idiopathic hypercalciuria, sickle-cell anemia, cystinosis, and tubular acidosis. Some of these conditions are familial, and a renal biopsy demonstrating normal kidney tissue is an essential prerequisite to the diagnosis of nephrogenic diabetes insipidus.

Mechanism[6]

Three renal abnormalities may be responsible for the failure to concentrate the urine: the arrival of too great a quantity of urine in the distal and collecting tubules, abnormality of the countercurrent mechanism, or inactivity of vasopressin. Studies of the renal architectonics have been undertaken as part of a study of the two first hypotheses. There is no evidence of an abnormal countercurrent mechanism, but shortening of the proximal tubules has been noted in some cases, and this raises difficult problems. For example, insufficient iso-osmotic reabsorption in the proximal tubule might cause a very exaggerated urinary flow in the beginning of the distal tubule that could result in "polyuria insipida."[70] A peculiar appearance of the mitochondria, showing myelinated structures, has been noted in the proximal and distal tubules.[67]

The primary disorder in NDI is generally discussed in terms of the action of vasopressin. Both the blood and urine contain normal amounts of antidiuretic substance, but the patients are insensitive to pitressin and to oxytocin. An abnormally rapid destruction of these hormones is unlikely, because they retain their vasomotor and gastrointestinal effects. The whole picture suggests that the renal tubule fails to respond to the action of vasopressin. Normally, vasopressin increases the water permeability of the distal and collecting tubules by increasing the porosity of one of the layers of the cell membrane. The vasopressin signal is recognized by a specific discriminator of the cytoplasmic membrane of the cells of the renal medulla. The recognition entails activation of the adenyl cyclase of this same membrane. Calcium ion concentration and a prostaglandin, PGE_1, are also concerned. The activation of adenyl cyclase leads to the synthesis of cyclic adenosine monophosphate (cyclic AMP), a "second messenger" that amplifies the order and triggers the response. Resistance to vasopressin or to cyclic AMP can be induced in vitro. The induced resistance to vasopressin is reversible, whereas the resistance to cyclic AMP is not.[68] It is not possible at the present time to define the primary abnormality of NDI or to be certain whether it concerns the discriminator, the second messenger, or the responding mechanism. Studies of cyclic AMP in the urine after the injection of vasopressin have failed to distinguish clearly between normal subjects and those affected by NDI.

Genetics

Nephrogenic diabetes insipidus is a hereditary disease transmitted as a sex-linked recessive trait. There is a great preponderance of males, and in published genealogies the condition is seen to be transmitted through the female line, most of the women involved being carriers who do not exhibit the disease. Transmission from father to son has not been seen, but this might be because most affected boys do not have children. Those affected men who have had progeny have never had a son who had the disease.[73]

A proper genetic analysis is in fact difficult for several reasons. First, sporadic cases are not uncommon in boys and girls, but as yet there is no information about their descendents. Second, the number of cases in girls is not negligible. These girls, like the boys, may have a null or "intermediate" response to vasopressin. Third, the carrier mothers may present a definite polyuric syndrome, also with a null or intermediate response to vasopressin. These mothers may be clinically normal but nevertheless have an inadequate response to water restriction or to vasopressin. No study of the response to water restriction or to vasopressin has yet been made in apparently healthy men in involved families. Fourth, there is now some evidence of transmission from father to son, and we ourselves have seen one such family.

Treatment

Water Supplementation.   All that is needed is to increase the fluid intake and to spread it equally throughout the 24 hours, especially in the infant. We have seen the blood sodium level rise from 135 to 160 mEq. per liter in an infant of 2 months when only a single drink was forgotten. It is often difficult to make infants of this age accept the necessary amount of fluid, especially when the infant is not thirsty. In serious cases, during the first months of life, it is essential to give water continuously throughout the 24 hours by gastric tube.

Diets of Low Osmotic Activity.   In infants below the age of 3 months, the food of choice is human milk or so-called "humanized" milk. Later, the diet is based on cow's milk with the sodium removed, supplemented by starch foods, butter, oil, and vitamins. Fruits and vegetables rich in mineral salts must be avoided. The calorie requirement is of the order of 100 to 150 cal./kg./day and the protein intake 2.5 g./kg./day. One third of the caloric requirements are given as fats and the remaining two thirds as carbohydrates. In older children and adults, the diet may be varied, but it should be salt-free, with only a limited amount of fruits and vegetables, and a protein intake of 1 to 2 g./kg./day.

Salt Diuretics.   Certain salt diuretics, in addition to their action on sodium diuresis, also have a water antidiuretic action. The most commonly used drug in this group is hydrochlorothiazide,[69] in doses of 1 to 2 mg./kg./day. The antidiuretic effect represents 30 to 40 per cent of the water output (Figure 19). This effect, which begins on the first day the drug is given, is a lasting one, and some of our patients have been on this treatment for more than five years. The effect depends on a decrease in the clearance of free water without significant alteration in the osmolar clearance. The clearance of free water never becomes negative. The action of hydrochlorothiazide is the same whether the diabetes insipidus is or is not sensitive to pitressin. This drug can cause potassium depletion, so potassium salts must be added. Aldosterone antagonists, such as spironolactone in doses of 15 mg./kg./day, increase the osmolar clearance without, in most

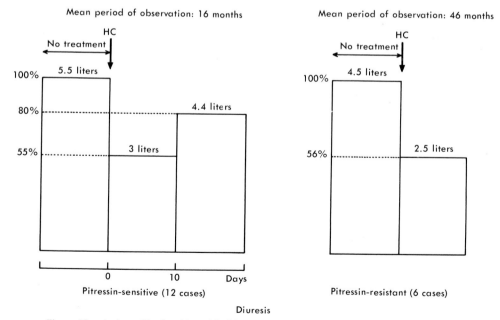

Figure 19.   Action of hydrochlorothiazide (HC) in a dose of 1.35 mg./kg./24 hours on urinary output in 12 cases of pitressin-sensitive diabetes insipidus and in 6 cases of pitressin-resistant diabetes insipidus. The percentage of diminution in urinary output is virtually identical.

cases, affecting the clearance of free water. It is sometimes useful to give both spironolactone and hydrochlorothiazide (each in average doses) in order to achieve increased osmolar clearance and diminished clearance of free water. Hydrochlorothiazide is particularly indicated in the neonate and young infant, and its use in these children will resolve most of the difficult dietetic problems. The drug may also be useful in older children in helping to prevent problems with schooling and for social convenience. Other salt diuretics, such as frusemide and ethacrinic acid, are equally effective but are used much less frequently. Chlorpropamide, carbamoyldibenzazepine (carbamazepine), and clofibrate produce negative clearance of free water in cases of diabetes insipidus sensitive to vasopressin, but they are ineffective in nephrogenic diabetes insipidus.

The results of treatment are good. In infants and young children, there is a rapid restoration of normal growth. Retardation of stature may be made up. When mental deficiency occurs, it may continue, improve, or be cured.

Pseudohypoaldosteronism

In 1958, Cheek and Perry described a salt-wasting syndrome in infants,[76] which seems to be very rare. There are many synonyms for this disorder, including pseudohypoadrenocorticism, pseudohypomineralocorticism, and pseudoaldosteronism.[76-80, 83, 84]

Genetics

The condition is apparently more common in boys. Many cases may occur in the same sibship. The mother of one patient had suffered from anorexia, vomiting, and defective growth until she reached the age of 6 months. In one of the affected families the parents were related. These few observations are as yet inadequate for satisfactory genetic interpretation.

Clinical Features

Pregnancy and delivery are normal, and so is the birth weight. From the first few days of life, there is anorexia, failure to gain weight, and occasional vomiting. There is insufficient subcutaneous fat, and signs of dehydration are present. The infants are sleepy, indifferent, and flaccid. The situation is complicated by attacks of cyanosis and acute dehydration crises. Intercurrent infections are common. On clinical examination, the lack of fat and the persistent skin fold contrast with a moist tongue. The external genital organs are normal, and there are no lumbar masses. Urinary output is usually normal, even during acute attacks of dehydration, and there may even be a moderate polyuria.

The biochemical picture is characterized by urinary loss of sodium chloride, hyponatremia, and hyperkalemia. The low blood sodium level may be partly masked by hemoconcentration, as revealed by an increased plasma protein level and hematocrit. In addition to the hyponatremia, there is hypochloremia and a low plasma osmolarity.

The state of renal function is variable. When dehydration and sodium deficiency are corrected, kidney function is completely normal except for the ability to conserve sodium chloride. Urinary infection and proteinuria do not occur. Intravenous urography and renal biopsy are normal. Attacks of sodium deple-

Table 12. Pseudohypoaldosteronism – Reported Cases

	Donnel et al.[78] (1959)	Lelong et al.[80] (1960)	Royer et al.[84] (1963)	Polonovski et al.[82] (1965)	Jeune et al.[79] (1967)	Pham-Huu-Trung et al.[81] (1970)	Proesmans (1972)	Proesmans (1972)
Sex of patient	M	M	M	F	F	F	M	M
Serum sodium (mEq./liter)	124	124	120	130	–	123	116	125
Serum potassium (mEq./liter)	7.0	7.1	6.7	5.9	–	7.2	7.4	7.1
Plasma cortisol (mg. per 100 ml.)	–	–	–	Normal	–	18	17.9	9.6
After ACTH	–	–	–	–	–	83	37.2	30
Urinary 17-hydroxysteroids (mg./day)	0.5	0.1	0.3	0.35	–	Trace	0.4	3.1
Urinary 17-ketosteroids (mg./day)	1.5	1.1	1.15	0.80	Normal	0.3	1.19	0.5
Urinary pregnanetriol (mg/day)	–	–	–	Normal	–	Trace amounts	0.19	0.12
Urinary aldosterone (mcg./day) N*	335	200	120	40		340	827	2050
S†	25	10	24	20		284	621	2037
Aldosterone secretion (mcg./day) N*					693			
S†					715			
G.F.R. (ml./min./1.73 m.²)	115	Normal	64	50	–	Normal	60	40
Maximal concentration	1038	–	1047 mOsm.	1027	–	1020	810 mOsm.	611 mOsm.
Proteinuria	0	–	0	0	–	0	0	0
Urography	Normal	–	Normal	Normal	–	Normal	Normal	Normal
Treatment (NaCl, g./day)	5	4	3–5	6	1.5–2	3	2	2–5

*With normal sodium intake.
†With high sodium intake.

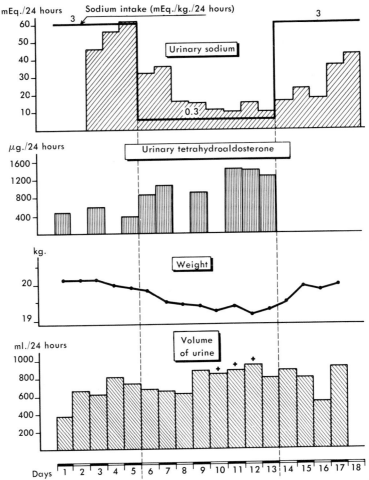

Figure 20. Pseudohypoaldosteronism. The daily sodium intake is 3 mEq./kg./24 hours during days 1 to 5, 0.3 mEq./kg./24 hours during days 6 to 13, and 3 mEq./kg./24 hours during days 14 to 18. Note the negative sodium balance during the period of sodium restriction despite a considerable rise in the urinary excretion of tetrahydroaldosterone, which reached as high as 1200 μg./24 hours.

tion lead to a moderate increase in the blood urea nitrogen, diminished clearance of endogenous creatinine, and diminished concentrating power (Table 12).

The urinary output of *tetrahydroaldosterone* is extremely high, between 200 and 350 micrograms (μg.) per 24 hours. On a low-salt diet, it may reach as much as 800 μg. per 24 hours (Figure 20). When a large amount of sodium chloride is added to the diet, the output may return to the normal level of 2.5 to 10 μg. per 24 hours. True aldosterone secretion is greatly increased. The mineralocorticoids, aldosterone, desoxycorticosterone, and α-fluorohydrocortisone have no effect on either the clinical condition or the biochemical abnormalities.

Diagnosis

Once it has been established that there is a urinary salt-losing syndrome, there remain two main problems in diagnosis.

The first problem is to rule out salt-wasting syndromes sensitive to mineralo-corticoids in the neonate and infant. Such syndromes — especially those resulting from a defect in 21-hydroxylase and in β-1-dehydrogenase — may be found in virilizing hyperplasia of the adrenals, and may also be seen in hereditary hypo-aldosteronism, which occurs in two forms: as an abnormality of 18-hydroxyla-tion, or as an abnormality of 18-dehydrogenation.[85] In hypoaldosteronism, the urinary output of tetrahydroaldosterone is almost nil, and the true aldosterone secretion is very low; in such cases, the injection of desoxycorticosterone is very effective in controlling the urinary sodium loss.

The second problem is to rule out complex nephropathies that may be ac-companied by salt loss in infants, including certain malformations of the urinary tract, hereditary polycystic disease, sometimes oligomeganephronia, and (usually at a later stage) nephronophthisis. In all these conditions, there are other signs of renal insufficiency in addition to the salt-losing syndrome.

Death may occur from collapse, dehydration, or secondary infection. In the majority of cases, the disease is increasingly well tolerated as the patient becomes older. We saw a boy suffering from this condition in 1963. He was treated for two years, and then his parents stopped giving the salt supplements. In 1971, his blood sodium and potassium levels were normal, but the urinary sodium loss persisted; the urinary output of tetrahydroaldosterone was more than 400 μg. per 24 hours, and the plasma renin level was very elevated. The metabolic ab-normality persisted, but the disorder was compensated for under basal condi-tions.[84]

Mechanism

There are complex bidirectional transfers of sodium in the renal tubule. There appear to be three principal regulatory factors involved — glomerular fil-tration, aldosterone, and the "third factor." The disease is generally attributed to a defective response by the renal tubule to aldosterone and to mineralocorti-coids. The principal targets of aldosterone are the epithelial cells, especially those of the colon and renal tubule. An aldosterone "receptor" has been identi-fied on the nuclear membrane, and there may be others in the cytoplasm and in the interior of the nucleus. In one of our cases, we studied the nuclear membrane "receptor" in a biopsy specimen of colonic mucosa and found it to be normal. In this child the Tm of glucose was lowered and the urinary sodium loss was in-creased by giving spironolactone. These observations suggest that the sodium loss may be independent of failure to respond to aldosterone.

Treatment

The condition is treated by giving a daily supplement of 3 to 6 g. of sodium chloride. The dose is regulated to restore the blood sodium, blood potassium, urinary tetrahydroaldosterone, and plasma renin to normal. The supplement may be reduced in the second year and is probably unnecessary after the age of 4 years.

Pseudohypoparathyroidism

In 1942, Albright and his colleagues[86] described a condition in which a dysmorphic state was associated with mental deficiency, and the biochemical picture was that of a parathyroid deficiency unresponsive to injections of parathormone. In 1952, the same author reported a similar syndrome without the biochemical features of parathyroid deficiency. The first type is called pseudohypoparathyroidism or type I of Albright's hereditary dystrophy; the second is pseudo-pseudohypoparathyroidism or type II hereditary dystrophy.

Clinical and Laboratory Features[91, 94, 95]

The symptoms appear very early, sometimes in the first year of life, but are not found at birth. The principal abnormalities are defective growth (in approximately 70 per cent of cases), with precocious fusion of the epiphyses, moon facies (80 per cent of cases), and obesity (65 per cent of cases), brachymetacarpia affecting particularly the first, fourth, and fifth fingers, brachymetatarsia (70 per cent of cases) with an epiphysis invaginated into the metaphysis, periarticular and muscular calcification, calcification of the central gray nuclei (20 to 30 per cent of cases), cataract (20 per cent of cases), and mental deficiency (50 per cent of cases). The teeth may be small and pointed, there may be exostoses at the bony attachment of fasciae and tendons, and various types of dysmorphia. There are three curious endocrine features—thyroid insufficiency,[95] which in three cases we have shown to result from a lingual ectopic thyroid; Turner's syndrome; and diabetes mellitus.

Type I hereditary dystrophy is characterized by hypocalcemia, hypophosphatemia, and hypocalciuria. Tetany, convulsions, and moniliasis are common clinical features. The blood calcium level rises slowly with perfusion of EDTA. Infusion of calcium may restore the percentage of tubular reabsorption of phosphorus to normal or may lower it.[95]

There is a normal lowering of the blood calcium level after injection of thyrocalcitonin. The intestinal absorption of calcium and the calcium balance are strongly positive, whereas the rapidly exchangeable calcium pool is diminished.

Mechanism

The pathophysiologic interpretation of Albright's hereditary dystrophy rests, at the moment, on five series of observations. The first concerns the parathyroids, which have been recorded as normal or hyperplastic in different reports.[86, 97, 99] The second concerns the effect of parathormone. The phosphodiuretic effect of 200 USP units of parathyroid hormone has been studied; whereas this effect is highly significant in hypoparathyroidism, it is slight or nil in hereditary dystrophy (the Ellsworth-Howard test). Because of many criticisms, the test has been modified, but it remains of uncertain value.[96] In another experiment, the effect on the blood calcium level of parathormone given in a dose of 150 USP units per day in two periods of five days was studied: the results were variable, but in most cases the blood calcium level was raised by the hormone.[94] The third observation is that there is no increase in the urinary level of cyclic AMP after injection of parathormone,[90] suggesting that the hormone does not activate the adenyl cyclase in the renal cortex. The fourth point is that thyrocalcitonin lowers the blood calcium level in the ordinary way. Fifth, it has been shown in two patients that the parathyroid glands secrete seven times as much biologically active parathormone and that the thyroid gland contains 50 times more thyrocalcitonin than the normal subject.[99]

Thus, it seems clear that the abnormal gene causes an abnormality of the membrane of the tubular cell of the renal cortex which in consequence can not "recognize" the hormone or fails to elaborate the second messenger, cyclic AMP. As in all cases of receptor failure, the hormone is produced in excess.

Hypo-hyperparathyroidism

The interpretation of the data may need to be modified in the light of the description by Costello and Dent[89] of a new variant, hypo-hyperparathyroidism, that combines renal resistance to parathormone, the bone lesions of osteitis fibrosa, and the presence or absence of the dysmorphic features characteristic of Albright's dystrophy. Frame and colleagues[92] have suggested distinguishing isolated renal resistance to parathormone (type I or hypo-hyperparathyroidism), renal and osseous resistance (type II), and isolated osseous resistance (type III) (Table 13). In all three types there is an elevated serum level of immunoreactive parathormone (PTH). It is interesting to note that vitamin D may restore a normal sensitivity to parathormone, and this suggests that the parathormone-adenyl cyclase system of the kidney or bone tissue may be vitamin D dependent.[98]

Genetics

Albright's osteodystrophy may be familial or sporadic. The following points emerge from the most recent studies.[93, 95, 97] The familial distribution is vertical,

Table 13. A Classification of Pseudohypoparathyroidism.*

	Type 1	Type 2	Type 3
Serum calcium	Lowered	Lowered	Lowered
Serum phosphorus	Raised	Raised	Normal
Serum alkaline phosphatase	Raised	Normal	Normal
Skeleton	Osteitis fibrosa	Normal	Normal
Parathyroid glands	Hyperplasia	Hyperplasia	Hyperplasia
Plasma PTH	Raised	Raised	Raised
Effect of PTH on blood calcium	Normal or diminished	Diminished	Diminished
Effect of PTH on blood phosphate	Nil	Nil	Normal or diminished
Effect of PTH on urinary cyclic AMP	Nil	Nil	Raised or nil
Effect of PTH on urinary phosphate	Nil	Nil	Raised or nil

*From Frame, B., et al.: Amer. J. Med. 52:311, 1972.
In type 1 there is renal resistance to parathyroid hormone, in type 3 bone resistance to parathyroid hormone, and in type 2 both kidney and bone resistance to the hormone.
PTH, Parathormone.

with involvement of many successive generations. Girls are affected twice as often as boys. Transmission has been noted from mother to daughter, from mother to son, and from father to son, but never from father to daughter. The degree of clinical expression of the disease varies, and in some patients there may be little more than minor dysmorphic signs, such as a round face or brachymetacarpia. At present, the data suggest a dominant transmission linked to chromosome X. The abnormal gene has variable penetrance and expressivity. An association with basal-cell nevus has been reported.[88]

Treatment

No specific treatment is known. In general, the treatment is similar to that of chronic hypoparathyroidism. Metallic calcium is given in doses of 0.5 to 1.0 g. per day, with 10,000 to 20,000 units of cholecalciferol daily, or one fifth the dose of 25-hydroxycholecalciferol. Some authors recommend thyroid extract.[95]

COMPLEX PRIMARY AND HEREDITARY TUBULAR INSUFFICIENCY

The simultaneous disturbance of many tubular functions in children was reported in 1933 by De Toni,[106] in 1934 by Debré and his colleagues,[5] and in 1936 by Fanconi.[107] The term "De Toni-Debré-Fanconi syndrome" or "Fanconi syndrome" has persisted to designate these complex tubular defects.

Some are *secondary to acquired disease.* Three such conditions are known in children: (1) Vitamin-deficiency *rickets* may be accompanied by hyperaminoaciduria and proximal loss of bicarbonate. (2) Some *serious nephrotic syndromes* progress to complex tubular deficiency, with glycosuria, hyperaminoaciduria, hypokalemia, hyposthenuria, hypophosphatemic rickets, hypocalcemia, and recurrent tetany, and these have a very poor prognosis.[129] (3) Many types of *poisoning* cause complex tubular defects, such as intoxications by lead, mercury, lysol, dichromate, cadmium, uranium, and calciferol. More recently, a transient picture of proteinuria, acidosis, glycosuria, hypophosphatemia, hyperaminoaciduria, and hypokalemia has been described following ingestion of out-of-date tetracycline containing degradation products; it seems that anhydroepitetracycline is the product responsible for the kidney damage.[102] This substance will induce the condition in experimental animals. In this context, it may be recalled that a De Toni-Debré-Fanconi syndrome can be reproduced experimentally by giving malic acid, a powerful inhibitor of Na-K-ATPase in dogs and rats,[115] and by orthodinitrocresol.[111]

Other complex tubular defects are *secondary to hereditary metabolic diseases,* such as galactosemia, fructose intolerance, Wilson's disease, tyrosinosis, and glycogenosis.[121] Cystinosis is the main cause of chronic De Toni-Debré-Fanconi syndrome in children.

Idiopathic De Toni-Debré-Fanconi Syndrome

This designation is applied to a primary, chronic, complex tubular insufficiency in which the main features are glycosuria, globulinuria, hyperaminoaciduria, raised phosphate clearance, acidosis, hyperuricuria, defective concentration of urine, and sometimes hypokalemia and a sodium-losing syndrome. An adult type, seen mainly in the fourth decade,[130] and also an infantile type, have been described. Only the infantile type will be considered here; it has been well reviewed by Illig and Prader.[112]

Clinical Features

The onset is between the ages of 1 and 2 years, usually with anorexia, vomiting, attacks of fever, episodes of dehydration, and especially retardation of growth and rickets. Glycosuria and generalized hyperaminoaciduria are constant findings. Acidosis, of the proximal tubular type with loss of bicarbonate, is common; it can be corrected by hydrochlorothiazide.[123] Exceptionally, there may be alkalosis, and in such cases there is sodium loss from the kidneys.[110] Hypophosphatemia with lowering of the tubular reabsorption of phosphate (TRP), which does not respond to calcium perfusion, and a normal blood calcium level with elevation of the serum alkaline phosphatase level, are usual findings. There is no intestinal malabsorption of calcium or phosphorus.[124] The urinary calcium output is normal or raised. Hypokalemia and hyperkaluria are found in 50 per cent of cases, with hyposthenuria and a high urinary level of uric acid. The proteinuria is of the tubular or mixed type. Often the tubular abnormalities increase to a phase of stabilization. The kidney appears normal on renal biopsy, except for changes owing to potassium deficiency. Histochemical studies in adults have shown a general diminution of the principal enzyme activities.[103] Treatment consists in giving phosphate, vitamin D, and bicarbonate, with supplements of sodium or potassium where indicated.

The condition continues into adult life, by which stage the patients may be dwarfed or deformed. Some cases of the Fanconi syndrome described in adults began in childhood, but the exact relationship between the infantile and adult forms of the disease is not clear. Glomerular insufficiency and uremia do not occur, although, in a family studied by Neimann and his colleagues,[118] in which four boys of 12 children were affected, one boy died of uremia and all showed severe glomerular, tubular, and interstitial lesions on renal biopsy.

Genetics

It is generally held that the disease is transmitted as an autosomal recessive trait. Many cases are sporadic. Brothers and sisters of patients may present glycosuria or hyperaminoaciduria, and in these cases the syndrome may become fully developed in adult life. It may be—though this is not certain—that a whole series of poorly classified conditions in which there is renal loss of glucose and amino acids,[114] of phosphate and amino acids,[119] or of glucose and phosphates[113] should be included in this syndrome. In a family studied by Sheldon and associates,[125] the transmission seemed to be dominant, with involvement of grandfather, father, and two twin sisters.

The Oculo-Cerebro-Renal Syndrome of Lowe

In 1952, Lowe and his colleagues described three boys who presented a syndrome of mental retardation, hydrophthalmos, high organic acid output in the urine, and diminished renal ammoniogenesis.[116] Further information was added in 1954 by Bickel and Thursby-Pelham[101] and in 1955 by Debré and associates.[105] Abbassi and his colleagues made an extensive review of the condition in 1968.[100]

Genetics

The disease is transmitted as a sex-linked recessive trait; only boys are affected. Genealogic studies reveal transmission by women who are carriers. The only point of debate is whether these carriers are normal or present abnormalities, such as hyperaminoaciduria, retinal detachment, and especially the early onset of cataract in adult life. Cataract is an almost constant finding, but it occurs at different ages in different carriers.[122]

Clinical Features[100]

Patients are first admitted to the hospital at an age that varies from 2 months to 19 years. The appearance of the patients is nearly always the same: The head is large, with a bulging forehead, saddle nose, large ears, and a pale skin, with visible venous network over the skull. There are also eye changes, such as cataract. Inconstant features include adiposity, dryness of the skin or eczema, and cryptorchidism. Deafness has been noted in three patients.

The effect on the *general condition* is often severe. The weight at birth is normal. A symptom noted frequently in the young child is thermal instability, with attacks of fever unexplained by any infection. Retardation of growth, sometimes amounting to dwarfism, is found in more than 50 per cent of cases. The weight is usually disproportionately low for the height. Osteoporosis is common, but rickets is less often seen. The blood calcium level is normal, with hypophosphatemia, hyperphosphaturia, and elevation of serum alkaline phosphatase level; when the urinary calcium level has been measured, it has been found to be normal or increased, never decreased as in ordinary rickets. The response of this type of rickets to treatment has been variable. Some patients respond to sodium bicarbonate or sodium citrate associated with vitamin D; other patients respond to bicarbonate alone or to large doses of vitamin D alone.

The *neurologic signs* are perhaps the most characteristic mark of the syndrome. Mental retardation is considerable and constant. Although the eye disorders make it difficult to assess, the IQ is below 50. There is also motor retardation. Neurological examination reveals two principal signs: Loss of muscle tone is always very accentuated, and tendon reflexes are completely or almost completely absent. On the other hand, there is no evidence of paralysis, pyramidal or extrapyramidal involvement, or of disturbances of sensation. Some children have motor agitation and emit piercing cries. Electromyography and muscle biopsy are normal. The electroencephalogram is normal or may show diffuse changes, with no special features. Air encephalography reveals moderate dilatation of the ventricular system.

The *eye signs* are constant. The most common is cataract, which is seen in almost every case. The description of the lens opacities is not always precise. It seems that the embryonic nucleus is usually affected, and that there are often opacities in the posterior pole. Some patients rub their eyes continually. Glaucoma is found in 33 per cent of cases and may appear after operation for cataract. Most often this is a simple glaucoma, but sometimes there is also a congenital hydrophthalmos. Nystagmus is extremely common; it is "searching" nystagmus owing to defective vision rather than a true nystagmus.

The *renal involvement* is remarkable. Whatever the age of the patient, evidence has never been found of significant disturbance of glomerular function. Blood pressure and intravenous urography are normal. Nephrocalcinosis is never seen. Exceptionally, there may be renal calculi, possibly owing to the high urinary calcium levels and high urinary pH. The most important kidney disturbances in Lowe's syndrome are related to *complex tubular dysfunction*. Proteinuria is moderate and of tubular type. Hypophosphatemia with a normal or elevated urinary phosphate level has often been noted. Phosphate clearance is elevated. The percentage of tubular reabsorption of phosphate is diminished but returns to normal with intravenous perfusion of calcium. Tubular acidosis has been found whenever it was sought. Urinary pH most often is between 6 and 7. The urinary bicarbonate level is elevated despite the low plasma pH and low plasma bicarbonate concentration. Hyperchloremia is common. The urinary ammonium level and the titratable acidity of the urine are within normal limits despite the metabolic acidosis. The reason for this acidosis is not quite clear. Bicarbonate titration studies in our patients have shown that the bicarbonate loss is fundamental and that the acidosis is of proximal tubular type. An acid load lowers the urinary pH, but the rise in titratable acidity and ammonium level are probably inadequate. The selective disturbance of ammoniogenesis emphasized in the earlier reports is doubtful. Hyperaminoaciduria is constant but may disappear after many years. Blood amino acid levels are normal. The hyperaminoaciduria is generalized, similar to that seen in the healthy premature infant.[109]

In his original description, Lowe emphasized that the organic acid output in the urine was even more significant than the aminoaciduria, but normoglycemic glycosuria is very rare; it has been found in only a few cases, and then only intermittently. If the absence of a defect in the concentrating ability of the kidney is confirmed, a matter that is as yet uncertain, it will be a very unusual finding in serious acidosis and in patients with a high urinary calcium level.

The disease *progresses* in three stages: a latent period in the first six months of life, with cataract the only sign present at birth; a period of evolution of the general, neurological, and renal manifestations, lasting five or six years; and finally a phase of stabilization. If the patients survive the metabolic disorders of the second stage, their expectation of life is probably good; some have experienced a normal puberty and have reached adult life.

Pathologic Anatomy

The appearance of the kidney on renal biopsy or at autopsy depends on the stage of the disease.[100, 108] In the beginning, the renal parenchyma is normal. Subsequently, discrete lesions are found in the glomeruli, and later there is marked atrophy and especially dilatation of the tubules, affecting both the loops of Henle and the collecting tubules. There are no vascular lesions. The most remarkable feature in most cases is the degree and diffuse nature of the tubular dilatation, accompanied by a fibrous or fibrocellular interstitial reaction. Serial biopsies have shown progression from the appearance of a normal kidney to gross tubular dilatation.[100] In the central nervous system, there may be diffuse changes, with demyelinization and appearance of fat in the perivascular spaces,

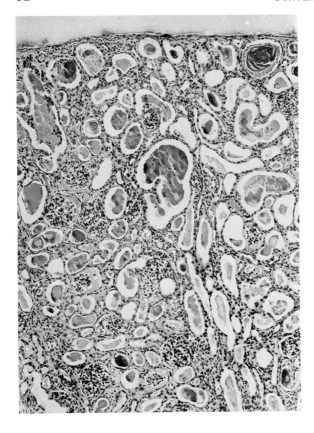

Figure 21. Lowe's syndrome. Note the severity of the tubular damage. The tubules are diffusely dilated, their epithelium is flattened, and they contain large hyaline casts. This is in contrast to the integrity of the glomeruli. ×60.

similar to the picture seen in familial leukodystrophy.[108] In other cases, there are no changes in the nervous system or only nonspecific ones[100] (Figure 21).

Treatment

The treatment is symptomatic, including general care, good hygiene, re-education when possible, surgery for cataract and glaucoma, administration of sodium bicarbonate to correct the acidosis, and administration of vitamin D either alone or with sodium bicarbonate when rickets is present.

Primary Disorder

Lowe's syndrome combines a particular involvement of the central nervous system, specific eye changes, and a unique complex tubulopathy with globulin-uria, generalized hyperaminoaciduria, and tubular acidosis of the proximal type, without any defect in the concentrating ability of the kidney. The primary disorder induced by the abnormal gene is unknown. Abnormality of organic acids[116] or of ornithine metabolism[125] has been suggested, but the question remains unresolved.

Variants

The characteristic feature of many variants is corneal opacity. In 1960, Scholten reported two sisters with the diagnosis of Lowe's syndrome who had both died at the age of 3 months.[126] Their syndrome included loss of muscle tone, absence of tendon reflexes, psychomotor retardation, hydrophthalmos with bilateral corneal opacities, glycosuria, proteinuria, and hyperaminoaciduria. Histological examination revealed dilatation of the proximal tubules. The rapidly fatal course, the corneal opacities, and the fact that the patients were girls all suggest that the disease was not Lowe's syndrome.

In 1960, McCance and his associates[117] described in two brothers a syndrome characterized by a serious growth defect, mental retardation, an intention tremor, corneal opacities with nystagmus, and hyperchloremic acidosis with high blood urea, very acid urine, and a marked defect in urinary ammonium excretion. Death ensued from progressive renal failure. Autopsy revealed cerebral, cortical, and cerebellar lesions, nephrocalcinosis, and the absence of testes.

In 1964, Oberiter and Najman[120] reported the case of a boy with mental deficiency, hypotonia, areflexia, glaucoma, cataract, corneal opacities, proteinuria, and acidosis, with deficient ammoniogenesis and hyperaminoaciduria.

REFERENCES

SINGLE ANOMALIES

Hereditary Normoglycemic Glycosuria

1. Berliner, R. W.: Outline of renal physiology. *In* M. B. Strauss and L. G. Welt: Diseases of the Kidney. Boston, Little, Brown & Co., 1963.
2. Gowaerts, P., and Lambert, P. P.: Pathogénie du diabète rénal. Acta Clin. Belg. *4*:341, 1949.
3. Krane, S. M.: Renal glucosuria. *In* J. Stanbury *et al.* (eds.): The Metabolic Basis of Inherited Disease. New York, McGraw-Hill, 1966.
4. Michon, P., Larcan, A., Rauber, G., and Huriet, C.: Étude biologique de 3 cas de diabète rénal étudiés par ponction-biopsie du rein. J. Urol. Med. Chir, *65*:643, 1959.
5. Monasterio, G., Oliver, J., Muiesan, G., Pardelli, G., Marizzoni, V., and Mac Dowell, M.: Renal diabetes as a congenital tubular dysplasia. Amer. J. Med. *37*:44, 1964.
6. Reubi, F.: Physiopathologie et diagnostic du diabète rénal. Rev. franç. Et. clin. biol. *1*:575, 1956.
7. Taggart, J. V.: Mechanisms of renal tubular transport. Amer. J. Med. *24*:774, 1958.

Idiopathic Chronic Hypokalemia (Bartter Syndrome)

8. Aarskog, D., Stoa, K. F., Thorsen, T., and Wefring, K. W.: Hypertension and hypokalemic alkalosis associated with underproduction of aldosterone. Pediatrics *39*:884, 1967.
9. Bartter, F. C., Pronove, P., Gill, J. R., and MacCardle, R. C.: Hyperplasia of the juxtaglomerular complex with hyperaldosteronism and kypokalemic alkalosis. Amer. J. Med. *33*:811, 1962.
10. Cannon, P. J., Leeming, J. M., Sommers, S. C., Winters, R. W., and Laragh, J. H.: Justaglomerular cell hyperplasia and secondary hyperaldosteronism (Bartter's syndrome). A reevaluation of the physiopathology. Medicine *47*:107, 1968.
11. Gall, D. G., Haddow, J., Vaitukaitis, J., and Klein, R.: Sodium flux across the red cell membrane in patients with Bartter's syndrome and with hyperaldosteronism (Abstract American Pediatric Society, Atlantic City, N.J., 1969, p. 21.
12. Gardner, J. D., Lapey, A., Simopoulos, A. P., and Bravo, E. L.: Abnormal membrane sodium transport in Liddle's syndrome. J. Clin. Invest. *50*:2253, 1971.
13. Liddle, G. W., Bledsoe, T., and Coppage, W. S.: A familial renal disorder simulating primary aldosteronism but with negligible aldosterone secretion. In Baulieu and Robel: Aldosterone. Oxford, England, Blackwell, 1964, p. 353.
14. McCredie, D. A., Blair-West, J. R., Scoggins, B. A., and Shipman, R.: Potassium-losing nephropathy in childhood. Med. J. Aust. *1*:129, 1971.
15. Royer, P., Delaitre, R., Mathieu, H., Gabilan, J. C., Raynaud, C., Pasqualini, J. R., Gerbeaux, S., and Habib, R.: L'hypokalemie chronique idiopathique avec hyperkaliurie de l'enfant. Rev. franç. Et. clin. biol. *9*:61, 1964.
16. Trygstad, C. L., Mangos, J. A., Bloodworth, J. M. B., and Lobeck, C. C.: A sibship with Bartter's

syndrome: Failure of total adrenalectomy to correct the potassium wasting. Pediatrics *44*:
234, 1969.

17. Wald, M. K., Perrin, E. V., and Bolande, R. P.: Bartter's syndrome in early infancy. Pediatrics
47:254, 1971.

Vitamin-Resistant Rickets

18. Albright, F., Butler, A. M., and Bloomberg, E.: Rickets resistant to vitamin D therapy. Amer. J.
Dis. Child. *54*:529, 1937.

19. Balsan, S., and Garabedian, M.: 25-Hydroxycholecalciferol. A comparative study in deficiency
rickets and different types of resistant rickets. J. Clin. Invest. *51*:749, 1972.

20. Balsan, S., Garabedian, M., and Le Bouadec, L.: Le rachitisme vitamino-résistant pseudo-
carentiel hypocalcémique. Arch. franç. Pédiat. *29*:287, 1972.

21. Cartier, P., Leroux, J. P., Balsan, S., and Royer, P.: Etude de la glucolyse et de la perméabilité
des érythrocytes aux ions orthophosphates dans le rachitisme vitamino-résistant hypophos-
phatémique héréditaire. Clin. Chim. Acta *29*:261, 1970.

22. Dent, C. E., and Harris, H.: Hereditary forms of rickets and osteomalacia. J. Bone Joint Surg.
38B:204, 1966.

23. Engfeldt, B., Zetterstrom, R., and Winberg, J.: Primary vitamin D resistant rickets. III. Bio-
physical studies of skeletal tissue. J. Bone Joint Surg. *38A*:1323, 1956.

24. Glorieux, F., and Scriver, C. R.: Loss of parathyroid hormone-sensitive component of phosphate transport in X-linked hypophosphatemia. Science *175*:997, 1972.

25. Prader, A., Illig, R., and Heierli, E.: Eine besondere Form der primären Vitamin D resistanten
Rachitis mit Hypocalcemie und autosomal dominant-Erbgang: die hereditäre Pseudo-Man-
gel-Rachitis. Helv. Paediat. Acta *16*:452, 1961.

26. Steendijk, R.: The renal tubular reabsorption of inorganic phosphate in primary refractory
rickets. Acta Paediat. (Uppsala) *49*:609, 1960.

27. Winters, R. W., Graham, J. B., Williams, T. F., McFalls, T. F., McFalls, V. W., and Burnett,
C. H.: A genetic study of familial hypophosphatemia and vitamin D resistant ricket, with a
review of the literature. Medicine *37*:971, 1958.

28. Witmer, G., and Balsan, S.: Biopsie osseuse dans quatre cas de rachitisme vitamino-résistant
idiopathique. Path. Biol. *16*:421, 1968.

Hypercalciuria

29. Albright, F., Henneman, P., Benedict, P. R., and Forbes, A.: Idiopathic hypercalciuria. J. Clin.
Endocr. *13*:860, 1953.

30. Beilin, L. J., Clayton, B. E.: Idiopathic hypercalciuria in a child. Arch. Dis. Child. *39*:409, 1964.

31. DeLuca, R., and Guzzetta, F.: L'ipercalciuria idiopatica infantile. La Pediatria *73*:613, 1965.

32. Dent, C. E., and Friedmann, M.: Hypercalciuric rickets associated with renal tubular damage.
Arch. Dis. Child. *39*:240, 1964.

33. Fanconi, A.: Idiopathische Hypercalciurie im Kindesalter. Helv. Paediat. Acta *4*:306, 1963.

34. Finn, W. F., Cerilli, G. J., Ferris, T. F.: Transplantation of a kidney from a patient with idiopathic hypercalciuria. New. Eng. J. Med. *283*:145, 1970.

35. Jeune, M., Gilly, R., Hermier, M., Frederich, A., Collombel, C., and Raveau, J.: I. hyper-
caliurie idiopathique de l'enfant. Pediatrie *22*:17, 1967.

36. King, J. S., Jackson, R., and Ashe, B.: Relation of sodium intake to urinary calcium excretion.
Invest. Urol. *1*:555, 1964.

37. Kleeman, C. R., Bohannan, J., Bernstein, D., Lind, S., and Maxwell, M. H.: Effect of variations
in sodium intake on calcium excretion in normal humans. Proc. Soc. Exp. Biol. N.Y. *115*:29,
1964.

38. Liberman, U. A., Sperling, O., Atsmon, A., Frank, M., Modan, M., and De Vries, A.: Metabolic
and calcium kinetic studies in idiopathic hypercalciuria. J. Clin. Invest. *47*:2580, 1968.

39. Nordio, S., Gatti, R., and Tambutti, M.: Il nanismo ipercalciurico. Mim. Pediat. *18*:1221, 1966.

40. Rosenkranz, A.: Ein eigenartiges Syndrom tubulärer Nierenstörungen mit Urolithiasis beim
Saügling. Helv. Paediat. Acta *13*:455, 1958.

41. Royer, P., Mathieu, H., Gerbeaux, S.: Hypercalciurie idiopathique avec nanisme et atteinte
rénale chez l'enfant. Ann. Pédiat. *38*:147, 1962.

42. Royer, P.: L'hypercalciurie idiopathique avec nanisme at atteinte rénale chez l'enfant. Acta
Paediat. Scand. Suppl. *172*:186, 1967.

43. Royer, P., and Balsan, S.: Effet d'un régime pauvre en chlorure de sodium dans le "syndrome
d'hypercalciurie idiopathique avec nanisme et troubles rénaux" de l'enfant. Schweiz. Med
Wschr. *96*:412, 1966.

44. Shieber, W., Birge, S. J., Avioli, L. V., and Teitelbaum, S. L.: Normocalcemic hyperparathyroidism with "normal" parathyroid glands. Arch. Surg. *103*:299, 1971.

45. Walser, M.: Calcium clearance as a function of sodium clearance in the dog. Amer. J. Physiol. *200*:1099, 1961.

46. Zetterstrom, R.: Idiopathic hypercalcemia and hypercalciuria. *In* Modern Problems in Paediatrics. New York, S. Karger, 1957, p. 478.

PRIMARY TUBULAR ACIDOSIS

47. Albright, F., Consolazio, W. V., Coombs, F. S., Sulkowitch, H. W., and Talbott, J. H.: Metabolic studies and therapy in a case of nephrocalcinosis with rickets and dwarfism. Bull. Johns Hopkins Hosp. *66*:7, 1940.

48. Butler, A. M., Wilson, J. F., and Farber, S. J.: Dehydration and acidosis with calcification in renal tubules. J. Pediat. *8*:489, 1936.

49. Donckerwolcke, R. A., Van Stekelenburg, G. J., and Tiddens, H. A.: Therapy of bicarbonate-losing renal tubular acidosis. Arch. Dis. Child. *45*:774, 1970.

50. Donckerwolcke, R. A., Van Stekelenburg, G. J., and Tiddens, H. A.: A case of bicarbonate-losing renal tubular acidosis with defective carboanhydrase activity. Arch. Dis. Child. *45*: 769, 1970.

51. Greenberg, A. J., McNamara, H., and McCrory, W. W.: Metabolic balance studies in primary renal tubular acidosis. Effects of acidosis on external calcium and phosphorus balances. J. Pediat. *69*:610, 1966.

52. Guibaud, P., Larbre, F., Freycon, M. T., and Genoud, J.: Ostéopétrose et acidose rénale tubulaire. Deux cas de cette association dans une fratrie. Arch. franç. Pédiat. *29*:269, 1972.

53. Mattenheimer, H., Pollak, V. E., Muehrcke, R. C., and Kark, R. M.: Quantitative biochemistry of the human nephron: the possible role of enzymes in proton and ammonia excretion. J. Lab. Clin. Med. *58*:941, 1961.

54. Morris, R. C.: Renal tubular acidosis. Mechanisms, classification and implications. New. Eng. J. Med. *281*:1405, 1969.

55. Nash, M. A., Torrado, A. D., Greifer, I., Spitzer, A., and Edelmann, C. M.: Renal tubular acidosis in infants and children. Clinical course, response to treatment, and progress. J. Pediat. *80*:738, 1972.

56. Rodriguez-Soriano, J., Boichis, H., Stark, H., and Edelmann, C. M.: Proximal renal tubular acidosis. A defect in bicarbonate reabsorption with normal urinary acidification. Pediat. Res. *1*:81, 1967.

57. Royer, P., Lestradet, H., Nordmann, R., Mathieu, H., and Rodriguez-Soriano, J.: Etudes sur quatre cas d'acidose tubulaire chronique idiopathique avec hypocitraturie. Ann. Pédiat. *38*:188, 1962.

58. Royer, P., and Broyer, M.: L'acidose rénale au cours des tubulopathies congenitales. *In* Actualités Néphrologiques de l'Hôpital Necker. Paris, Flammarion, 1967, p. 73.

59. Vert, P., Marchal, C., Neimann, N., and Pierson, M.: Traitement symptomatique des acidoses rénales par administration orale de citrate de THAM. Arch. franç. Pédiat. *25*:91, 1968.

60. Schwartz, W. B., Faibriard, A., and Lemieux, G.: The kinetics of bicarbonate reabsorption during acute respiratory acidosis. J. Clin. Invest. *38*:939, 1959.

61. Seldin, D. W., Rector, F. C., Portwood, R., and Carter, N.: Pathogenesis of hyperchloremic acidosis in renal tubular acidosis. *In* Proceedings of the First International Congress of Nephrology. Paris, S. Karger, 1960, p. 175.

62. Seldin, D. W., and Wilson, J. D.: Renal tubular acidosis. *In* J. Stanbury et al. (eds.): The Metabolic Basis of Inherited Disease. New York, McGraw-Hill, 1966.

63. Vainsel, M., Fondu, P., Cadranel, S., Rocmans, C., and Gepts, W.: Osteopetrosis associated with proximal and distal tubular acidosis. Acta Paediat. Scand. *61*:429, 1972.

64. Wilson, D., Williams, R. C., and Tobian, L.: Renal tubular acidosis. Three cases with immunoglobulin abnormalities in the patients and their kindreds. Amer. J. Med. *43*:356, 1967.

65. Wrong, O., and Davies, H. E. F.: The excretion of acid in renal disease. Quart. J. Med. *28*:259, 1959.

66. Yaffe, S. J., Craig, J. M., and Fellers, F. X.: Studies on renal enzymes in a patient with renal tubular acidosis. Amer. J. Med. *29*:168, 1960.

PSEUDOENDOCRINOPATHIES

Hereditary Diabetes Insipidus Resistant to Pitressin

67. Abelson, H.: Nephrogenic diabetes insipidus. Pediat. Res. *2*:271, 1968.

68. Brown, E., Clarke, D. L., Roux, V., and Sherman, G. H.: The stimulation of adenosine 3,5 - monophosphate production by antidiuretic factors. J. Biol. Chem. *238*:852, 1963.

69. Crawford, J. D., Kennedy, G. C., and Hill, L. E.: Clinical results of treatment of diabetes insipidus with drugs of the chlorothiazide series. New Eng. J. Med. *282*:737, 1960.
70. Darmady, E. M., Offer, J., Prince, J., and Stawack, F.: The proximal convoluted tubule in renal handling of water. Lancet *2*:1254, 1964.
71. Gorden, P., Robertson, G. L., and Seegmiller, J. E.: Hyperuricemia, a concomitant of congenital vasopressin-resistant diabetes insipidus in the adult. New Eng. J. Med. *28*:1057, 1971.
72. Orloff, J., and Burg, M. B.: Vasopressin resistant diabetes insipidus. *In* M. B. Strauss and L. G. Welt: Disease of the kidney. Boston, Little, Brown & Co., 1963, p. 961.
73. Walker, N. F., and Rance, C. P.: Inheritance of nephrogenic diabetes insipidus. Amer. J. Hum. Genet. *6*:354, 1954.
74. Waring, A. J., Kajdi, L., and Tappan, V.: A congenital defect of water metabolism. Amer. J. Dis. Child. *69*:323, 1945.
75. Williams, R. H.: Nephrologic diabetes insipidus occuring in males and transmitted by females. J. Clin. Invest. *25*:937, 1946.

Pseudohypoaldosteronism

76. Cheek, D. B., and Perry, J. W.: A salt wasting syndrome in infancy. Arch. Dis. Child. *33*:252, 1958.
77. Corbeel, L.: Diabète salin du nourrisson sans insuffisance surénalienne. Pédiatrie *18*:557, 1963.
78. Donnell, G. N., Litmann, N., and Roldau, M.: Pseudohypoadrenalocorticism. Renal sodium loss, hyponatremia and hyperkalemia due to renal tubular insensitivity to mineralocorticoid. Amer. J. Dis. Child. *97*:813, 1959.
79. Jeune, M., Lamit, J., Coras, and Do, Mme.: Un cas de pseudo-hypoadrenalocorticisme. Arch. franç. Pédiat. *24*:714, 1967.
80. Lelong, M., Alagille, D., Philippe, A., Gentil, C., and Gabilan, J. C.: Diabète salin par insensibilité congénitale du tubule à l'aldostérone. Pseudohypoadrenocorticisme. Rev. franç. Et. clin. biol. *5*:558, 1960.
81. Pham-Huu-Trung, M. T., Piussan, C., Rodary, C., Legrand, S., Attal, C., and Mozziconacci, P.: Etude de taux de sécrétion de l'aldostérone et de l'activité de la rénine plasmatique d'un cas de pseudo-hypoaldosteronisme. Arch. franç. Pédiat. *27*:603, 1970.
82. Polonovski, C., Zittoun, R., and Mary, F.: Hypocorticisme global, hypoaldostéronisme et pseudo-hypoaldostéronisme du nourrisson: trois observations. Arch. franç. Pédiat. *22*:1061, 1965.
83. Raine, D. N., and Roy, J.: A salt losing syndrome in infancy: pseudohypoadrenocorticism. Arch. Dis. Child. *37*:548, 1962.
84. Royer, P., Bonnette, J., Mathieu, H., Gabilan, J. C., Klutchong, and Zittoun, R.: Pseudo-hypoaldosteronisme. Ann. Pédiat. *39*:2612, 1963.
85. Royer, P.: L'hypoaldosteronisme congénital. Rev. franç. Et. clin. biol. *12*:111, 1967.

Pseudohypoparathyroidism

86. Albright, F., Burnett, C., Smith, O. H., and Parsons, W.: Pseudohypoparathyroidism, an example of "Seabright bantam syndrome." Endocrinology *30*:992, 1942.
87. Albright, F., Forbes, A. L., and Henneman, P. H.: Pseudopseudohypoparathyroidism. Trans. Ass. Amer. Phys. *65*:337, 1952.
88. Chopra, I. J., and Nugent, C. A.: Concurrence of features of pseudohypoparathyroidism, pseudo-pseudohypoparathyroidism and basal-cell nevus syndrome. Amer. J. Med. Sci. *260*:171, 1970.
89. Costello, J. M., and Dent, C. E.: Hypo-hyperparathyroidism. Arch. Dis. Child. *38*:397, 1963.
90. Chase, L. R., Melson, G. L., and Aurbach, G. D.: Metabolic abnormality in pseudohypoparathyroidism: defective renal excretion of cyclic 3',5'-AMP in response to parathyroid hormone. Amer. Soc. Clin. Invest. Abstract No. 58, 1968.
91. Elrich, H., Albright, F., Bartter, F. C., Forbes, A. P., and Reeves, J. D.: Further studies on pseudo-hypoparathyroidism: report of 4 new cases. Endocrinology *5*:199, 1950.
92. Frame, B., Hanson, C. A., Frost, H. M., Block, M., and Arnstein, A. R.: Renal resistance to parathyroid hormone with osteitis fibrosa. Amer. J. Med. *52*:311, 1972.
93. Mann, J. B., Auterman, S., and Hills, G.: Albright's hereditary osteodystrophy comprising pseudohypoparathyroidism and pseudo-pseudohypoparathyroidism. Ann. Intern. Med. *56*:315, 1962.
94. Rosenberg, D., Moreau, P., Salle, B., Gauthier, J., and Monnet, P.: Ostéodystrophie héréditaire d'Albright. Observation familiale sur deux generations. Ann. Pédiat. *14*:757, 1967.
95. Royer, P., Lestradet, H., and de Menibus, C. H.: Les syndromes d'insuffisance parathy-

roïdienne sans hypoparathyroïdie anatomique. Les hypoparathyroïdies de l'enfance. *In* 17ᵉ Congrès des Pédiatres de langue française, Montpellier. Montpellier, 1959, Dehan Paul, p. 311.

96. Royer, P., Lestradet, H., de Menibus, C. H., and Frederich, A.: L'épreuve de phosphodiurèse provoquée par la parathormone et le diagnostic de pseudohypoparathyroïdie chez l'enfant. Rev. franç. Et. clin. biol. *4*:1007, 1959.

97. Schwartz, G., and Bahner, F.: Die Genetic des Pseudohypoparathyroidismus und Pseudo-pseudohypoparathyroidismus. Deutsch. Med. Wschr. *88*:240, 1963.

98. Suh, S. M., Fraser, D., and Kooh, S. W.: Pseudohypoparathyroidism: responsiveness to para-thyroid extract induced by vitamin D therapy. J. Clin. Endocr. *30*:609, 1970.

99. Tashjian, A. H., Frantz, A. G., and Lee, J. B.: Pseudohypoparathyroidism: assays of parathy-roid hormone and thyrocalcitonin. Proc. Nat. Acad. Sci. (Wash.) *56*:1138, 1966.

PRIMARY AND HEREDITARY COMPLEX TUBULAR DEFICIENCIES

100. Abbassi, V., Lowe, C. U., and Calcagno, P. L.: Oculocerebrorenal syndrome. Amer. J. Dis. Child. *115*:145, 1968.

101. Bickel, H., and Thursby-Pelham, D. C.: Hyperamino-aciduria in Lignac-Fanconi disease, in galactosemia and in obscure syndrome. Arch. Dis. Child. *29*:224, 1954.

102. Cleveland, W. W., Adams, W. C., Mann, J. B., and Nyhan, W. L.: Acquired Fanconi syndrome following degraded tetracycline. J. Pediat. *66*:333, 1965.

103. Corvilain, J., Gepts, W., Beghin, P., Vis, H., Verbank, M., and Verniory, A.: Exploration rénale fonctionnelle et histoenzymologique d'un cas de syndrome de De Toni-Debré-Fanconi. J. Urol. Néphrol. *71*:354, 1965.

104. Debré, R., Marie, J., Cléret, F., and Messimy, R.: Rachitisme tardif coexistant avec une néphrite chronique et une glycosurie. Arch. Med. Enfants (Paris) *37*:597, 1934.

105. Debré, R., Royer, P., Lestradet, H., Straub, W.: L'insuffisance tubulaire congénitale avec arrieration mentale, cataracte et glaucome (syndrome de Lowe). Arch. franç. Pédiat. *12*:337, 1955.

106. De Toni, G.: Remarks on the relation between renal rickets (renal dwarfism) and renal diabetes. Acta Paediat. *16*:470, 1933.

107. Fanconi, G.: Der frühinfantile nephrotischglykosurische Zwergwuchs mit hypophosphate-mischer Rachitis. Jahrb. Kinderhlk. *147*:299, 1936.

108. Habib, R., Bargeton, E., Brissaud, H. E., Raynaud, J., and LeBall, J. C.: Constatations anato-miques chez un enfant atteint d'un syndrome de Lowe. Arch. franç. Pédiat. *19*:945, 1962.

109. Hambraeus, L., Pallisgaard, G., and Kildeberg, P.: The Lowe syndrome. Acta Paediat. Scand. *59*:631, 1970.

110. Houston, I. B., Boichis, H., and Edelmann, C. M.: Fanconi syndrome with renal sodium wast-ing and metabolic alkalosis. Amer. J. Med. *44*:638, 1968.

111. Huguenin, A., Monier, J. C., and Aiache, J. M.: Diabète glucophosphoaminé expérimental chez le rat albinos par ingestion d'orthodinitrocrésol. Path. Biol. *10*:1707, 1962.

112. Illig, R., and Prader, A.: Ein Fall von idiopatischem Gluko-amino-phosphat-Diabetes. Helv. Paediat. Acta *16*:622, 1961.

113. Jacobson, N.: Hypophosphatemic glycosuric rickets (Fanconi syndrome): radiological features. Calif. Med. *70*:25, 1949.

114. Juillard, E., and Piguet, C.: Glucosurie et aminoacidurie familiale. Ann. Paediat. (Basel) *183*:257, 1954.

115. Kramer, H. J., and Gonick, H. C.: Experimental Fanconi syndrome. J. Lab. Clin. Med. *76*:799, 1970.

116. Lowe, C. U.: Terrey, M., MacLachlan, E. A.: Organoaciduria, decreased renal ammonia pro-duction, hydrophthalmos, and mental retardation; a clinical entity. Amer. J. Dis. Child. *83*:164, 1952.

117. McCance, R. A., Matheson, W. J., Gresham, G. A., and Elkinton, J. R.: The cerebroocular re-nal dystrophies: a new variant. Arch. Dis. Child. *35*:240, 1960.

118. Neimann, M., Pierson, M., Marchal, C., Rauber, G., and Grignon, G.: Néphropathie familiale glomérulo-tubulaire avec syndrome du De Toni-Debré-Fanconi. Arch. Franç. Pédiat. *25*:43, 1968.

119. Nicoll, P., Ambrosino, C., Pavesio, D., and Campadello, G.: Diabete fosfo-aminico. Min. Pediat. *17*:87, 1965.

120. Oberiter, V., and Najman, E.: Das oculo-cerebro-renale Syndrom mit Hornhauttrübung. Ann. Paediat. *203*:413, 1964.

121. Odièvre, M.: Glycogénose hépatorénale avec tubulopathie complexe. Rev. Intern. Hepato-logie *16*:21, 1966.

122. Pallisgaard, G., and Goldschmidt, F.: The oculo-cerebro-renal syndrome of Lowe in four generation of one family. Acta Paediat. Scand. *60*:146, 1971.

123. Rampini, S., Fanconi, A., Illig, R., and Prader, A.: Effect of hydrochlorothiazide on proximal renal tubular acidosis in a patient with "idiopathic de Toni-Debré-Fanconi syndrome." Helvet. Paediat. Acta 23:13, 1968.
124. Rodriguez-Soriano, J., Houston, I. B., Boichis, H., and Edelmann, C. M.: Calcium and phosphorus metabolism in the Fanconi syndrome. J. Clin. Endocr. 28:1555, 1968.
125. Sheldon, W., Luder, J., Webb, B.: A familial tubular absorption defect of glucose and amino-acids. Arch. Dis. Child. 36:90, 1961.
126. Scholten, H. G.: Een meisje met het syndroom van Lowe. Maandschr. Kindergeneesk. 28:251, 1960.
127. Streiff, E. B., Straub, W., and Golay, L.: Les manifestations oculaires du syndrome de Lowe. Ophtalmologica (Basel) 135:632, 1968.
128. Schwartz, R., Hall, P. W., and Gabuzda, G. J.: Metabolism of ornithine and other amino-acids in the cerebro-oculorenal syndrome. Amer. J. Med. 36:778, 1964.
129. Tegelaers, W. H. H., and Tiddens, H. W.: Nephrotic-glucosuric-aminoaciduric dwarfism and electrolyte metabolism. Helv. Paediat. Acta 10:269, 1955.
130. Wallis, L. A., and Engle, R. L.: The adult Fanconi's syndrome. Amer. J. Med. 22:13, 1957.

For recent additions to the literature, see:

a. Brodehl, J., Franken, A., and Gelissen, K.: Maximal tubular reabsorption of glucose in infants and children. Acta Pediat. Scand. 61:413, 1972.
b. Chaimovitz, C., Levi, J., Better, O. S., Oslander, L., and Benderli, A.: Studies on the site of renal salt loss in a patient with Bartter's syndrome. Pediat. Res. 7:89, 1973.
c. Coe, F. L., Canterbury, J. M., Firpo, J. J., and Reiss, E.: Evidence for secondary hyperparathyroidism in idiopathic hypercalciuria. J. Clin. Invest. 52:134, 1973.
d. Godard, C., Vallotton, M. B., Broyer, M., and Royer, P.: A study of the inhibition of the renin-antiotensin system in renal potassium wasting syndromes, including Bartter's syndrome. Helv. Paediat. Acta 27:495, 1972.
e. Greene, M. L., Lietman, P. S., Rosenberg, L. E., and Seegmiller, J. E.: Familial hyperglycinuria. Amer. J. Med. 54:265, 1973.
f. Lewy, J. E., Cabana, E. C., Repetto, H. A., Canterbury, J. M., and Reiss, E.: Serum parathyroid hormone in hypophosphatemic vitamin D resistant rickets. J. Pediat. 81:294, 1972.
g. White, M. G.: Bartter's syndrome. Arch. Int. Med. 129:41, 1972.

Chapter Six

NEPHROPATHIES
SECONDARY TO OR
ASSOCIATED WITH
HEREDITARY DISEASES

Some nephropathies present as complex tubular insufficiencies similar to cystinosis, the principal cause of the De Toni-Debré-Fanconi syndrome in children; others present like oxalosis, with progressive uremia; and some are latent, as, for example, most of those seen in association with the sphingolipidoses.

CYSTINOSIS

Cystinosis was described by Abderhalden in 1903.[1] A classic study was made in 1952 by Bickel and his associates.[2] Three major varieties are recognized: infantile cystinosis causing serious damage to the kidneys, which has a very poor prognosis; juvenile cystinosis;[5] and adult cystinosis.[10] The relationship among these three diseases is not clear. The following observations concern our experience with 21 cases of infantile cystinosis (Table 14).

Genetics

Cystinosis is transmitted as an autosomal recessive trait. The condition is familial in one third of the cases, and in one sixth of the cases the parents are consanguineous. The incidence of the condition is estimated at one in 40,000 population and the incidence of the abnormal gene at one in 200.

Symptomatology

The clinical presentation of cystinosis is that of a nephropathy in which tubular insufficiency predominates for a long time (Table 15).

Onset. The *onset* is in the first months of life. Systematic study of infants in an affected sibship reveals that the first pathologic sign is usually hyperaminoaciduria appearing between two and four months after birth. This is followed by thirst, polyuria, thermal instability, constipation, vomiting, retardation of

99

Table 14. Infantile Cystinosis (Personal Series)

Case	Age at Onset (years)	Sex	Familial Character	Height, cm. (S.D.)	Rickets	Osteoporosis	Depigmentation	Photophobia	Retinopathy
1	1 year 4 months	F	0	65 (−5)	+	+	+	+	?
2	1 year 1 month	M	0	72 (−3)	+	0	?	0	?
3	6	M	+	115 (−4)	+	+	?	+	?
4	2/12	F	+	(−6)	+	+	+	0	?
5	7/12	F	+	96 (−4)	+	+	+	+	?
6	1	F	?	77 (−4)	0	+	+	0	?
7	1	F	+	79 (N)	+	+	+	+	?
8	9/12	F	0	70 (−3)	+	+	?	+	?
9	8/12	F	?	72 (−0.5)	+	0	+	?	?
10	7/12	M	0	75 (N)	+	0	+	?	?
11	3/12	M	+	84 (−4)	0	+	0	+	?
12	11/12	F	+	81 (−4)	0	+	+	+	+
13	2/12	F	+	77 (−3)	+	+	+	+	+
14	4/12	M	+	70 (N)	+	+	+	+	0
15	2	F	C+	71 (−6)	+	+	+	+	0
16	3/12	M	0	75 (−2)	0	+	+	0	+
17	9/12	M	0	85 (−4)	0	+	+	0	?
18	6/12	M	+	67 (−1)	0	+	+	0	0
19	7/12	M	+	66 (−1)	0	+	+	0	0
20	1	M	0	66 (−4)	+	+	+	0	0
21	9/12	M	C	76 (−1.5)	+	0	0	+	0

C, Consanguinity; S.D., standard deviations: TRF, terminal renal failure.

Table 14.   Infantile Cystinosis (Personal Series)—*Continued*

Fanconi Syndrome	Uremia (at Onset)	Cystine in Leukocytes (μM./g. proteins)	Cornea	Marrow	Kidneys	Follow-up (years)	Death	Present Condition
				Cystine Crystals				
+	+	?	+	+	?	8	+	
+	0	?	+	+	?	7	+	
+	+	?	+	+	?	4	+	
+	+	?	+	+	?	12	+	
+	0	?	+	+	?	9	+	
+	+	?	+	+	+	?	?	?
+	0	?	−	+	?	1/12	+	
+	0	9.5	−	+	?	7	0	Poor
+	0	?	?	+	+	6/12	+	
+	0	5.5	+	?	?	10/12	+	
+	+	8.7	+	+	?	8	0	TRF
+	+	23	+	+	?	7	0	Hemodialysis
+	+	13.4	+	+	?	7	0	TRF
+	+	9.7	+	+	?	4	0	TRF
+	+	12.7	+	+	?	2	0	Mediocre
+	+	7.1	+	+	0	3	0	Mediocre
+	0	14	0	+	0	4	0	Mediocre
+	0	13	0	+	?	6/12	+	
+	0	20	+	+	?	10/12	0	Fair
+	0	5	+	0	?	3	0	Mediocre
+	0	?	+	+	?	11	0	Hemodialysis

Table 15.   Infantile Cystinosis
(Summary of Findings in 21 Personal Cases)

Age at apparent onset	2 months to 6 years
Sex	10 F, 11 M
Familial character	11/21
Height (in S.D.)	−0.5 to −6
Rickets	14/21
Osteoporosis	17/21
Depigmentation	16/18
Photophobia	11/19
Retinopathy	5/9
Fanconi syndrome	21/21
Uremia at onset	10/21
Hypokalemia	17/21 (3 with paralysis)
Age at death	1 month to 12 years

growth, and attacks of dehydration—all signs common to various pathologic states in the infant. The failure to grow becomes more and more obvious. There is a lack of pigmentation of the skin and hair. Photophobia may develop early.

Early Signs.   In the first two years of life, skeletal and renal disorders are prominent. Dwarfism is obvious. Clinical and radiologic examination of the skeleton may reveal normal bones, osteoporosis, or moderate rickets or osteomalacia resistant to vitamin D. The children are prone to infection. Decoloration of the hair, cutaneous depigmentation, and photophobia are marked. Renal function studies show a normal or slightly lowered clearance of inulin and endogenous creatinine, whereas tubular insufficiency is of considerable proportions—though sometimes it is only an isolated hyperaminoaciduria or metabolic acidosis with defective urine concentration. In one of our cases, the disease presented as a hypokalemia with defective urine concentration, and the picture resembled a Bartter syndrome. In most cases, cystinosis causes a secondary De Toni-Debré-Fanconi syndrome, with proteinuria, normoglycemic glycosuria, hypophosphatemia with lowering of the percentage of tubular reabsorption of phosphorus, acidosis, defective concentration of urine, and severe hypokalemia with hyperkaluria. Urinary sodium loss may occasionally be seen.

The proteinuria is often of tubular type, with triple globulinuria, or it may be of mixed character. The tubular acidosis is of proximal type and results from renal loss of bicarbonate. The calciuria is variable; it has been said to be low in cases of cystinosis, and this is true in the uremic stage of the disease, but in the earlier stage, when tubular insufficiency predominates, the urinary calcium output in most cases is increased, and calciuria may be considerable. We have seen a urinary calcium output of more than 15 mg./kg./24 hours. The hyperaminoaciduria is of the generalized type and involves particularly glycine, alanine, serine, glutamine, valine, leucine, isoleucine, phenylalanine, lysine, arginine, and proline. Taurine is not found, and the urinary histidine level is normal. The cystine is normal or almost normal. Blood amino acid levels are normal but there are increased amounts of citric acid, α-ketoglutaric acid, and especially pyruvic acid.

It is not always possible to interpret the chemical disorders in terms of a simple tubular dysfunction. The sugar in the urine may be lactose or a pentose. It has been suggested that malabsorption of phosphorus and calcium in the intestine may play a part.[2]

Diagnosis.   *The diagnosis of cystinosis* is not difficult to suspect. There may be a family history of a probable case or a certain case in a sibling. The first step in confirming the diagnosis is to look for cystine crystals in a specimen of bone marrow. It is important not to use formol or cedar oil, which might dissolve the crystals. These hexagonal or rectangular crystals are birefringent in polarized light. It has long been known that crystals may be found in the conjunctiva and the subepithelial part of the cornea, where they are revealed as thousands of shining specks on slit-lamp examination. A recent advance is the demonstration of alterations of pigment epithelium in the peripheral zones of the fundus of the eye; these pigment changes increase with age.[14] The diagnosis can be made with absolute certainty by measuring the cystine content of leukocytes or cultured fibroblasts. The cystine levels in these cells is more than 100 times as great as in normal subjects.[9] This technique is a very valuable one. Heterozygotes can be identified by the fact that their intracellular cystine levels are intermediate between the normal and those found in children with cystinosis; in fibroblast cultures, the cystine level is six times greater than normal. During pregnancy, amniocentesis can be practiced at an early stage and the amniotic cells cultured to determine if the child will be normal, heterozygotic, or affected with cystinosis; the technique has been greatly refined by using radioactive cystine in cultures of the amniotic cells.[12] Measurement of cystine levels in leukocytes and fibroblasts is helpful also in assessing the value of treatment.

Course.   In the past, the disease usually progressed to death in the first two years of life from acute dehydration, acidosis, hypokalemia, and intercurrent infection. These complications now are more easily controlled.

Typically, the nephropathy develops in three stages over a period of years. Initially tubular insufficiency is the dominant feature. Rickets may become very severe. An occasional complication is periodic hypokalemic paralysis. At this stage, glandular enlargement and hepatomegaly may appear. The photophobia is often intense, and some patients have to wear dark glasses continually or live in a darkened room. It is apparently the retinopathy rather than the crystals in conjunctiva and cornea that is responsible for the photophobia. At a later stage, glomerular insufficiency appears or increases. Some of the biochemical and skeletal signs may seem to improve at this stage, when there is less glomerulotubular imbalance. The last stage is one of progressive uremia, with extreme dwarfism — much more marked than in any other chronic renal failure. Renal osteodystrophy is the rule. Death ensues from acidosis, uremia, or intercurrent infection, usually between the ages of 6 and 12 years.

Cystinosis may follow a different pattern. In rare cases, the onset may be very early, in the first year of life, with global renal failure and uremia, but subsequent progress is no more rapid than in the typical case.

Pathologic Anatomy

The body content of cystine is more than 500 times the normal amount. The cystine crystals occur extracellularly or are found in the histiocytes or the reticuloendothelial system. There are abundant deposits in the lymph nodes, thymus, spleen, liver, gastrointestinal submucous tissue, cornea, and bone marrow. Crystals are not deposited in cortical bone.

The nephropathy in cystinosis may appear in various forms. The kidney may be normal, there may be atrophy of the proximal tubule, with a "swan neck" appearance in the postglomerular part, or there may be extensive changes in glomeruli, tubules, and interstitial tissue, with atrophied kidneys. The amount of cystine in the kidney is very variable and does not seem to be related directly to the intensity of the renal lesions. Even when no cystine crystals can be detected in the kidney, there may be major tubular lesions, especially in the proximal tubules, characterized by swelling and hyperchromatism of the tubular cells, with some of these cells grouped in multinucleate masses (Figure 22). Ultrastructural studies have shown that the cystine is localized in a subcellular compartment of the leukocytes, fibroblasts, and reticuloendothelial cells, and rarely in hepatocytes, thyroid cells, and the cells of the renal epithelium. It is possible that the lysosomes form the particular subcellular compartment.[11] However, with both light and electron microscopy, dark cells with a high sulfur content have been found with no membrane bounding the dark zone. These are interstitial cells and podocytes, but no such cells have been found in the proximal tubular epithelium.[13]

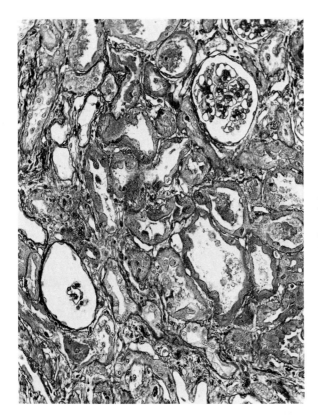

Figure 22. Cystinosis. Note the irregularity of the cells in the epithelium of the proximal convoluted tubules; some are flattened, others are very large, some are vacuolated, and others are strongly chromophilic. ×175.

Pathogenesis

The pathogenesis of cystinosis remains obscure. Attempts have been made in vain to demonstrate a simple metabolic failure of conversion of cystine to cysteine. The cystine reductase is normal, as is the utilization of ^{35}S. The gluta- thione-cysteine dehydrogenase in the liver is normal. Current thinking concerns the possibility of the initial accumulation of cystine in the lysosomes, explaining the presence of cystine outside the lysosomes in some dark cells on the basis of macrophage phenomena. It is suggested that the accumulation in the lysosomes is the result of a hydrolase defect breaking the disulfide bonds of cysteine,[11] or a failure of egress of the lysosomes.

It has long been thought that most of the manifestations of cystinosis are secondary to the cystine deposits in the tissues. However, the extreme dwarfism suggests that there is a more profound metabolic disorder. It is known that a deficit in free SH groups can diminish the activity of certain enzymes,[7] especially the succinic dehydrogenase in the Krebs cycle, and produce a deficit in cell energy. The nephropathy of cystinosis probably can be traced to some general phenomenon of this type, but there may be other, unknown abnormalities. It is quite clear that the deposits of cystine in renal parenchyma do not become signi- ficant in pathogenesis until a late stage.

Treatment

The treatment of cystinosis is currently directed along several lines. Two measures have been applied, with the object of reducing the cystine deposits.

A diet with low methionine and cystine content has been used. The diet may be based on pure amino acids or on lentil flour, which is poor in sulfur-containing amino acids, or a more varied diet, with restriction of substances with a high con- tent of these amino acids, may be used. The short-term effects on the general condition[8] are sometimes good, probably because they correct the acidosis – the sulfated amino acids are responsible for some 80 to 90 per cent of the intake of H^+ ions. Actually, the corrective effect may be so marked as to produce an alka- losis, with aggravation of the hypokalemia. The long-term value of this dietary treatment is nil, and we have found no reduction of the cystine levels in the leukocytes and fibroblasts in our patients after continuing the treatment for 6 to 18 months.

D-*Penicillamine* can convert cystine into soluble penicillamine-cysteine that can be eliminated by the kidney. However, trials with a dose of 10 to 30 mg. three or four times a day, alone or in combination with a special diet, have not been successful.[3] We have continued the treatment for six months without any good response (Table 16).

Dithiothreitol is under trial,[4] but it is probably too toxic for clinical use.

Symptomatic Treatment. This type of treatment is very important and will often ensure prolonged survival and sometimes even normal activity and well-being. The most important aspects are correction of the hypokalemia by large doses of potassium (3 to 6 mEq./kg./day), correction of the acidosis by giving bicarbonate, usually potassium bicarbonate, and improvement of the state of the bones by prescribing phosphate and cholecalciferol. The hypercal- ciuria that is frequently present is a contraindication to the use of high doses of cholecalciferol, and in such cases it may be better to give phosphate (300 to 750

Table 16.   Cystine Concentration in Leukocytes During Treatment
for Cystinosis (in μM./g. of Protein)*

Case	Before Treatment	After Diet Poor in Sulfur-Containing Amino Acids for Six Months	After Penicillamine for Six Months
1	5.6	9.7	7.5
2	8.5		
3	2.7	9.5	12.5

*Normal value: 0.08 ± 0.06.

mg. per day added to the diet). The osteodystrophy of the uremic stage does not respond to treatment. Because of the defect in urine concentration, the osmotic load of the diet should be reduced, and considerable amounts of water should be drunk day and night. In our experience, the use of anabolic steroids, especially norethandrolone and oxandrolone, in nonvirilizing doses, is helpful in improving the activity and the muscle mass of the children.

Treatment has little effect on growth, on the development of the nephropathy, on the amount of cystine in the leukocytes, or on the osteodystrophy of the uremic stage.

Kidney Transplantation.   A considerable number of children afflicted with cystinosis have been put on maintenance hemodialysis and have undergone kidney transplantation. Cystine accumulates in the transplanted kidneys, but the crystals are found only in the interstitial tissue and not in the cells of the glomerular and tubular epithelium. Lengthy survival has been obtained without recurrence of the complex tubular insufficiency.[6]

Adult Cystinosis

Cystinosis of the adult type is asymptomatic and is often discovered by chance during ophthalmological examination. There are crystalline deposits in the conjunctiva and cornea, and cystine crystals can be found in the bone marrow. There is no retinopathy or renal lesions. The cystine content of leukocytes and fibroblasts is 30 to 50 times greater than normal, intermediate between the amount in heterozygotes and that in homozygotes with infantile cystinosis.[8] An intermediate form, *adolescent cystinosis*, has recently been described.[5] This begins in the second decade, with a late Fanconi syndrome and corneal cystine deposits but no retinopathy, and is transmitted as an autosomal recessive trait (Table 17).

Table 17.   Types of Cystinosis

Type	Kidney	Retina	Crystals in Conjunctiva and Bone Marrow	Leukocyte Cystine
Infantile	+++	+++	+++	100 times normal
Juvenile	Fanconi syndrome	0	++	30–50 times normal
Adult	0	0	++	30–50 times normal

HEREDITARY HYPEROXALURIA OR OXALOSIS

Primary hyperoxaluria or oxalosis is a rare and very serious condition, often recognized before the age of 10. It may even present in the first weeks of life, but some cases develop only at a much later age. Death occurs from uremia before the age of 20. It is a hereditary disease transmitted as an autosomal recessive trait. We have seen 10 cases (Table 18).

Symptomatology

The symptoms have been described in detail in two recent reviews (Buri[15] and Hockaday and his colleagues[18]). It presents in early childhood with recurrent calcium oxalate calculi causing pain, hematuria, and pyuria. There is also severe renal failure with progressive uremia, owing to the deposition of calcium oxalate in the kidney, as well as intense nephrocalcinosis. Variants include an appearance of severe tubular acidosis in early life,[17, 20] and isolated renal failure without nephrocalcinosis or visible calculi on radiologic examination. Rare extrarenal manifestations include retinitis pigmentosa and atrioventricular block owing to oxalate deposits in the atrioventricular bundle or its branches. The prognosis is poor. The disease begins before the age of 5 years in 65 per cent of cases, and 80 per cent of the patients have died by the age of 20 (Table 19). Calcium oxalate crystals can be found in the kidney and many other viscera (Figure 23).

Diagnosis

The association of calcium oxalate stones, nephrocalcinosis, and progressive uremia is very suggestive. There may be a family history of definite or probable involvement of another sibling. Only rarely can characteristic crystals be found in the bone marrow or in a renal biopsy specimen. The basic step in diagnosis is measuring the oxalate level in the urine. Archer's method, as modified by Dent,[17] or measurement by an isotope dilution technique,[4] gives comparable results. The normal adult output is 15 to 30 mg./24 hours, and the output in children is similar if related to a body surface area of 1.73 m.[2] Patients eliminate more than 50 mg./24 hours—often as much as 100 or even 200 mg./1.73 m.[2]— but these figures fall when there is advanced renal failure.

Pathogenesis

The metabolic error is a deficit in α-ketoglutarate-glyoxylate-carboligase. Patients with the disease excrete glycolic acid and glyoxylic acid in the urine in addition to excessive amounts of oxalate. A less common variety, with identical clinical features, has been described, but in this type there is an output of L-*glyceric acid* in the urine in the region of 300 to 400 mg./24 hours instead of the normal 5 mg./24 hours. In this form, the metabolic block is between glycolate and glyoxalate.

Table 18.   Oxalosis (Personal Series)

Case	Age at Onset (years)	Sex	Familial Character	Lithiasis	Nephrocalcinosis (on X-ray)	G.F.R. (ml./min./1.73 m.²)	Blood Pressure (mm. Hg)	Urinary Oxalate (mg./24 hours/1.73 m.²)
1	1/12	M	C	0	0	?	?	?
2	3	M	C 1 sister	+	+	42	100/70	?
3	6	F	C 1 brother	+	0	108	90/50	173
4	3	M	C	+	+	45	90/50	560
5	9	F	0	+	+	?	110/60	200
6	10	F	0	+	+	10	120/?	149
7	4	F	1 brother	+	+	64.35 −2	100/60	250
8	5	M	1 sister	+	+	89	110/70	353
9	5	F	1 sister	+	+	74	100/70	331
10	1	F	1 sister	+	0	89	120/80	242

C, Consanguinity; N, oxalate nephrocalcinosis; G.F.R., glomerular filtration rate.

Treatment

Many treatment plans, including the use of calcium carbamide, disulfiran, glutamic acid, allopurinol, malonate, and pyridoxine, have been tried without success. Dent and Stamp have found some benefit in nine patients from the continuous administration of magnesium hydroxide and sodium phosphate, along with a low-calcium diet (less than 400 mg./day).[17] Kidney transplantation has been tried in cases of oxalosis. Deposits of calcium oxalate do recur in the transplanted kidney, but sufficiently slowly for this not to be a contraindication to placing a patient on a dialysis-transplantation program.

OTHER NEPHROPATHIES SECONDARY TO OR ASSOCIATED WITH HEREDITARY DISEASES

Hereditary Diseases of Metabolism

Various renal abnormalities, functional or structural, serious or benign, affecting principally the renal tubule or leading to progressive uremia, may

Table 18.   Oxalosis (Personal Series) — *Continued*

Oxalate Crystals	Renal Biopsy	Treatment	Interval (years)	Present Condition
?	N	0	3/12	Dead
0	N	0	6	Dead
?	?	0	4	G.F.R. normal; no calculi
Marrow	?	Calcium carbamide	4	Dead
0	?	0	0	Advanced uremia
Marrow	?	0	6	Advanced uremia
0	N	0	6/12	Advanced uremia
0	N	0	2	G.F.R. normal; stones
?	?	Magnesium	3	G.F.R. stable; stones
?	?	Magnesium	6	G.F.R. stable; No stones

Table 19.   Oxalosis (Summary of 10 Personal Cases)

Familial character	8/12
Consanguinity	4/10
Age at onset	1 month to 10 years
Lithiasis	9/10
Nephrocalcinosis on x-ray	7/10
Nephrocalcinosis on biopsy	4/4
G.F.R. (ml./min./1.73 m.^{2})	10 to 108
Urinary oxalate (mg./24 hours/1.73 m.^{2})	149 to 560
Crystals in bone marrow	2/6
Dead	3 (3 months, and 4 and 6 years)
Living:	
With advanced uremia	3
With stable renal function	4

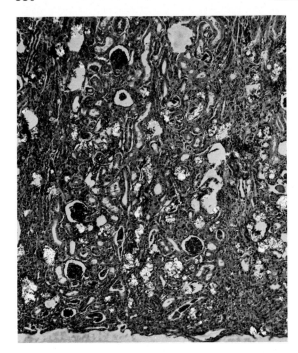

Figure 23. Oxalosis. The entire renal parenchyma is encrusted with crystalline formations of varying size, having the morphology of oxalate crystals. ×65.

occur secondary to various hereditary diseases of metabolism. In *galactosemia* and *hereditary fructose intolerance,* in addition to the generalized hyperamino-aciduria and sugar in the urine, there is proteinuria of the tubular type, and sometimes also a tubular acidosis of proximal type and hypokalemia. These disorders disappear when the relevant sugar is withheld from the diet, but recur on an unrestricted diet. *Tyrosinosis* presents as a congenital cirrhosis with hepatomegaly and complex tubular insufficiency, including hyperamino-aciduria, hypophosphatemia, defective concentration of urine, hypokalemia, proximal tubular acidosis, and sometimes gross hypercalciuria. Dwarfism and skeletal disorders are often marked. *Wilson's disease* produces a similar picture, with cirrhosis, complex tubular insufficiency, neurologic signs, a green peri-corneal ring, and cataract. The ceruloplasmin level is low, with a very high urinary copper output. A certain number of cases of renal disorder have been reported in children. Another condition that remains to be clarified is the association of hereditary nephropathy with deafness and *hyperprolinemia* or hyperhydroxyprolinemia. All these conditions are transmitted as autosomal recessive traits. Much more severe renal disorders can be found in the heredi-tary metabolic diseases to be considered below.

Lesch-Nyhan Syndrome[27]

This disease is transmitted as a sex-linked recessive trait. It results from a defect in hypoxanthine-guanine-phosphoribosyl-transferase, the enzyme that catalyzes the formation of purine nucleotides from hypoxanthine and guanine. The clinical features include mental retardation, a tendency to self-mutilation, and extrapyramidal signs. A megaloblastic or macrocytic anemia cured by the administration of adenine has been described. Blood and urinary levels of uric acid are very high. Renal signs, with deposits of uric acid crystals in the kidney, interstitial nephropathy, and lithiasis, have been observed in childhood. In one of our patients, a renal disorder (a polyuria insipida resistant to pitressin) was the presenting feature (see page 180).[32]

Hepatorenal Glycogenosis with Complex Tubulopathy

This very rare disease, presenting as an idiopathic De Toni-Debré-Fanconi syndrome, was described by Fanconi and Bickel in 1949.[22] Several additional cases have since been reported.[26, 29] The disease is present from the first months of life. There is severe dwarfism, polyuria, polydipsia, marked hepatomegaly, and a variable degree of rickets. There is a gluco-amino-phosphate diabetes associated with defective reabsorption of uric acid and a proteinuria of tubular type. Histologically, there is an overload of glycogen in some of the epithelial cells in both the proximal and the distal tubules. There is also a glycogen overload in the liver, but no abnormality of the enzyme systems, such as may be found in other glycogenoses, is present (Figure 24).

Fabry's Disease

Fabry's disease is a hereditary sphingolipidosis transmitted as a sex-linked recessive trait. It results from lack of a lysosomal acid hydrolase, trihexosyl-1-ceramide-galactosyl-hydrolase, that leads to deposition in the viscera of tri-hexosyl and dihexosyl ceramide. These substances may be found in the urine

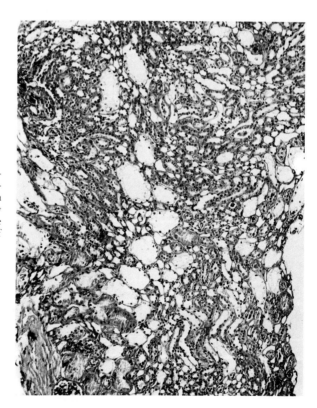

Figure 24. Hepatorenal glycogenosis with De Toni-Debré-Fanconi syndrome without a detectable enzyme abnormality (Bickel-Fanconi syndrome). Note the excess of glycogen in some of the tubules. ×80.

before the onset of clinical symptoms. Clinically, there are three stages: (1) arthralgia, fever, myalgia, acroparasthesia, angiokeratoma, corneal opacities, and sometimes proteinuria during childhood and adolescence; (2) lessening of the preceding features and renal deterioration; (3) serious uremia and cardiac and cerebral signs. The renal lesions are characteristic. There is vacuolization and distention of the cells of the glomerular tuft and of the cells of the distal tubule. These cells are overloaded with lipid, as are the smooth muscle fibers of the blood vessels, the myocardium, the corneal epithelium, and the reticulo-endothelial system.[23] It has been shown recently that renal transplantation, carried out to treat the uremia, partly compensates for the metabolic disorder.

Lesions with varying degrees and types of overload have been found in the mucopolysaccharidoses and other sphingolipidoses, such as the sulfa-tidoses, the sphingomyelinoses of Niemann-Pick, and the GM_1 gangliosidoses of Landing. The renal lesions are latent, but a case of nephrotic syndrome has been reported as a complication of Niemann-Pick disease.[33]

Lipodystrophies

The total or partial lipodystrophies are complicated by renal manifestations. More than half of the cases of facial lipodystrophy or faciotruncal lipodystrophy are affected in this way. In the total lipodystrophies, because of the associated diabetes, the principal renal lesion is a diabetic glomerulosclerosis, but there are sometimes more complex features. In the partial lipodystrophies, the clinical presentation is one of acute glomerulonephritis, or a rapid onset of severe uremia with hypertension, or sometimes proteinuria with recurrent hematuria. Various types of glomerulonephritis have been found on renal biopsy or at autopsy, including focal glomerulonephritis, diffuse glomerulo-nephritis with simple endocapillary proliferation, or membranoproliferative disease.[25] Our own three cases had a membranoproliferative glomerulonephritis with dense deposits in the basement membranes and a lowered serum complement level.

Sickle Cell Anemia

Defective concentration of urine with hyposthenuria is found in the majority of homozygote and heterozygote subjects with hemoglobinosis S. The same finding is noted in double S-C heterozygotes. The concentration disorder presents early and does not respond to vasopressin or water deprivation. During mannitol diuresis, the clearance of free water may become negative. Transfusions of fresh blood sometimes restore the concentrating ability of the kidney, at least in young children.

Microscopic and sometimes gross hematuria has been noted in patients with sickle-cell anemia and adults with S-C trait. There is an increased incidence of abacterial leukocyturia and proteinuria. Renal infarction and the nephrotic syndrome are rare. Urographic abnormalities have been reported, including enlargement of the kidney and calyceal irregularity. Histological findings may include juxtaglomerular congestion, infarcts and necrosis in the medulla, and increased weight of the kidney.[27] Most of these features are probably secondary to intravascular stasis and thrombosis caused by the sickling, owing to the low oxygen concentration and hyperosmolarity of the medulla.

Renal Abnormalities and Phakomatoses

The phakomatoses result from an abnormal gene with an incompletely dominant expression. Renal abnormalities are not uncommon.

Neurofibromatosis

Patients with neurofibromatosis may have simple cysts of the kidney, ganglioneuromas compressing the renal vessels, and in particular the characteristic abnormalities of the trunk and main branches of the renal artery. The walls of these vessels are infiltrated with very characteristic fusiform and stellate cells, which obliterate the vascular lumina to a variable extent. Sometimes associated abnormalities, such as aneurysm and stenosis, affect many of the renal, mesenteric, and iliac vessels. These problems are considered in more detail in Part IV, Chapter 4 (see page 412).

Tuberous Sclerosis of Bourneville

Renal manifestations are second only to those affecting the nervous system. They account for 50 per cent of instances of visceral involvement. The condition may be found in infants and older children. Presenting signs include proteinuria, hematuria (which may be massive), pain and urinary infection, and the presence of an abdominal or lumbar mass. Malformations of the urinary tract are common, as are the presence of horseshoe kidney and renal agenesis. Cysts and malignant tumors are very rare. The tumors that usually occur include hamartoma, angiolipoma, myolipoma, and angiolipoma with tortuous, thick-walled vessels. Hamartoma may be unilateral or bilateral and may invade the renal vein, but it does not produce metastases.

Von Hippel-Lindau disease is very commonly complicated by kidney cysts.

Nephropathies and Hereditary Diseases of the Skeleton

Renal complications may occur in many hereditary diseases of bone. In *hereditary hypophosphatasia*, the hypercalcemia produces serious renal complications. Renal failure may develop in other hereditary bone diseases, such as *essential acro-osteolysis*, which may occur sporadically or as a familial disease with dominant transmission.[21] *Onycho-osteodysplasia* is an autosomal dominant condition in which nephropathies have been reported which nearly always take the form of a chronic glomerulonephritis progressing to death from uremia in adolescence or early adult life.[28] *Thoracic asphyxiant dystrophy* may also be complicated by major kidney lesions. This disease is usually transmitted as an autosomal recessive trait, but there are some reports suggesting dominant transmission with variable expressivity.[24] Renal lesions may also be associated with *Cockayne's dwarfism*. In two cases of Cockayne syndrome presenting with dwarfism, tapetoretinal degeneration, deafness, mental retardation, and precocious senility, renal biopsy has revealed thickening of the basement membrane and of the mesangium, glomerular hyalinization, tubular atrophy with thickening of the basement membranes, and interstitial fibrosis.[30]

REFERENCES

CYSTINOSIS

1. Abderhalden, E.: Familiäre Cystindiathese. Hoppe Seylers Z. Physiol. Chem. *38*:557, 1903.
2. Bickel, H., Baar, H. S., and Smellie, J. M.: Cystine storage disease with aminoaciduria and dwarfism. Acta Paediat. Uppsala *42* (suppl. 90): 1952.
3. Clayton, B., and Patrick, A. D.: Use of dimercaprol or penicillamine in the treatment of cystinosis. Lancet *2*:909, 1961.
4. Goldman, H., Scriver, C. R., Aaron, K., and Pinski, L.: Use of dithiothreitol to correct cystine storage in cultured cystinotic fibroblasts. Lancet *1*:811, 1970.
5. Goldman, H., Scriver, C. R., Aaron, K., Devlin, E., and Canlas, Z.: Adolescent cystinosis: comparisons with infantile and adult forms. Pediatrics *47*:979, 1971.
6. Mahoney, C. P., Striker, G. E., Hickman, R. O., Manning, T. L., and Marchioro, T. L.: Renal transplantation for childhood cystinosis. New Eng. J. Med. *283*:397, 1970.
7. Patrick, A. D.: Deficiencies of SH-dependent enzymes in cystinosis. Clin. Sci. *28*:427, 1965.
8. Schärer, K., and Antener, I.: Zur Therapie und Biochemie der Cystinose. Ann. Paediat. (Basel) *203* (suppl. 1): 1964.
9. Schneider, J. A., Bradley, K., and Seegmiller, J. E.: Increased cystine in leucocytes from individuals homozygote and heterozygote for cystinosis. Science *157*:1321, 1967.
10. Schneider, J. A., Wong, V., Bradley, K., and Seegmiller, J. E.: Biochemical comparisons of the adult and childhood forms of cystinosis. New Eng. J. Med. *279*:1253, 1968.
11. Schulman, J. D., Wong, V., and Olson, W. H.: Lysosomal site of crystalline deposits in cystinosis as shown by ferritine uptake. Arch. Path. *90*:259, 1970.
12. Schulman, J. D., Fujimoto, W. Y., Bradley, K., and Seegmiller, J. E.: Identification of heterozygous genotype for cystinosis *in utero* by a new pulse-labeling technique. J. Pediat. *77*:468, 1970.
13. Spear, G. S., Slusser, R. J., Tousimis, A. J., Taylor, C. G., and Schulman, J. D.: Cystinosis. An ultrastructural and electron-probe study of the kidney with unusual findings. Arch. Path. *21*:206, 1971.
14. Wong, V. G., Lietman, P. S., and Seegmiller, J. E.: Alterations of pigment epithelium in cystinosis. Arch. Ophth. *77*:361, 1967.

OXALOSIS

15. Buri, J. F.: L'oxalose. Helv. Paediat. Acta *17* (Suppl. 2), 1962.
16. Deodhar, S. D., Tung, K. S. K., and Nakamoto, S.: Renal homotransplantation in a patient with primary familial oxalosis. Arch. Path. *87*:118, 1969.
17. Dent, C. E., and Stamp, T. C. B.: Treatment of primary hyperoxaluria. Arch. Dis. Child. *45*: 735, 1970.
18. Hockaday, T. D. R., Clayton, J. E., Frederick, W. E., and Smith, L. H.: Primary hyperoxaluria. Medicine (Baltimore) *43*:315, 1964.
19. Hockaday, T. D. R., Clayton, J. E., and Smith, L. H.: The metabolic error in primary hyperoxaluria. Arch. Dis. Child. *40*:485, 1965.
20. Royer, P., L'Hirondel, J., Habib, R., Lestradet, H., and Corbin, J. L.: Acidose rénale hyperchlorémique du nourrisson due à une oxalose. Arch. franç. Pédiat. *15*:1371, 1958.

OTHER NEPHROPATHIES

21. Berthoux, F., Robert, J. M., Zech, P., Fries, D., and Traeger, J.: Acro-ostéolyse essentielle a début carpien et tarsien avec néphropathie. Arch. franç. Pediat. *28*:615, 1971.
22. Fanconi, G., and Bickel, H.: Der chronische Aminoacidurie bei der Glykogenose und der Cystinkrankheit. Helv. Paediat. Acta *4*:359, 1949.
23. Hamburger, J., Dormont, J., Montera, H., and Hinglais, N.: Sur une singulière malformation de l'épithélium rénal. Schweiz. Med., Wschr. *94*:871, 1964.
24. Herdman, R. C., and Langer, L. O.: The thoracic asphyxiant dystrophy and renal disease. Amer. J. Dis. Child. *116*:192, 1968.
25. Hamza, M., Levy, M., Broyer, M., and Habib, R.: Deux cas de glomérulonéphrite membranoproliférative avec lipodystrophie partielle de type facio-tronculaire. J. Urol. Néphrol. *76*: 1032, 1970.
26. Lampert, F., and Mayer, H.: Glykogenose der Leber mit Galaktoseverwertungstörung und schwerem Fanconi-Syndrome. Z. Kinderheilk. *98*:133, 1967.

27. Lesch, M., and Nyhan, W. L.: A familiar disorder of uric acid metabolism and central nervous system function. Amer. J. Med. *36*:561, 1964.
28. Miller, H. T.: Hereditary osteo-onychodysplasia. Calif. Med. *108*:377, 1968.
29. Odièvre, M.: Glycogénose hépatorénale avec tubulopathie complexe. Rev. Int. Hepat. *16*:1, 1966.
30. Ohno, T., and Hirooka, M.: Renal lesions in Cockayne's syndrome. Tohoku J. Exp. Med. *89*:151, 1966.
31. Plunket, D. C., Leiken, S. L., and LoPresti, J. M.: Renal radiologic changes in sickle cell anemia. Pediatrics *35*:955, 1965.
32. Royer, P.: L'encéphalopathie hyperuricémique héréditaire avec troubles neurologiques et rénaux. Rev. Pédiat. *17*:1927, 1967.
33. Zoepffel, H.: Eine Niemann-Picksche Krankheit unter dem Bild der Lipoïdnephrose. Arch. Kinderheilk. *171*:271, 1964.

For recent additions to the literature, see:

a. Bennett, W. M., Musgrave, J. E., Campbell, R. A., Elliot, D., Cox, R., Brooks, R. E., Lovrien, E. W., Beals, R. K., and Porter, G. A.: The nephropathy of the nail-patella syndrome. Amer. J. Med. *54*:304, 1973.
b. Boquist, L., Linqvist, B., Östberg, Y., and Steen, L.: Primary oxalosis. Amer. J. Med. *54*:673, 1973.
c. Krivit, W., Desnick, R. J., and Bernlohr, R. W.: Enzyme transplantation in Fabry's disease. New Eng. J. Med. *287*:1248, 1972.

THE KIDNEY
IN THE NEWBORN

The neonate, whether premature or full term, shows a significant incidence of renal problems. There are three aspects which give these problems a special character. The renal physiology of the fetus and newborn infant has certain unique characteristics owing to the progressive maturation of the kidney; most of the conditions encountered are peculiar to this period of life and many urgently need diagnosis; treatment must take into account the special requirements of the neonate. The renal disorder may be accompanied by various types of neurologic or respiratory distress, or it may be complicated by metabolic disorders, such as hyperglycemia or hypocalcemia. Accounts have been published of urologic[12] and renal[4] emergencies in the newborn, and of neonatal kidney diseases.[22]

DEVELOPMENT OF RENAL FUNCTION IN THE NORMAL NEONATE

Fetal Kidney

The mammalian kidney secretes *before birth* a urine that has a very low osmolar concentration, high sodium and chloride contents, and small amounts of potassium, urea, and phosphates. Up to 20 per cent of the glomerular filtrate is excreted to the bladder by the fetal kidney. This excretion begins about the fourth month of fetal life and contributes to the formation of the amniotic fluid.

Urine in the Neonate

The first micturition occurs in the first 24 hours of life in 92 per cent of neonates, during the second day in 7 per cent, and later in the remaining 1 per cent. In the earliest urine, the osmolar concentration rises to 400 mOsm./liter; urea is the principal constituent, followed by sodium chloride. There are considerable amounts of phosphate and potassium. In the first few days of life, the urine is often cloudy and reddish, owing to an excess of urate, which persists to the sixth day. Indeed the crystalluria may cause hematuria in 1 or 2 per cent of neonates. In 25 per cent of children at this age, there may be moderate glycosuria and a urinary protein output of 0.10 to 0.70 g./liter. Physiologic hyperaminoaciduria persists for several weeks. Examination of the urinary sediment often reveals round cells that may be confused with altered polymorphonuclear leukocytes. During this period, the diuresis increases progressively, but the amounts are variable (Table 20).

Table 20. Urinary Output in the Newborn

Day	ml./24 Hours
1	0–20
2	20
3	30
4	60
5	100
6	120
8	150
10	200
12	200–250

Limitations of Renal Homeostasis

Much work has been done on renal function in the neonate, both premature and full term. This work has been summarized in various critical reviews,[2,13,14,20,21] and some of the findings are given in Table 21. The practical consequences of the limitations of renal homeostasis in the newborn child, especially the premature infant, may be summed up under four headings.

Function Studies

The results of function studies in the neonate are difficult to interpret for many reasons. There is certainly a considerable possibility of technical error in measurement. The range of normal values is much wider than in adults. The time of maturation of each function varies considerably from one child to another. Comparison with adult figures requires the adoption of a reference system such as kidney weight, body surface area, total body water, or extracellular water. Particular points to note are the low glomerular filtration rate, with consequent risk of sudden azotemic crisis; the glomerulotubular disequilibrium, which explains in part the physiologic hyperaminoaciduria; the ease with which glycosuria may appear; the frequency of hyperphosphatemia; and the defective concentration, contrasting with a good diluting ability.

Neonatal Pathology

Some of the problems of the neonate, such as certain types of edema in the premature infant, acidosis, neonatal hypocalcemia, and some features of acute dehydration in the newborn, can be explained in part by the renal immaturity. At this stage of life, acute dehydration very easily gives rise to serious functional renal failure, because in these conditions it is very easy for the glomerular filtration rate to fall to very low levels.

Diet

If a newborn infant is fed on cow's milk without any carbohydrate supplement, the amount of milk needed to provide the necessary calories contains a

Table 21.   Functional Development of the Kidney

	Full-term Neonate	Premature Infant	Adult	Age of Maturation (in months)
Glomerular filtration rate (ml./min./1.73 m.²)	40–60	30–50	120	12–24
Renal plasma flow (ml./min./1.73 m.²)	120–150		630	3–6
Filtration fraction (per cent)	30–40		20	6–36
Tm PAH (mg./min./1.73 m.²)	12–30		75	12–24
Tm glucose (mg./min./1.73 m.²)	35–100		300	12–24
Urea clearance (ml./min./1.73 m.²)	20–50	15–30	75	12–24
Extreme dilution of urine (mOsm./liter)	50	50	50	
Maximal concentration of urine (mOsm./liter)	400–600	400–600	1400	3
Maximal U/P osmolar ratio		2.5	4	3
Ammoniogenesis	Normal	Lowered		
Lowering of urinary pH	Normal	Normal		
Hydrogen ion excretion	Normal or lowered	Lowered		

Tm, Maximal tubular reabsorption; PAH, para-aminohippurate; U/P, urine/plasma.

Table 22.   Amount of Water Necessary for Excretion of Dietary Osmotic Residues Corresponding to 100 Calories for Different Milks

Milk	mOsm./liter	mOsm./100 cal.	Milliliters of Water for Urine at 300 mOsm./kg.	Milliliters of Water for Urine at 600 mOsm./kg.
Undiluted cow's milk	220	31	102	51
Half-cream powdered milk (13 per cent)	265	36	118	59
SMA–S 26	93	14	46	23
Similac	104	15.5	51	25.5
NAN	100	14	46	23
Human milk	80	11	36	18

quantity of salt and proteins that may exceed the ability of the kidney to excrete dissolved substances, leading to salt retention, whereas the same child, if fed on mother's milk, is not exposed to this problem. Because of the slow maturation of the concentrating ability, especially in some children, an excess of water is used to eliminate the surplus of dissolved substances (Table 22). This water is no longer available for heat control, which, at this age, depends more on sweating than on radiation, and fever results. It is sufficient to increase the water intake to restore the ratio between water and urinary solute to normal; the fever then disappears. In other cases, especially in premature infants, the salt overload may cause hypernatremic edema.

Treatment

Methods of rehydration in full term or premature neonates must be adapted to the data just provided. There is a definite relationship between the urinary volume, the urinary solute concentration, and the amount of solute to be excreted. This ratio is variable, and its limits are defined by the ability of the kidneys to concentrate and to dilute, which differs from that in the normal adult. In the case of dehydration owing to salt loss, if only water and sugar are provided, the premature infant, lacking salt, cannot excrete excess water and rapidly develops signs of water intoxication. Conversely, in dehydration with hypernatremia, if isotonic saline is given, the adult kidney can retain 80 ml. of water from each 100 ml. of solution, but the neonatal kidney can retain only 60 ml. On the other hand, the ability of the premature infant to excrete potassium is such that very large amounts of this electrolyte can be used therapeutically.

RENAL PATHOLOGY IN THE NEWBORN

This will be considered from a practical viewpoint.

Retention of Urine[4, 12]

Undue delay in the first micturition, an abnormal urinary stream, and the presence of a palpable bladder are alarm signals. Urethral catheterization should be avoided. It is better to use suprapubic puncture—better still, suprapubic cystography—for diagnosing the cause of the trouble. The most common cause is a posterior urethral valve, and this is usually an urgent indication for bilateral ureterostomy. Less common causes include atresia of the urethra or meatus, "neurogenic bladder," or compression by a fibrosarcoma of the urogenital sinus, which can be felt on rectal examination. Another possible cause is ureterocele, and in a girl this may even appear at the vulva.

Anuria

Primary Anuria

No urine is passed. There are two causes of this disorder.

Bilateral Renal Agenesis.[16] This is a rare condition, which is three times as common in boys as in girls. Both kidneys, ureters, and renal vessels, and sometimes even the gonads, are absent. The bladder is rudimentary and may be little more than a cord. The condition has been found in two siblings, but there are discordances in identical twins.[18] There is total congenital anuria, with no or little amniotic fluid, and a peculiar facies with hypertelorism and a fold running from the inner canthus of the eye to the malar region, flattening of the bridge of the nose, retrognathism, and long, folded ears containing little cartilage (Potter's syndrome). In some cases, there may also be clubfoot, congenital dislocation of the hip, and hypoplasia of the lungs. There is nothing to feel in the lumbar fossae, and there are no ureteric orifices in the bladder. No kidney shadow is detectable on radiography or scintiscanning. Autopsy reveals no trace of the renal blastema and no ureteral bud. Early death is inevitable. There have been reports of association with sirenomelia and monomelia[1] and with sacro-coccygeal agenesis and esophageal atresia.[10]

Bilateral Aplasia and Multicystic Dysplasia. This is more common than bilateral renal agenesis (see page 23). There may be presence (dysplasia) or absence (aplasia) of renal blastemal tissue. The ureters are present but often are no more than fibrous cords. Renal arteries are present, and a variable number of cysts occur in place of the kidneys. When the condition is bilateral, there is total congenital anuria with early death. The clinical features are identical to those of bilateral renal agenesis, but associated abnormalities of the face and limbs are less common. It may be possible to feel cystic masses in the lumbar fossae, and ureteric orifices can be seen on cystoscopy. The diagnosis is often possible only at autopsy.

Secondary Oliguria or Anuria

Oliguria or anuria develops in a neonate who in most cases has had normal diuresis for one or more days. The condition develops in the context of serious anoxia, dehydration with collapse, or bacteremic shock. The kidneys are not enlarged. The exact diagnosis is not always easy; it may be an acute functional renal failure resulting from hypovolemia, an acute tubular necrosis, or a bilateral cortical necrosis.

Symmetrical Cortical Necrosis of the Kidneys.[3] This may be seen in older children, but more often it occurs in infants, in whom it is likely to be secondary to shock or to a hemolytic-uremic syndrome. The greatest incidence of the condition is in the newborn.

The cause is ischemia of the renal cortex due to anoxia or shock, which may be the result of a prenatal accident, such as eclampsia or antepartum hemorrhage, or a postnatal incident, such as dehydration, anoxia, septicemia, or hemolytic disease.

The clinical features depend on the causal condition and the subsequent water and electrolyte disorders. The anuria is more or less total, and any small quantity of urine that may be produced contains red cells and protein. Diarrhea and abdominal distention are common. There may be rapid development of severe hypertension which does not respond to hypotensive drugs or to peritoneal dialysis. The condition is generally fatal, and cortical necrosis is confirmed or discovered at autopsy (Figure 25).

However, recovery is possible. In such cases, there is often, though not always, chronic renal insufficiency or hypertension. In these patients, the necrosis is only patchy, and the diagnosis therefore is difficult to confirm even with renal biopsy. Nephrocalcinosis may appear after some months (Table 23).

Acute Tubular Necrosis.[19] Acute tubular necrosis causes acute renal fail-

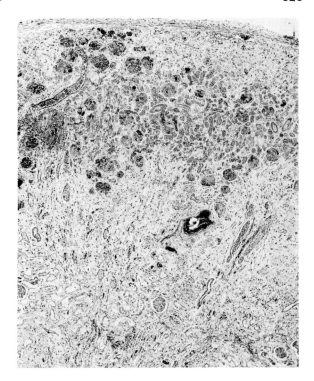

Figure 25. Bilateral symmetrical cortical necrosis. This infant died at the age of 10 months after 18 days of anuria preceded by severe diarrhea. The glomeruli and tubules in the necrotic zone appear as if rubbed with an eraser. A narrow subcapsular band retains its blood supply. In the necrotic zone, an arcuate artery with fibrinoid necrosis of its wall and partial thrombosis can be seen. ×35.

Table 23. Cases of Cortical Necrosis of the Kidney with Prolonged Course (Diagnosis Proved by Renal Biopsy)

Age at Onset	Interval from Onset (years)	G.F.R.* (ml./min./1.73 m.²)	Maximal Urine Concentration	Hypertension	Nephrocalcinosis
8 months	2/12	19		0	0
	2	18		0	0
	2 years 4 months	24	500 mOsm./kg.	0	+
9 months	2/12	14		0	0
	1	39		0	0
	2	47	560 mOsm./kg.	0	0
12 months	2/12	28		0	0
	8/12	51		0	0
5 months	2	38	1.016 (S.G.)	+	0
	8	Blood urea, 25 mg. per 100 ml.		0	+
18 months	2	32	1.010 (S.G.)		0
	5	58	1.010 (S.G.)	+	0
	10	113	—		0
	12	46	1.008 (S.G.)		0
	13	55	—	0 (with treatment)	0

*Glomerular filtration rate estimated by clearance of creatinine and/or inulin.
S.G., Specific gravity.

ure that is usually reversible after a period of oliguria or anuria, which may last from 10 to 15 days. Characteristically, this type of nephropathy is found in newborn infants who have suffered neonatal anoxia or have a hemolytic disease. The condition may be caused by some drugs such as colistin or gentamicin. Water intoxication can also cause transient renal failure with tubular changes.

Functional Renal Failure.[4] This is by far the most common complication of the conditions already mentioned that can cause acute tubular or cortical necrosis, and the common denominator is anoxia and hypotension. In these circumstances, it is difficult to be sure that a reversible renal failure results simply from functional disorder, even though satisfactory diuresis sets in when the respiratory, circulatory, or metabolic disorder is put right. There is often hematuria or proteinuria, which is evidence of organic disturbance of the kidney.

Infants born after a high-risk pregnancy, even if there have been no serious complications, for the first 10 or 15 days may have oliguria with an elevated blood urea level, low glomerular filtration rate, microscopic hematuria, and proteinuria.

The "Large Kidney-Hematuria" Syndrome

This syndrome merits special consideration. Hematuria may be the first sign, but generally there is serious general disturbance and oliguria with hematuria and proteinuria. Abdominal palpation reveals enlargement of one or both kidneys. Many pathological conditions must be considered.

Renal Vein Thrombosis

Renal vein thrombosis is the most common cause of this syndrome. It is generally a complication of severe dehydration owing to diarrhea. Some cases have been reported as complications of congenital nephrotic syndrome or occurring in newborn infants of a diabetic mother. The condition may even be primary. The onset is sudden, with oliguria, hematuria, enlargement of one or both kidneys, shock, vomiting, and abdominal distention. In unilateral forms, intravenous urography may be possible, and the large kidney is radiologically silent. Thrombocytopenia is often found. This condition formerly was regarded as almost certainly fatal. Because in some cases of unilateral disease diuresis set in after removal of the affected kidney, it was suggested that the kidney should be removed as soon as the diagnosis was made. In fact, it seems that such surgery is pointless if not dangerous during the anuric period, because it does not prevent the contralateral kidney from becoming involved. There have been several reports of cure, either spontaneous or after administration of heparin; in these cases, the enlarged kidney diminished progressively in size at the same time that diuresis set in, but subsequently renal atrophy was found. The thrombosis may affect either the main renal vein or the intrarenal tributaries, or both. It is generally associated with zones of hemorrhagic infarction[24-27] (Figure 26).

Thrombosis of the Renal Artery

Thrombosis of the renal artery is much rarer than thrombosis of the renal vein. The clinical picture is much the same in both conditions, which often occur in the same context of dehydration. Arterial thrombosis commonly occurs also

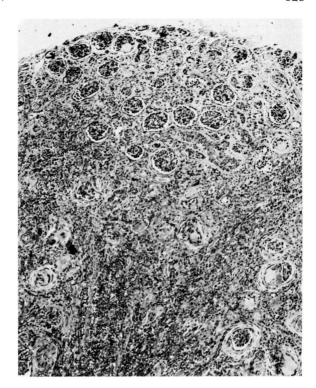

Figure 26. Unilateral renal vein thrombosis in a child aged 6 months who had had recurrent hematuria from birth. Intravenous urography had shown no secretion from the left kidney. Because of the degree of tubular atrophy and interstitial fibrosis, the glomeruli are much closer together than is normal. Some of the glomeruli display pericapsular fibrosis with more or less complete hyalinization of the tuft. Note the hemorrhagic infarction of the renal parenchyma. In the renal vein and its tributaries were found old thromboses that had become recanalized. ×75.

in other parts of the body: there may be mesenteric thrombosis with melena, or thrombosis of limb vessels with gangrene of the toes. If the infant survives, the kidney atrophies and hypertension may follow.[27]

Intense Renal Vasodilatation

Intense vasodilatation in the kidney occurs without hemorrhage or thrombosis and may also be a cause of the "large kidney-hematuria" syndrome. Because there is no irreversible inorganic lesion, uneventful recovery should be possible.[7]

Perirenal Hematoma and Adrenal Hematoma with Renal Disorders[23]

In both of these conditions, there may be a lumbar mass, anemia, a history of obstetric trauma, overweight at birth, or a hemorrhagic syndrome. In both conditions, there may be hematuria, oliguria, and a rising blood urea level. It may be virtually impossible to distinguish between perirenal hematoma and adrenal hematoma, but the treatment is not the same for the two cases. A perirenal hematoma must be evacuated, or it will organize, and the resulting perirenal sclerosis will cause atrophy of the kidney and hypertension. Adrenal hematoma, on the other hand, should be left alone, but exploratory surgery may be considered if the diagnosis is in doubt. The critical point is to distinguish these hematomas from thrombosis of the renal vein, especially if the latter is to be treated with anticoagulant drugs.

The "large kidney-hematuria" syndrome of the newborn creates immediate and late problems.[22] The *immediate problem* is that of treatment. Treatment includes antibiotics and peritoneal dialysis. If some kidney function persists, urography will distinguish between perirenal hematoma and other conditions, and will give information about the contralateral kidney. When neither kidney is producing urine, heparin should be given. When the disease is unilateral and the condition deteriorates, and if hypertension is serious and there is no return of diuresis after two weeks, a nephrectomy should be performed. When the probable diagnosis is perirenal hematoma and there is persistent oliguria, hypertension, or a deteriorating general condition, heparin is not given and surgery is performed to evacuate the hematoma.

The *late problems* require further study. In most cases, the "large kidney-hematuria" syndrome of the newborn recovers rapidly without surgery. Diuresis returns and the blood urea level begins to drop in a matter of days. The kidney returns to normal size in two to four weeks, and macroscopic hematuria disappears in about the same time. Proteinuria and microscopic hematuria may persist for weeks or months. In the long run, the simple vasodilatations and the thromboses that recanalize are doubtless cured. After some months, renal function and the urographic appearance have returned to normal. The unilateral forms may recover or go on to renal atrophy, which may give rise to hypertension and necessitate secondary nephrectomy. Radiologic study will show the absence of function and in some cases calcification in the kidney itself, in the perirenal space, or in the adrenal gland.

Large Kidneys Without Hematuria[22]

The problems posed by these large kidneys differ in unilateral and bilateral cases.

Unilateral Cases

Congenital hydronephrosis presents as a more or less regular, soft, ill-defined mass that is not easy to feel. Wilms' tumor may be enormous and may occupy virtually the entire abdomen. Unilateral cystic disease may appear in many forms — simple cysts, unilateral multicystic dysplasia, and multilocular cysts.

A plain radiograph of the abdomen shows an opacity displacing the intestine. Intravenous urography may reveal enormous hydronephrosis or may indicate the distortion characteristic of Wilms' tumor or a multilocular cyst. A renal scan will give evidence of renal tissue, especially in nephroblastoma and large cysts. Cystography through a suprapubic puncture may also provide valuable information. The exact diagnosis may not be made until the mass is explored surgically. A special problem is the unilateral large kidney resulting from a cyst or tumor compressing the opposite ureter and causing anuria. In these cases, surgery is clearly indicated.

Bilateral Cases

All the conditions just described may be bilateral, although this is exceptional in the newborn.

Bilateral masses are nearly always due to *infantile polycystic disease* (see page 20).

Urinary Infections in the Newborn

These are considered with pyuria (see page 136) in their common forms[11] and also in the less common forms of microabscesses in septicemia, congenital subacute interstitial nephritis,[15] and acute papillary necrosis.[9]

Neonatal Glomerulopathies

These constitute a problem that remains poorly understood.

Glomerulosclerosis

This term is used to describe an appearance of the glomeruli found at autopsy or biopsy in newborn infants suffering from many different diseases. These lesions affect fewer than one glomerulus in five. The glomeruli are small but not contracted. There is some proliferation of cells which are arranged in a corona around the glomerular tuft. Partial or complete hyalinization of the tuft develops. The afferent arteriole may be obliterated. This picture may represent normal involution of a population of primitive glomeruli, which may last from 1 to 15 months or even longer.[8]

Congenital Glomerulonephritis

There have been reports of glomerulonephritis with endocapillary and extracapillary proliferation, formation of epithelial crescents and hyalinization. The condition is very serious, but it is rare and its cause is unknown, although it has been suggested recently that German measles in the mother may be responsible.[5, 6]

Acute Glomerular Thrombosis

This entity is a complication of septicemic states and is characterized by multiple thromboses of the glomerular tufts. Its exact significance in the renal pathology of the newborn is not at all clear.[27]

Miscellaneous Conditions

Newborn infants may present the signs of a congenital nephrotic syndrome, of metabolic disorders due to primary tubular acidosis, of pitressin-resistant diabetes insipidus, or of pseudohypoaldosteronism. Two particular conditions merit emphasis.

Uriniferous ascites may be found in newborn infants with obstructive uropathy. It may result from rupture of bladder or renal pelvis, but more often surgical exploration reveals no communication between the urinary tract and the peritoneal cavity.

Hypertension is rare, but it may complicate thrombosis of the renal vessels or aorta or a malformation of the aorta.

CONCLUSIONS

Renal pathology is varied and relatively specific in the newborn. From a practical point of view, there are three important things to remember.

First, any urinary tract abnormality or renal malformation should be diagnosed as soon as possible so that suitable treatment can be instituted. A delay in the onset of micturition, an abnormal urinary stream, a large, palpable bladder, or a large, palpable kidney constitute alarm signals that must not be missed. Renal insufficiency should specifically be sought in all serious illnesses or whenever there are suggestive signs, such as gastrointestinal disorders or convulsions.

Second, some things are to be avoided, including the passage of a urethral catheter in cases of retention, and ill-considered intravenous perfusion to "provoke" diuresis when there is no proven dehydration. In addition, when dehydration is present, the clinician must keep a careful watch on the urinary output for early recognition of organic renal insufficiency, in order to avoid water intoxication.

Finally, if acute renal failure is confirmed, close clinical and laboratory observations may indicate the need for peritoneal dialysis, especially if there are signs of vascular overload, convulsions owing to hyponatremia, a blood potassium level above 7.5 mEq./liter, severe metabolic acidosis, or a blood urea level higher than 200 mg./100 ml.

REFERENCES

1. Bain, A. D., Beath, M. M., and Flint, W. F.: Sirenomelia and monomelia with renal agenesis and amnion nodosum. Arch. Dis. Child. 35:250, 1960.
2. Barnett, H., and Vesterdal, J.: The physiologic and clinical significance of immaturity of kidney function in young infants. J. Pediat. 42:99, 1953.
3. Bouissou, H., Régnier, C., and Hamousin-Metregiste, R.: La nécrose corticale symétrique des reins du nourrisson. Ann. Pédiat. 39:523, 1963.
4. Broyer, M., and Alizon, M.: Les urgences rénales chez le nouveau-né et le nourrisson. Revue Prat. (Paris) 19:4243, 1969.
5. Cocuzza, S., and Perfetto, V.: Su due casi di glomerulonefrite neonatale. Min. Pediat. 20:559, 1968.
6. Collins, R.: Chronic glomerulonephritis in a newborn child. Amer. J. Dis. Child. 87:478, 1964.
7. Fleury, J., de Menibus, C. H., Evreux, R., and Bohu, D.: Sur les infarctus hémorragiques du rein: guérisons spontanées. Arch. franç. Pediat. 18:331, 1961.
8. Friedli, B.: Le glomérule hyalin du nouveau-né. Biol. Néonat. (Basel) 10:359, 1966.
9. Kössling, F. K.: Über Nierenmark-bzw. Papillenspitzennekrosen bei Saüglingen unter besonderer Berücksichtigung gleichzeitiger, heterotoper, ischämischer Organnekrosen beim sog "Neugeborenen-Schock." Z. Kinderheilk. 89:131, 1964.
10. Kucera, J., and Lenz, W.: Caudale Regression mit oesophagus Atresie und Nierenagenesie — ein Syndrome. Zeitschr. für Kinderheilk. 98:326, 1967.
11. Laplane, R., Lasfargues, G., Roy, C., and Etienne, M.: L'infection urinarie du nourrisson. Ann. Méd. Interne (Paris) 121:205, 1970.
12. Lattimer, J. K., Uson, A. C., and Melicow, M. M.: Urological emergencies in newborn infants. Pediatrics 29:310, 1962.
13. McCance, R. A., and Widdowson, E. M.: Renal function before and after birth. J. Physiol. 118:61, 1952.
14. Metcoff, J.: Some aspects of renal structure and function of body fluids. Pediat. Clin. N. Amer. 6:1, 1959.
15. Porter, K. A., and McGiles, H.: A pathological study of five cases of pyelonephritis in the newborn. Arch. Dis. Child. 31:303, 1956.
16. Potter, E. L.: Bilateral renal agenesis. J. Pediat. 29:68, 1946.
17. Potter, E. L.: Pathology of the Fetus and the Newborn. Chicago, Year Book Medical Publishers, 1952.
18. Rizza, J. M., and Downing, S. E.: Bilateral renal agenesis in two female siblings. Amer. J. Dis. Child. 121:60, 1971.
19. Robinson, G. C., and Wong, L. C.: Acute tubular necrosis in infancy and childhood. Am. J. Dis. Child. 95:417, 1958.
20. Royer, P.: Régulation rénale chez le nouveau-né. Arch. Sci. Physiol. 8:225, 1954.

21. Royer, P.: Physiologie rénale. *In* Pédiatrie. Paris, Encyclopédie médico-chirurgicale, Fascicule 4083 A 10, 1966.
22. Royer, P.: Maladies du rein chez le nouveau-né et le nourrisson. Päd. Fortbildungskurse. Vol. 27. Basel, S. Karger, 1970, p. 55.
23. See, G., Chavannes, L., Jurkovitz, P., and Mézard, P.: Hématome surrénal du nouveau-né associé à des troubles rénaux. Arch. franç. Pédiat. *22*:1093, 1965.
24. Smith, B. A.: Renal vein thrombosis in the newborn. J. Urol. (Baltimore) *73*:765, 1955.
25. Verhagen, A. D., Hamilton, J. P., and Genel, M.: Renal vein thrombosis in infants. Arch. Dis. Child. *40*:214, 1965.
26. Warren, H., Birdsong, M., and Kelley, R. A.: Renal vein thrombosis in infants. J.A.M.A. *152*: 700, 1953.
27. Zuelzer, W., Charles, S., Kurnetz, R., Newton, W., and Fallon, R.: Circulatory diseases of kidney in infancy and childhood. Amer. J. Dis. Child. *81*:1, 1951.

PART
II

Urinary Infection and the Pathology of Interstitial Tissue

HENRI MATHIEU

Chapter One

URINARY INFECTION

Urinary infection may be acute, recurrent, or chronic. It is characterized by the presence of large numbers of bacteria and leukocytes in the urine, and may be caused by various microbial organisms.

Urinary infection is the most common condition in pediatric nephrology. It occurs in 1 per cent of all newborn infants and in 30 per cent of newborn infants who are admitted to hospital,[18, 19] and at this age there is a marked preponderance of boys. It affects 2 to 4 per cent of older infants and children, involving girls 10 times as often as boys, and accounting for 0.3 to 5.8 per cent of admissions to a general pediatric service.[13, 19] It is second only to respiratory disorders as the source of disease in children.

The diagnosis of pyuria must be made with great care, including paying strict attention to the technique of collecting urine and examining it for the presence of cells and bacteria. There are two real difficulties: failing to make the diagnosis, with delay in starting treatment, or overdiagnosing and prescribing useless treatment, which, as well as overlooking the true cause of the trouble, may cause alarm to the family.

The significance of a urinary infection is not a simple matter to determine. Its origin, nature, localization to different levels of the urinary tract,[13, 22, 26] effect on the kidneys, and long-term danger to life have been and still are interpreted in extreme fashions. Some authors are alarmists and equate any urinary infection with acute or chronic pyelonephritis, which suggests a poor prognosis in every case of recurrent or chronic pyuria.[9] Others are lulled into a false sense of security by the large number of easy cures and the absence of late complications in many cases, and as a result they may give inadequate treatment and neglect follow-up. It is important to avoid any dogmatic approach and to regard every instance of pyuria as a symptom to be evaluated in detail. It is important also to realize that there is still much to be learned about the mechanisms and the consequences of recurrent and chronic pyuria.

ETIOLOGY
Type of Organism[20]

The organism most commonly found is *Escherichia coli*, especially serotypes 04, 06, 02, 01, and 75. This species usually is sensitive to many antibiotics. In chronic and recurrent pyuria, *E. coli* is less commonly found, and then it is often resistant to one or more antibiotics. In the majority of these cases, one or more other organisms, such as *Proteus, Pseudomonas aeruginosa, Enterobacter, Klebsiella,* or *Streptococcus faecalis,* are usually responsible (Figure 27). In one third of

131

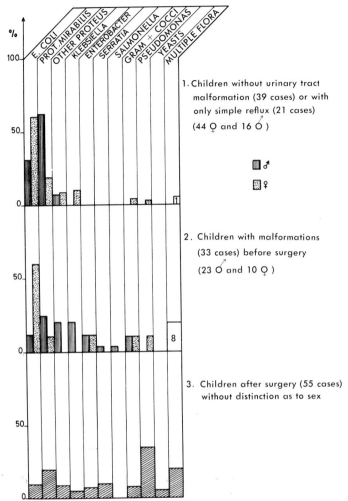

Figure 27. Organisms found in urinary infection in children. *1* (top graph), Children with simple vesicoureteral reflux. *2* (center graph), Children with urinary tract malformations before surgery. *3* (lower graph), Children with urinary tract malformations after surgery.

cases, these organisms are resistant to a single antibiotic, and in one third they are resistant to several antibiotics.

Routes of Infection

Organisms may reach the urinary tract by the ascending route or from the bloodstream.

Ascending Infection

This is by far the most common means of infection.[14] The responsible organism is often found in the urethra, vagina, and perineum, and also in the feces.[7] In the case of *E. coli,* the serotype of the organisms is the same in all these sites.[3] The antibiotic resistance profile is identical in organisms collected from different sites.[3] The fundamental importance of infection beginning in the ano-genital region would seem to account for the much greater frequency of infection in girls, especially since the female urethra is so short. This can be noted in the pyuria secondary to polycystic kidneys.[17] Another significant factor may be the powerful bactericidal activity of prostatic fluid.[23]

Blood-borne Infection

In the experimental animal, pyelonephritis can be induced by the intra-venous injection of various organisms, especially if associated with massage of the kidney or after potassium depletion. The sequence of events is: (1) localization of bacteria in the medulla, (2) involvement of the papilla and pelvic mucosa, and (3) two days later, the appearance of organisms in the urine. It is unlikely that this route is significant in children except in cases of septicemia (owing to E. coli,[15] for example) or in the newborn.[19]

Predisposing Causes

The existence of predisposing causes is suggested by the fact that age (newborn), sex (female), and individual characteristics in certain patients are significant and determine a recurrent or chronic course of urinary infection.

General Predisposing Causes

In children it is very rare to find an immunoglobulin deficiency, potassium depletion, or lack of vitamin A. Diabetes mellitus is a rare cause of pyuria in childhood. On the other hand, one cannot overemphasize the importance, for reasons that are far from clear, of four factors: (1) the neonatal period per se; (2) acute respiratory or intestinal infection, and certain eruptive fevers involving the vulva, such as herpes and chicken pox; (3) serious metabolic disorders; and (4) the most important of all—severe malnutrition. Kwashiorkor and maras-mus very commonly are complicated by pyuria that is often recurrent and un-responsive to treatment. It should be noted that the nephrotic syndrome is often complicated by pyuria. An interesting problem, as yet unresolved, con-cerns a deficiency of the systems that normally protect the urinary tract against multiplication of organisms excreted by the kidney in the physiologic state.[18]

Local Predisposing Causes

Local causes, which may be of two types, must be sought with care for the proper diagnosis and treatment of pyuria.

The first concerns the external genital organs and the perianal region. Malformations, infections, mycoses, worm infestations, the use of crude soap, foreign bodies, and masturbation predispose to contamination of urethra and bladder. The importance of meatal stenosis in girls has been emphasized, but meatotomy does not cure urinary infection.

The second group includes obvious abnormalities of the kidneys and uri-nary tract, among them tumors, cysts, calculi, neurogenic bladder, and in partic-ular urinary malformations, whether obstructive or not. Three abnormalities are thought to encourage persistence or recurrence of urinary infection. The first is *vesicoureteral reflux*; this may be primary, owing to congenital abnormality of the ureterovesical junction, or secondary to infection, disappearing after cure of the infection. This disorder is discussed in the section on pyelonephritis (see page 154). The second is *pyelocalyceal atony,* often characteristic of recognized reflux but sometimes secondary to the action of bacteria or their toxins on the ureters.[25] The third is *residual urine in the bladder* in girls with chronic or recurrent urinary infection; it doubtlessly occurs secondarily to urinary infection due to inflammation of the bladder neck. Beginning as a functional lesion, this condition may progress to organic fibrosis of the bladder neck or urethrotrigonitis, and it then becomes another cause of stasis and infection.

SYMPTOMATOLOGY

In the young infant, vomiting, anorexia, fever, and loss of weight are the usual signs. In addition, in the newborn, a transient or lasting icterus, respiratory distress, and neurologic signs are often present. In the older child, more suggestive signs include a fluctuating fever with rigors, general malaise, pain on micturition, frequency, dysuria, an abnormal urinary stream, pubic pain, and hematuria. Urinary infection may be present even though the urine is clear and, conversely, a cloudy urine may result not from infection but from an excess of phosphates.

At any age, urinary infection may be asymptomatic, or the only indication may be simple fatigability or a change in behavior. This is particularly true of recurrence after treatment. In such cases, the diagnosis can be made only by discovering leukocytes and bacteria in the urine.

Every case of pyuria in the newborn, in a boy, or recurring despite adequate treatment on more than two occasions in a girl is an absolute indication for careful investigation to discover general or local predisposing causes, including first of all intravenous urography with cystography before, during, and after micturition. Suprapubic cystography and cystoscopy may also be indicated.

In all these conditions, a precise study must be made of renal function, including as a minimum determinations of blood urea and creatinine levels, urine concentration tests, blood and urine chemistry, and tests of endogenous creatinine clearance. Repeated studies will indicate the true danger to kidney function, such as associated dysplasia or atrophy resulting from stasis or infective pyelonephritis.

DIAGNOSIS

Diagnosis depends on the demonstration of leukocyturia and bacteriuria. Organisms and pus cells may be seen on direct examination of a fresh specimen of urine. Bacteria and white cells may be revealed by examination of the centrifuged deposit. If bacteria are noted in this way, the bacterial count must be more than 10^5 per ml. (Table 24).

The leukocyturia may be quantified by counting the white cells per microscopic field or per milliliter of fresh, uncentrifuged urine. We prefer to determine the cell output per minute, and we regard a figure over 1500 cells per minute as pathologic. It should be noted that in 20 per cent of cases, bacteriuria

Table 24.   Leukocyturia and Bacteriuria
(Normal Values from Our Laboratory)

Leukocyturia/min. (Percentage of Cases)		500	500–1000	1000–1500	
Boys (23 cases)		71.5	21.5	8	
Girls (23 cases)		50	43	7	

Bacteriuria/ml. (Percentage of Cases)	Sterile	100	100–200	200–300	500–1000	1000–10,000
Boys (36 cases)	55	14	11	5.5	5.5	9
Girls (41 cases)	56	#15	#10	#5	#10	#5

exists without leukocyturia, and that leukocyturia can occur without urinary infection (as in glomerulonephritis, nephrocalcinosis, or vaginal infection). The urine can be cultured to identify the organism and establish its antibiotic sensitivity. The bacteria can be counted by culture techniques. In the child who can control micturition, a figure higher than 10^5 per ml. is pathologic, a figure less than 10^3 is normal, and a count between 10^3 and 10^5 is suspect. In the normal infant, the normal count is rarely below 10^5. These figures refer to urine obtained after washing the genitalia. Urine obtained by suprapubic puncture is sterile. In fact, with patent infection, there is rarely any difficulty in diagnosis. It should be noted, however, that in cases of urinary infection, false negative results may be produced by recent antibiotic therapy, by a urinary pH below 5 or above 8, by a very high urinary output, or by complete ureteral obstruction on the infected side. During treatment, the presence of bacteriuria even below 10^3 per ml. remains significant if the organism is identical to the original organism causing the infection.

Various tests have been suggested to simplify the search for bacteriuria.[5] Microscope slides coated with culture medium* can be used for bacterial counting with very good results. Less satisfactory are the results obtained with tests that use a color change caused by bacterial metabolism as an indicator, or those that measure glucose concentration, with a figure below 2 mg. per 100 ml. indicating bacterial metabolism. Tests of this type give too many false negatives.

CLASSIFICATION

Although any classification must be arbitrary, it is useful from a practical point of view to divide cases of bacteriuria in children into five groups.

Occasional Pyuria

Occasional pyuria most often is a urinary infection with *E. coli*. Generally it occurs without apparent cause in an otherwise healthy infant or child. The

---

*Uricult.

septicemic or local complications that often were seen in former times no longer occur unless there is gross negligence in diagnosis and treatment. A short course of treatment is effective, and there is no recurrence. Nevertheless, particular care should be taken if such a pyuria occurs in a child suffering from malnutrition, infection, or a serious disorder such as cystic fibrosis of the pancreas, insulin-dependent diabetes, or a nephrotic syndrome. In such cases, the pyuria may be more difficult to cure and may prove a serious complication of the underlying disease.

Idiopathic Recurrent Pyuria in Girls

This is an extremely common condition that usually presents about the age of 2 or 3 years. The frequency of attacks may vary from one to 10 per year. The symptoms are usually clear-cut. At the outset, the causative organism most often is *E. coli*, but later another organism may be involved. The attacks respond to treatment. On investigation, the kidneys and urinary tract appear normal, at least during the first years. It is common, though not universal, to find oxyuriasis, vaginitis, some minor malformation of the external genitalia, such as meatal stenosis, or possibly mycosis. Renal function is normal.

Idiopathic recurrent pyuria in girls, when correctly treated from the beginning of each attack, is nearly always a benign disease, as shown by follow-up studies of more than 20 years in some of our cases.

However, when the recurrences are frequent, two problems may arise.

First, the frequent recurrences may cause serious fatigability and frequent absences from school, as well as psychologic problems related to the recurrent attacks and an unduly pessimistic prognosis by the family and the physician. The situation may be complicated by obsessions with special diets and nonmedical treatment. When the girl reaches adolescence, she may reject surveillance and treatment, so that more serious, untreated attacks occur.

Second, various complications are possible. We have only very rarely seen chronic pyelonephritis, but the condition may be complicated by chronic hypertrophic urethrotrigonitis, with very disagreeable urinary symptoms, and there may be secondary stenosis of the bladder neck and vesicoureteral reflux, predisposing to recurrent infection. In such cases, urologic treatment may be indicated, including cauterization of urethral vegetations, plastic operations on the bladder neck, and antireflux operations on the ureter.

Recurrent and Chronic Pyuria Secondary to Abnormalities of the Kidney and Urinary Tract

In patients with stone, tumor, congenital renal dysplasia, or malformations of the urinary tract, the urine may remain sterile for a long time or even throughout life. However, secondary urinary infection is common. The pyuria may be occasional, but more often it is recurrent or chronic, persistent, and often difficult to treat. Organisms other than *E. coli* are common, and in many cases there are two or more different organisms.

This type of urinary infection is often difficult to manage. Three factors contribute to the gradual onset of chronic renal failure: cortical hypoplasia and dysplasia that may have preceded the infection; urinary stasis; and atrophy owing to pyelonephritis (see page 152). This redoubtable form of urinary infection is found in both sexes. Vesicoureteral reflux, ureteral atony, and organic obstruction all play a part. The renal involvement may be unilateral or bilateral, symmetrical or asymmetrical.

Urinary Infection of the Newborn

Pyuria due to various organisms, *E. coli* in particular, is common in the newborn. It differs from the pyuria of the older infant or child in many ways, including the predominance in boys, the intensity of general signs (fever, gastrointestinal disorders, dehydration), the high incidence of acidosis and hyponatremia, the not uncommon association with icterus, the rarity of urinary tract malformations, and the good long-term prognosis. It must be remembered, however, that pyuria in the newborn may actually be a manifestation of four other, much more serious conditions. The first of these is medullary microabscess complicating a septicemia, resulting perhaps from umbilical sepsis. This condition has become rare. The second is acute pyelonephritis complicating a urinary tract malformation, with or without renal dysplasia—for example, urethral valves in a boy. Third is congenital subacute interstitial nephritis, sometimes familial, with a serious prognosis owing to diffuse interstitial cellular infiltration, tubular atrophy, and periglomerular fibrosis. This condition is still often unrecognized. The fourth condition, acute papillary necrosis, is rare in the newborn. It presents with fever, gastrointestinal disorders, proteinuria, hematuria, an elevated blood urea level, and pyuria. It may proceed to a fatal outcome in a few days. If the child survives, the prognosis is good, and urography may reveal amputation of the tips of the papillae. At autopsy, papillary necrosis, sometimes with deposits of urate or bilirubin, is found. In some cases, there is necrosis in other organs. Three types have been distinguished: (1) papillary necrosis associated with a generalized shock state, multiple necroses, and hemorrhages; (2) papillary necrosis associated with hemolytic jaundice of the newborn; and (3) specific infections of the papilla.

Asymptomatic Bacteriuria

Because of the real risks of urinary infection, infants and schoolchildren have been studied to determine the incidence of asymptomatic bacteriuria. Bacterial colony counting and the measurement of glucose concentration are the tests most often employed. In infants, asymptomatic bacteriuria has been found in 2 to 4.5 per cent of girls and in 0 to 0.5 per cent of boys. In schoolchildren, the condition has been found in 1.2 per cent of girls and in 0.03 per cent of boys.[18] The figure rises to 5 per cent in adolescent girls. Urographic examination of children with asymptomatic bacteriuria has revealed varying percentages of urologic abnormalities in the different studies. In cases of treated urinary infection, asymptomatic bacteriuria is common.

The urinary infection may be classified as benign or as potentially serious, owing to its localization and to the risk of pyelonephritis (see page 149).

The criteria for *benign pyuria* are: occurrence in girls over the age of 1 year, a single attack or few recurrences, a single organism involved, which is sensitive to antibiotics, symptoms restricted to the lower urinary tract, and the absence of any abnormality on urographic examination.

The signs of potential seriousness are: occurrence in the newborn, occurrence in males, pyuria that is recurrent or resistant to treatment, multiplicity of infecting organisms, significant renal or general signs, depression of renal function, and in particular abnormalities discovered on intravenous urography and cystography.

TREATMENT
Benign Pyuria

The treatment of this type of pyuria is relatively simple. The chosen antibiotic or antibacterial agent should be well tolerated, of low toxicity, and highly concentrated in the urine, because the infection is localized to the lower urinary tract. The choice is made on the result of sensitivity tests. The most useful drugs are the sulfonamides, nitrofurantoin (Furadantin), nalidixic acid (Negram), the hydroxyquinolines, and ampicillin. The response to treatment should be confirmed after some days. This response should include the disappearance of symptoms and signs, the elimination of bacteriuria, and the return of the urinary leukocyte count to normal. When the urine becomes sterile, treatment should be continued for about two weeks. There is no advantage to more prolonged treatment.[4, 26, 27]

Predisposing conditions, such as vaginitis or worm infestation, should also be treated.

If the treatment is not effective immediately, the antibiotic therapy may have to be changed. If infection persists, the pyuria must then be regarded as potentially serious.

Potentially Serious Pyuria

This is not the place to consider the surgical measures for the treatment of calculi and malformations, or the special treatment of any renal insufficiency that may develop. Whenever there is a general predisposing cause, the urinary infection cannot be cured until that cause has been treated.

In cases of ureterovesical reflux, in which the ureters are contractile and not dilated and there is no renal damage, surgical treatment should not be considered until conservative treatment has been tried, because in many cases the reflux will disappear with suitable antibacterial therapy.

Initial Treatment

Choice and Mode of Administration of Antibiotics (Table 25). The choice of antibiotic is based on sensitivity studies. These are usually performed by the disk method. If the pyuria persists, it may be necessary to study the bactericidal power of the antibiotic. The problem is whether the activity of the antibiotic should be tested at its concentration in the serum or at its concentration in the urine. Many authors consider that only the plasma concentration is significant.[1, 2] According to these authors, the tissue concentration of the drug is close to the blood concentration. Other authors consider that it is better to focus on the concentration in the urine and to adapt the dosage accordingly.[21, 24] The concentration of antibiotic in the renal medulla is probably close to that in the urine and lymph.[8] The results are better correlated with tests of sensitivity in vitro in urine than with tests of sensitivity in vitro in serum.[21]

(*Text continued on page 142*)

139

Table 25. Antibiotics and Chemotherapy Used in Urinary Infection

Family	Antibiotics	Action	Blood	Urine	Optimal pH
			Concentration		
Beta lactamines	Penicillin G	Bactericidal	+ +	+ + +	>7
	Ampicillin	Bactericidal	+ +	+ + +	>7
	Cephalothin	Bactericidal	+ +	+ + +	>7
	Cephaloridine	Bactericidal	+ +	+ + +	>7
	Cephaloglycin	Bactericidal	±	+ + +	>7
Aminoglycosides	Streptomycin	Bactericidal	+	+ + +	>7
	Kanamycin	Bactericidal	+	+ + +	>7
	Gentamycin	Bactericidal	+	+ + +	>7
Polymyxins	Colimycin	±	+	+ + +	?
Chloramphenicol	Chloramphenicol	Bacteriostatic	+	±	Variable
	Thiamphenicol	Bacteriostatic	+	+ + +	Variable
Cyclines	Oxytetracycline	Bacteriostatic	+	+ +	<7
	Tetracycline base	Bacteriostatic	+	±	<7
	Chlortetracycline	Bacteriostatic	+	±	<7
Macrolides	Erythromycin	Bacteriostatic	+	±	>7
Synergistines	Rovamycin	Bacteriostatic	+	±	>7
	Pristinamycin	Bacteriostatic	+	±	?
	Vingimycin	Bacteriostatic	+	±	?
Rifamycins	Rifampin	Bactericidal	+	+	?
Sulfonamides	Various	Bacteriostatic	+	+	Variable
Nitrofurantoin	Furadantin	Bacteriostatic	±	+ + +	Immaterial
Nalidixic Acid	Negram	Bacteriostatic	±	+ + +	?
Nitro-hydroxyquinoline (nitroxoline)	Nibiol	Bacteriostatic	±	+ + +	?

Table 25. Antibiotics and Chemotherapy Used in Urinary Infection *(Continued)*

Sensitive Organisms		Routes of Administration			Doses per 24 Hours
Gram-Positive	Gram-Negative	Oral	Intramuscular	Intravenous	
+++	±		+	+	2–4
+++	+++	+	+	+	2–4
+++	+++		+	+	2–4
+++	+++		+	+	2–4
+++	+++	+			4
+	+++		+		3
+	+++		+		3
++	+++ (*pyocyaneus sp.*)		+		3
0	+++ (*pyocyaneus sp.*)		+		2–3
+++	+++	+			4
+++	+++	+	+	+	3–4
++	++	+			4
++	++	+			4
++	++	+			4
+++	±	+			4
+++	±	+			4
+++	±	+			4
+++	±	+			4
+++	+++	+			4
++	++	+			4–6
0	++	+			4–6
0	++	+			4–6
0	++	+			4–6

Table 25. Antibiotics and Chemotherapy Used in Urinary Infection *(Continued)*

Change of Dosage in Renal Failure				
No Change	Lower Dose	Avoid	*Principal Complications*	*Dosage*
	+		Allergy	50,000 to 100,000 I.U.
	+		Allergy	50 to 100 mg.
	+		Allergy	50 to 100 mg.
		+	Renal insufficiency	20 to 50 mg. (average)
				50 to 100 mg. in serious infection
+			−	50 to 100 mg.
	+ +		Kidneys?	50 mg.
			Ear	
	+ +		Kidneys?	10 to 20 mg.
			Ear	
	+ +		Kidneys?	2 to 4 mg. in 3 injections
			Ear	
	+ +		Kidneys	50,000 I.U.
			Brain	
+			Aplasia of bone marrow	50 to 100 mg.
+			Aplasia of bone marrow	30 to 50 mg.
+			Dental dysplasia before 6 years	50 mg.
+			Dental dysplasia before 6 years	50 mg.
+			Dental dysplasia before 6 years	20 to 50 mg.
+			0	50 mg.
+			0	50 mg.
+			0	50 to 100 mg.
+			0	50 to 100 mg.
+			Hepatic cytolysis	10 to 20 mg.
	+ +		Hematuria Anuria	100 to 150 mg.
	+ +		Diarrhea Polyneuritis	5 mg.
	+ +		Acidosis	60 mg.
	+		0	10 mg.

As this problem has not been resolved, the best practice is to choose an antibiotic with a good plasma concentration and a very good urine concentration. Because of the poor concentration of active products in the urine, chloramphenicol, tetracyclines, macrolides, synergistines, and cephalothin are little used. Cephaloglycin, sulfonamides, nitrofurantoin, nalidixic acid, and the hydroxyquinolines are not indicated because of their low plasma concentrations. The antibiotics used most often are the beta lactamines, the aminoglycosides, the polymyxins, thiamphenicol, and cephaloridine.[2]

Another factor to be considered is whether the antibiotic is bactericidal or bacteriostatic. When possible, a bactericidal antibiotic should be preferred, but bactericidal power varies both with organism and with dosage.

In some cases, it is necessary to adapt chemotherapy to the urine pH, or vice versa. Using this method, Brumfitt succeeded in increasing his therapeutic success from 64 to 91 per cent.[6]

It is essential to use two antibiotics, since often more than one organism is involved in this type of urinary infection. The use of two antibiotics diminishes the risk of development of a resistant mutant organism, and in addition the two drugs may act synergistically. It is difficult to predict the most effective bactericidal combination, but as a general rule there is synergism between the beta lactamines and the aminosides, and synergism is common between the aminoglycosides and colimycin. Conversely, the beta lactamines and thiamphenicol, and also the tetracyclines and macrolides, are generally antagonistic.

The choice of antibiotic is influenced also by its general toxicity and its nephrotoxicity, and by the state of renal function.[17, 22] Some particularly nephrotoxic antibiotics, such as kanamycin, should be used only in cases of absolute necessity. Antibiotic dosage may have to be adapted to defective renal function, and this is particularly important with drugs such as streptomycin, colimycin, gentamycin, nitrofurantoin, and cephaloridine. Some drugs may be contraindicated because of previous sensitization.

Dosage should be adapted to the concentration judged desirable as a result of in vitro sensitivity tests. Some antibiotics have to be administered parenterally to achieve an adequate plasma concentration, and it may be necessary to increase the dosage when treatment is unsuccessful.[1]

Monitoring Progress and the Duration of Initial Treatment. Progress is monitored by bacteriologic examination because only rarely is there clinical evidence of early relapse while the patient is being treated. The bacterial colony count and the urinary leukocyte output per minute should be estimated on the third day of treatment. When treatment is effective, the number of bacteria is reduced 100 times in 6 to 10 hours, and the mean sterilization time is 10 to 20 hours.[1] The slower the initial elimination of bacteria, the less effective the treatment is.

If infection persists on the third day, this means, in most cases, that there has been a rapid substitution of a new bacterial species resistant to the particular treatment. This occurs especially when the initial infection is caused by more than one organism. In these cases, the treatment must be changed, and attempts must be made to find antibiotics that are effective against both the original and the new organism (Table 26).

Persistent infection may result from the selection of a resistant mutant, a phenomenon that is particularly likely to happen with rifampin and nalidixic

Table 26.   Changes in Causal Organism During the Course of Treatment
of Chronic Urinary Infection in a Girl Born April 10, 1958*

Date	April 24, 1970	April 28, 1970	May 5, 1970		May 12, 1970
Organism	*Klebsiella*	*Proteus vulgaris*	*Enterococcus*	*Proteus morgani*	0
Bacteriuria	32×10^5	1.5×10^5	1.6×10^5		
Sensitive to	Colimycin Nibiol Streptomycin Gentamycin Furadantin Negram	Nibiol Streptomycin Gentamycin Negram	Gentamycin Furadantin	Gentamycin Furadantin Negram	
Resistant to		Colimycin	Streptomycin	Streptomycin	
Treatment	Colimycin Nibiol	Streptomycin Negram	Gentamycin Furadantin		

*Ileal loop urinary diversion and calculi in left kidney. This record of a case of infection from multiple organisms shows the value of rapid changes of antibiotic. It is important to use antibiotics that have high concentrations in both plasma and urine.

acid. In most cases, this can be avoided by using a combination of antibiotics. Another possibility is the selection of resistant bacteria carrying an R factor (a type of extrachromosomal resistance). The sensitive strain is very rapidly replaced by a strain resistant to many antibiotics, including the antibiotic used. According to Acar[1] this suggests the existence in the first instance of two strains of bacteria, one antibiotic-sensitive and the other belonging to the same species but carrying the factor R. On the other hand, the bacterial flora may remain unchanged because the antibiotic had not attained an adequate concentration at the site of the infection. This may result from renal insufficiency, or the organism may have an intermediate sensitivity to the antibiotic used, the ratio between required antibiotic concentration and minimal inhibitory concentration being diminished. In such cases, when possible, the antibiotic dosage should be increased.[1]

In most cases, treatment is effective, and the question then concerns how long treatment should be continued.

Duration of Treatment and Early Relapse.   There is no definite evidence of the optimum duration of initial treatment. It is our practice to continue the chosen combination of antibiotics for 10 days.[20] Treatment is then continued with the safest antibiotic for three weeks. Three days after discontinuing this treatment, we confirm that the urine remains sterile. This regimen is effective in the initial instance in 80 per cent of cases.

Early relapse may follow cessation of treatment. In such cases, therapy must be recommenced with a combination of bactericidal drugs, at a higher dosage and for a longer time.

This type of relapse may result either from true persistence of organisms in some focus that has not been reached by the antibiotic, or from the renaissance of degraded bacterial forms, particularly the L forms.[10]

Maintenance Treatment and Recurrence

Having cured the urinary infection, the problem is to prevent recurrence. Some authors recommended prolonged antibacterial therapy for several months.[11, 12] Other authors take the opposite view, considering such treatment useless and ineffective, and holding that it may be responsible for the appearance of resistant strains. It is our experience that prolonged antibacterial therapy is indispensable.

The majority of reinfections occur by the ascending route. Hence, it is important to choose an antibiotic with a high concentration in the urine, one that is well tolerated and not toxic, that is not subject to extrachromosomal resistance, and that produces little change in the fecal and periurethral flora.[27] Suitable agents include nitroxoline (Nibiol), nalidixic acid (Negram), and nitrofurantoin (Furadantin). Possibly it is better to use urinary antiseptics such as mandelamine.

Many measures are helpful in preventing recurrence. Above all, any predisposing cause must be eliminated. This obviously applies to malformations of the urinary tract and to reflux. However, it is also helpful to seek to prevent vulvovaginitis by insisting on strict genital and perineal hygiene. It is also helpful to maintain a high throughput of fluid.

A special problem is the prevention of infection in children who have had the urine diverted to the skin surface. Nonrefluxing collecting bags have proved to be a great advance in this field. When catheterization is essential, the use of the three way catheter, allowing immediate local disinfection, has greatly diminished the incidence of complicating infection and septicemia. The ureters should be brought onto the skin as high as possible, so that an appliance can be fitted more easily and with less risk of fecal contamination.

SPECIFIC INFECTIONS

Apart from diffuse microabscesses of the renal parenchyma complicating septicemia, now a very rare condition, we may cite renal tuberculosis, infection with *Staphylococcus aureus*, and renal candidiasis.

Renal Tuberculosis

This has always been uncommon in children and now is very rare. It develops months and years following the primary infection, sometimes at the same time as a miliary tuberculosis or as tuberculosis of bones and joints.

The tubercle bacilli are carried by the bloodstream and produce a large number of tiny lesions in the cortex of both kidneys. The majority of these lesions heal, but a few may persist to form a caseous focus or even a calcified lesion in the medulla. This lesion may ulcerate into a calyx, with subsequent infection of the ureter, bladder, and, in some cases, prostate and epididymis.

Clinical evidence of the disease may include pyuria, leukocyturia, hematuria, and disorders of micturition, and there may be a history of primary or other tuberculous lesions. Radiologic evidence includes irregularity and deformity of the calyces, cavity formation, and calcification. The definitive diagnosis is made by identifying the tubercle bacillus in the urine. Good results are usually obtained by using suitable antituberculous drugs for two or three years.

Staphylococcal Disease of the Kidney

Hematogenous infection of the kidney by *Staphylococcus aureus* may produce a renal abscess or carbuncle, and there may be secondary perinephritis or perinephric abscess. Fever, pain, psoas irritation, pyuria, and inflammatory reactions in the neighboring pleurae and lung may suggest the diagnosis. Staphylococci may be isolated on culture of urine or blood. X-ray studies may show perirenal edema, displacement of the kidney, and scoliosis. Suitable antibiotic therapy gives very good results.

Renal Infection with *Candida*

Renal candidiasis is rare. It is seen mainly in the newborn and young infants. Predisposing factors include antibiotic therapy and various hereditary immune disorders.

CONCLUSIONS

The demonstration that urinary infection may remain localized to the bladder and urethra[14, 24] has laid open to question the postulate that every instance of pyuria is indicative of pyelonephritis. The distinction between benign pyuria localized to the lower urinary tract and a potentially dangerous infection involving the kidney must rest on precise criteria. For benign cases, treatment is simple, but it must prove effective, and follow-up is essential. For potentially serious cases, extensive treatment is needed. This treatment is often difficult and may have to be adapted nearly from day to day to the needs of the particular patient. We need more information about the metabolism of many antibiotics in the kidney.[8] Further studies are needed also to determine what concentrations of antibiotic are required in urine, plasma, and kidney tissue.

REFERENCES

1. Acar, J. F.: Dynamique de la bactériurie dans les infections urinaires à bacilles gram négatif traitées par les antibiotiques. Path. Biol. *17*:859, 1969.
2. Bastin, R., Acar, J., and Pechère, J. C.: Les principaux antibiotiques utilisables au cours de l'infection urinaire du nourrisson et de l'enfant. *In* Antibiothérapie des infections urinaires du nourrisson et de l'enfant. Paris, Chaix-Defossés, 1970, p. 39.
3. Bergstrom, R., Lincoln, K., Orokov, I., and Winberg, J.: Studies of urinary tract infection in infancy and childhood. VIII. Reinfection vs. relapse in recurrent urinary tract infections. Evaluation by means of identification of infecting organisms. J. Pediat. *71*:13, 1967.
4. Bergstrom, T., Lincoln, K., Redin, B., and Winberg, J.: Studies of urinary tract infections in infancy and childhood. X. Short or long term treatment in girls with first or second time urinary tract infections uncomplicated by obstructive urological abnormalities. Acta Paediat. Scand. *57*:186, 1968.
5. Bouvier, L. M., Vaux, G., and Bessis, F.: Une méthode simple et précise de numération des bactéries dans l'urine. Gaz. méd. France *80*:353, 1973.
6. Brumfitt, W.: Adjustment of urine pH in the chemotherapy of urinary tract infections. Lancet *1*:186, 1962.
7. Cox, C. E., Lacy, S. S., and Hinman, F., Jr.: The urethra and its relationship to urinary tract infection. II. The urethral flora of the female with recurrent urinary infection. J. Urol. *99*:632, 1968.
8. Currie, G. A., Little, P. J., and McDonald, S. J.: The localisation of cephaloridine and nitrofurantoin in the kidney. Nephron *3*:282, 1966.
9. Le Luca, F. C., Fischer, J. H., and Swenson, O.: Review of recurrent urinary tract infection in infancy and early childhood. New Eng. J. Med. *268*:75, 1963.
10. Domingue, G. J., and Schegel, J. U.: The possible role of microbial L-forms in pyelonephritis. J. Urol. *104*:790, 1970.
11. Freeman, B., Bromer, L., Brancato, F., Cohen, S., Garfield, C. F., Griep, R. J., Hinman, F. J.,

Richardson, J. A., Thurm, R. H., Urner, C., and Smith, W.: Prevention of recurrent bacteriuria with continuous chemotherapy. Ann. Intern. Med. *69*:655, 1968.

12. Gardaz, P. C.: Prophylaxie et traitement des infections urinaires en urologie infantile. Importance et modalités de la chimiothérapie antiinfectieuse dans la chirurgie plastique des voies urinaires et la guérison de la pyélonéphrite chronique. Helv. Paediat. Acta *1*:91, 1968.

13. Grenet, P., and Gallet, J. P.: Fréquence et gravité de l'infection urinaire chez l'enfant. *In* Antibiothérapie des infections urinaires du nourrisson et de l'enfant. Paris, Chaix-Desfossés, 1970, p. 7.

14. Hutch, J. A., Chisholm, E. R., and Smith, D. R.: Summary of pathogenesis and new classification for urinary tract infection (and report of 381 cases to which this classification has been applied). J. Urol. *102*:758, 1969.

15. Kenny, J., Medearis, D., Klein, W., Drachman, R., and Gibson, L.: An outbreak of urinary tract infections and septicemia due to *E. coli* in male infants. J. Pediat. *68*:530, 1966.

16. Kleeman, C. R., Hewitt, W. L., and Guze, L. B.: Pyelonephritis. Medicine *39*:3, 1960.

17. Kunin, C. M.: Nephrotoxicity of antibiotics. J.A.M.A. *202*:204, 1967.

18. Kunin, C. M.: Epidemiology and natural history of urinary tract infection in school age children. Pediat. Clin. N. Amer. *18*:509, 1971.

19. Laplane, R., Lasfargues, G., Roy, C., and Etienne, M.: L'infection urinaire du nourrisson. Ann. Méd. Interne *21*:205, 1970.

20. Mathieu, H., Bouvier, S., and Moreono, J. L.: Le traitement des infections urinaires chez les enfants atteints de malformations des voies excrétrices. Gaz. Méd. France Suppl. *38*:117, 1972.

21. McCabe, W. R., and Jackson, G. G.: Evaluation of factors influencing therapeutic response in chronic pyelonephritis. *In* E. H. Kass, Progress in Pyelonephritis. Philadelphia, F. A. Davis, 1965, p. 728.

22. Richet, G., Fabre, J., Freudenreich, J., and Podevin, R.: La tolérance médicamenteuse au course de l'insuffisance rénale. J. Urol. Nephr. *72*:257, 1966.

23. Stamey, T. A., Fair, W. R., Timothy, M. M., and Chung, H. K.: Antibacterial nature of prostatic fluid. Nature *218*:444, 1968.

24. Stamey, T. A., Gouan, D. E., and Palmer, J. M.: The localisation and treatment of urinary tract infections: the role of bactericidal urine levels as opposed to serum levels. Medicine *44*:1, 1965.

25. Teague, N., and Boyarsky, S.: Further effects of coliform bacteria on ureteral peristalsis. J. Urol. *99*:720, 1968.

26. Whitaker, J., and Hewstone, A. S.: The bacteriologic differentiation between upper and lower urinary tract infection in children. J. Pediat. *74*:364, 1969.

27. Winberg, J.: Round table conference on non-obstructive urinary tract infections in children. Acta Paediat. Scand. Suppl. *177*:42, 1967.

28. Winberg, G., Lincoln, K., and Lindin-Janson, G.: Le terapia della infezioni delle via urinaire infantili non malformative. Prosp. Pediat. *2*:165, 1972.

Chapter Two

BACTERIAL
PYELONEPHRITIS

Writing about pyelonephritis poses a problem in semantics,[4] but here we shall use the term in its strict sense, meaning lesions involving both renal pelvis and renal parenchyma, which are primarily interstitial and only secondarily involve the tubules and glomeruli. These histologic disorders are in accord with an inflammation of bacterial origin. This definition implies that a urinary infection is not a pyelonephritis if it involves only the urinary tract and not the kidney. It implies also that by this measure interstitial nephritis is not a pyelonephritis when it is not of bacterial origin or when the pelvis is not involved. The great practical difficulty in any particular case is knowing whether the lesions of pyelonephritis are present or absent; it is often impossible to be certain, and the diagnosis of pyelonephritis often remains only a probable diagnosis.

Pathology[13]

From the histologic point of view, pyelonephritis may be acute, subacute, or chronic. In all three varieties, there is a common characteristic, the alternation of healthy zones of tissue with diseased zones that are often arranged in a roughly triangular, radiating fashion, with the base of the triangle situated under the kidney capsule and the apex reaching the mucosa of the renal pelvis.

In acute pyelonephritis, the interstitial tissue in both cortex and medulla is infiltrated with polymorphonuclear cells, most marked in the subcapsular region, at the corticomedullary junction and at the tip of the papilla. The polymorphonuclear cells are found also in the lumina of the tubules. Sometimes there is actual microabscess formation which in places destroys the renal parenchyma. The mucosa of the renal pelvis is also infiltrated with polymorphonuclear leukocytes. The principal elements of the kidney parenchyma, the glomeruli and tubules, are not affected.

In subacute pyelonephritis, the infiltration comprises round cells, mainly plasmocytes. The same zones are affected, but here again there is no involvement of the glomeruli or tubules. In fact, the difference between the subacute and acute forms is not great. There are no polymorphonuclear cells in the lumina of the tubules. In a matter of days the polymorphonuclear inflammatory infiltrate of the acute form may be replaced by a predominantly round-cell infiltration, and both the acute and subacute forms may co-exist side by side.

Chronic inflammatory pyelonephritis (Figure 28) is characterized by a diffuse inflammatory infiltration of the interstitial tissue, consisting of round

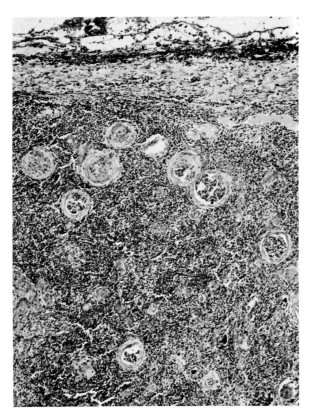

Figure 28. Chronic pyelo-nephritis. Interstitial nephritis characterized by gross inflammatory infiltration, virtually complete disappearance of the tubules, and periglomerular and glomerular fibrosis. ×70.

cells which in places are grouped into lymphoid islands. Within the infiltrated area, the glomeruli are small, fibrous, and encircled by a fibrous thickening of Bowman's capsule. They rarely remain normal. The tubules are atrophic. At an advanced stage, the kidney is contracted by intense interstitial fibrosis.

Changes in the arteries are, in our experience, relatively rare.

Pathogenesis

Type of Organism

There is no systemic study of the organisms found within the kidney in pyelonephritis, but correlation with the organisms found in the urine is very good.[7] There is no evidence that any one variety of bacteria is more likely than another to provoke pyelonephritis in man, unlike the situation in experimental animals, in which it is found that various species are susceptible to different organisms.

Route of Infection

The ascending route is the principal route of infection of the renal parenchyma. Blood-borne infections and infections via the lymphatics are much more debatable (see page 132). It is generally agreed that bacteria reach the ureters and kidney from the bladder by ascending the column of urine. Experimentally, massive infection of the bladder in rats by *Proteus* produces pyelonephritis in 60 per cent of animals. If, however, the ureter on one side is tied or divided, the kidney above that ureter becomes involved in only 9 per cent of cases. If a model is constructed with two communicating compartments, upper and lower, organisms introduced into the lower compartment can reach the upper compartment provided that the rate of urine flow is not more than 25 ml. per hour. Infection of the renal pelvis is an obligatory step in infection of the kidney.

Predisposing Factors

Sensitivity of Kidney Tissue to Infection. It has been found experimentally that kidney tissue is less resistant to infection than other tissues. In the hours following intravenous injection of *E. coli* in rabbits, the number of organisms diminishes rapidly in liver and spleen but remains unchanged or increases in the kidney. This is the result of many factors, which have been studied extensively in recent years. For one thing, the kidney is poor in reticuloendothelial tissue. For another, the mobilization of granulocytes in the renal medulla after various types of stimulation is not very active. In addition, the kidney has an anticomplementary activity that inhibits the bactericidal power of serum, affecting especially the fraction IV of complement. Local physicochemical factors also are involved, including high tissue concentrations of ammonium and urea and hypertonicity, all of which favor infection.

The Role of Abnormalities in the Urinary Tract. In cases of urinary tract malformation and lithiasis, urinary infection produces a very high incidence of pyelonephritis. The same applies to renal abnormalities such as cysts, precalyceal canalicular ectasia and calyceal diverticula. Conversely, in our experience, pyelonephritis is rare in the absence of malformations of the urinary tract. To produce hematogenous pyelonephritis in the experimental animal, it is necessary to restort to various artifices, such as mechanical, chemical, or electrical trauma to the kidney, ischemia, or transient obstruction.

General Factors. All the general factors that render the body more receptive to urinary infection will predispose to pyelonephritis. Diminished immune adherence of lymphocytes toward *E. coli* has been noted in certain patients with chronic pyelonephritis.

ACUTE PYELONEPHRITIS

It is obviously not practical to insist on histologic criteria in order to distinguish between pyuria localized to the lower urinary tract and pyelonephritis. It is thus necessary to consider the validity of the various other criteria of acute pyelonephritis in the light of various studies correlating histologic with clinical and laboratory findings.

Clinical Features

Symptoms suggesting pyelonephritis in the presence of pyuria include a body temperature rise (102 to 104° F.) with chills and sweating, general symptoms of bacteremia, abdominal pain, and gastrointestinal upsets. Even more indicative features include loin pain, renal tenderness, and, rarely, a swollen kidney that is palpable. Another suggestive feature is reflux pain: during micturition the patient feels pain radiating from the bladder up to the kidney on one or both sides. All these signs are undoubtedly valuable, and their presence suggests acute pyelonephritis.

Some authors place great emphasis on hypertension as a sign of acute pyelonephritis, but in our experience this symptom is extremely rare.

Laboratory Findings

The association of hematuria with the pyuria is a presumptive but not absolute indicator of renal involvement. Signs of disordered renal function are very helpful. The first disorder is diminished concentrating power of the kidney.[22] Then there may be hyperchloremic acidosis and decrease in glomerular filtration. Diminished renal plasma flow is common and occurs early. Urinary protein output greater than 1 g./24 hours is also a valuable sign. Further evidence may be furnished by analyzing the type of proteinuria by immunoelectrophoresis and starch gel electrophoresis. The proteinuria will be of the tubular type, with relatively moderate albuminuria, triple globulinuria, and especially the presence of a protein that migrates more slowly than the gamma-globulins or "post gamma globulins." Some authors have suggested that leukocytes of renal origin (consequently indicative of renal infection) have a particular appearance. This is described as increased size on staining with gentian violet and safranin, with a globular and vacuolated nucleus that stains pale blue or pink instead of the usual deep blue. It is said that when viewed with the oil-immersion lens these cells are seen to exhibit intense Brownian movement. In fact, the cells, described by Steinheimer and Malbin, do not appear to be specific for renal involvement and can be found in any pyuria.

Radiologic Signs

The discovery of urinary tract or renal malformations and the demonstration of reflux are important. When such findings occur in conjunction with urinary infection they constitute a presumption in favor of pyelonephritis. Reflux should be looked for in every case.[19] Retrograde cystography is performed with strict asepsis, using a fine catheter. The study is carried out after all dye from intravenous urography has disappeared, or preferably before the intravenous urograms. The films must cover the entire urinary tract and should be taken at various stages of bladder filling and during micturition, under the control of an image intensifier.

Pyelotubular reflux is suggestive but not positive evidence of pelvic involvement.[12] Changes in the tone of calyces and ureters are difficult to interpret. The kidney may at times be increased in size, but this parameter too is difficult to measure. Special attention should be paid to the calyces and renal contours, but the changes occur late in the course of the disease and are found principally in chronic pyelonephritis. There may be localized irregularity of the renal contour, forming a notch. The outline of the papilla may disappear, so that the calyx is cupped and convex instead of concave. The distance between the calyx and cortex is diminished. These findings, associated with pyuria, suggest pyelo-

nephritis. They are found, in fact, in acute exacerbations of chronic pyelonephritis.

Serum Antibodies

Various types of antibodies have been studied, including hemagglutinating
antibodies against E. coli O-antigen from organisms found in urine, antibodies
of the same type against a polyvalent antigen, and precipitating antibodies.
There is a good correlation between the level of hemagglutinating antibodies
and various other criteria, such as clinical signs of pyelonephritis and diminished
renal concentrating ability,[1, 17] and the presence of bacteria in ureteric urine[11]
and in the kidney.[6] It is suggested that precipitating antibodies to E. coli O-
antigens will be found in recurrent pyelonephritis and indicate the onset of
chronic disease.[10] These conclusions are valid only insofar as all other paren-
chymatous infections by the same organism have been excluded — for example,
prostatitis. Some authors extrapolate these results and describe pyelonephritis
complicating asymptomatic bacteriuria purely on the basis of a rise in the antibody level.[1, 17] These authors diagnose pyelonephritis in cases in which the
clinical picture was suggestive but there was no evidence of urinary infection.[1]
However, it would seem premature to come to any conclusions.

The Value of Biopsy

Because of the radial arrangement of the lesions of pyelonephritis, with
alternation of healthy and diseased zones, it is obvious that the diagnosis cannot be excluded with certainty merely on the evidence of negative renal
biopsy findings. However, in many cases, the diagnosis of pyelonephritis may
be proved by biopsy.[21] Culture of the kidney fragment may yield the same
organisms that are found in the urine.[6, 7]

Course and Prognosis of Acute Pyelonephritis

In cases of urinary tract malformation or lithiasis, the prognosis should
be guarded. Actually, provided that the condition is treated effectively, the immediate course of acute pyelonephritis in the absence of urinary tract malformation is usually very favorable. The temperature falls to normal, and local and
general signs disappear. The urine becomes sterile in one or two days. The
renal concentrating power returns to normal in a matter of weeks.[22] The
antibody level drops over a period of months, or a year at the most.[1]

It has been shown that in some very exceptional cases, there may be sequelae
of a single attack of pyelonephritis in the absence of any urinary tract malformations. In these cases, at the time of the initial attack, which is rapidly
brought under control, the kidneys are normal on intravenous urography. In
the following months, although there is no new infection, the radiological
changes of pyelonephritis appear, and hypertension has been reported in one
case.[1] We have never seen this sequence of events, but one should be alert for
it if the antibody levels remain high.[1, 17]

In the absence of urinary malformation, what is the risk of repeated attacks of acute pyelonephritis? There is no doubt that progression to chronic
pyelonephritis has been described in neglected cases of urinary infection.[1, 17]

Here it is worth distinguishing between a *recurrence* (i.e., a totally new infection) and a *relapse* of the same infection owing to persistence of some bacterial focus. Apart from determination of the type of causal bacteria, the distinction may be made by studying the serum antibodies and finding, for example, either a high titer of antibodies against one or several antigens or a second rise in the level of specific antibodies.[17] It is suggested that precipitating antibodies rather than hemagglutinating antibodies will indicate recurrence and a risk of developing chronic pyelonephritis.[10] It is even more difficult to define the risks from latent, asymptomatic infection. Many authors think that such infection is a serious matter,[1, 17, 18] but in our experience this is not so.

Treatment

The treatment is the same as that for urinary infection (see page 138). The proper treatment and its success determine the prognosis of acute pyelonephritis and the prevention of chronic pyelonephritis.

In conclusion, it seems that in the presence of an acute urinary infection the arguments in favor of a diagnosis of acute pyelonephritis are: heavy proteinuria, disturbance of renal function (especially tubular), and the presence of hemagglutinating antibodies against the O-antigen of the *E. coli* in the urine. Radiographic evidence of malformation of the urinary tract or of stone indicates a high risk in any urinary infection and makes the diagnosis of acute pyelonephritis very probable. However, one should not rush to any conclusions merely on finding an isolated vesicoureteral reflux.

CHRONIC PYELONEPHRITIS

Chronic bacterial pyelonephritis may present in various ways.

Bilateral Chronic Pyelonephritis

Bilateral chronic pyelonephritis in children presents as a slowly progressive renal insufficiency. In this clinical situation, many features may suggest the diagnosis. Among the first is the presence of bacteriuria with leukocyturia that can appear as an isolated instance or in infrequent attacks, but which more commonly occurs in recurrent attacks or persists chronically. The urinary infection may or may not be accompanied by fever, abdominal pain, gastrointestinal upsets, and disturbances of micturition. A second point is that over a long period, the renal insufficiency affects principally tubular function, with diminished concentrating power, tubular acidosis, and, rarely, a salt- or potassium-losing syndrome. Later, the urea, sulfate, and phosphate levels rise and other features appear, including anemia, dwarfism, and renal osteodystrophy. Hypertension is rare in the earlier stages but may appear with terminal uremia. A third diagnostic feature, in cases in which there is adequate glomerular filtration, is evidence obtainable from intravenous urography, such as reduction in the thickness of the kidney between the kidney capsule and the calyces, dilatation of the calyces, deformity of the calyceal stems, and atrophy (often asymmetrical) of the kidney, with irregular notches on the convex border[12] (Figure

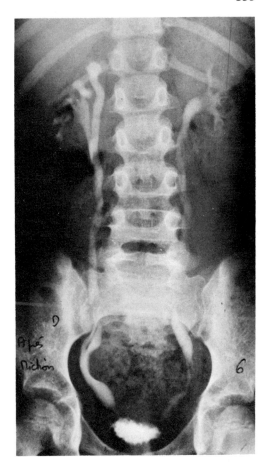

Figure 29. Intravenous urogram in chronic pyelonephritis in a patient born November 10, 1966. There was a five-year history of recurrent urinary infection. In April 1967, both kidneys were normal on intravenous urography; the height of the right kidney was 5.8 cm. and of the left kidney 6.2 cm. In November 1972, the height of the right kidney was 5.8 cm. and of the left kidney 7.5 cm.

29). As in acute pyelonephritis, some immunologic evidence may be helpful. If a renal biopsy specimen is taken from a characteristic zone, it will reveal infiltration with inflammatory cells, tubular atrophy, and pericapsular glomerular sclerosis. Culture of the kidney fragment yields the same organism that is found in the urine.

The chronic renal insufficiency of pyelonephritis is homogeneous when there is no urinary obstruction, and corresponds to the picture of a reduced nephron population.[5] The treatment is that of urinary infection and of renal failure, and this ultimately implies hemodialysis and transplantation. The dominant factor in treatment is the state of the urinary tract and the possibilities of surgical cure. In this regard, bilateral chronic pyelonephritis can be divided into four groups, each with specific problems.

Bilateral Chronic Pyelonephritis with Urinary Tract Malformations and/or Lithiasis

This group includes the great majority of cases of chronic pyelonephritis in childhood. The renal insufficiency often is not homogeneous, and the problem is to determine how much of the renal insufficiency is the result of bacterial pyelonephritis that may respond to antibacterial therapy, how much results from urinary obstruction that may be relieved by surgery, and how much results from associated malformations of the kidney, such as dysplasia, cortical hypoplasia, or segmental hypoplasia. This problem is discussed in more detail in Chapter 3 (see page 160).

Bilateral Chronic Pyelonephritis with Isolated Vesicoureteral Reflux

There are conflicting opinions on the significance of isolated vesicoureteral reflux in the development of chronic pyelonephritis. Some authors place great emphasis on the serious dangers of reflux.[19] This opinion may have to be modified, however, in the light of recent evidence. Köllermann and Ludwig[14] studied 102 healthy children between the ages of 2 days and 5 years and found reflux in 30 per cent of cases; the incidence was 65 per cent at 6 months, 47 per cent at 1 year, and 30 per cent at 2 years, dropping to zero at 5 years. This physiologic reflux had no ill effects. Blank and Girdany[3] followed for a minimum of 5 years 115 children who exhibited symptomatic bacteriuria with reflux. They found radiographic evidence of renal damage in only one case. We have performed renal biopsy on four children who had bacteriuria with isolated reflux. In two cases the kidney was normal within the limits of the biopsy specimen, and in two cases there was interstitial nephritis. Further study of this question is needed.

Chronic Bacterial Pyelonephritis Without Uropathy, Lithiasis, or Reflux

This type of pyelonephritis is probably very rare in children. We have seen only three cases. Neumann and Pryles found only two cases in 1999 autopsies on children under the age of 16 years; one was in a girl aged 15 years and the other in a boy aged 10 years.[18]

Chronic Pyelonephritis Without Urinary Infection ("Abacterial" Pyelonephritis)[2]

It is possible that chronic pyelonephritis may originate in a single attack of urinary infection, or in an asymptomatic infection, or even in a bacteriuria that can be demonstrated only by provocative tests with pyrogens or steroids. A search for bacteria in kidney tissues may prove negative when the organisms are in the L form. Finally pyelonephritis may be an immune process resulting from the persistence of a bacterial antigen such as has been found in both animals and men. Further information is needed on this important point.

Unilateral Chronic Bacterial Pyelonephritis

Unilateral chronic pyelonephritis with urinary infection may be the consequence of unilateral lithiasis or a urinary tract malformation. It may affect only one pole of the kidney, especially when there is renal duplication. It is not a common cause of hypertension in children. Such hypertension most often results from segmental hypoplasia that is frequently confused with chronic pyelo-nephritis (see page 14).

XANTHOGRANULOMATOUS PYELONEPHRITIS*

This is a chronic pyelonephritis characterized by the presence of yellow nodules in the kidney consisting of granulomata in which xanthomatous cells predominate. It may be diffuse or localized to one pole of the kidney. It is very rarely bilateral, and is even rarer in children than in adults. We have seen six examples of the diffuse variety, and these are summarized in Table 27.[9]

Diffuse Form[8, 9, 16, 20]

Some dozen cases have been recorded in children, and these form the basis of the following description.

Clinical Features

A particular feature is the early age at which the urinary symptoms appear—before 8 months in three of the cases and before the age of 2 years in five

---

*This section was written by Dr. Micheline Lévy.

Table 27.   Xanthogranulomatous Pyelonephritis
(Summary of Six Personal Cases)

Case	1	2	3	4	5	6
Sex	M	F	M	M	F	M
Age at onset (years)	2 years 6 months	1/12	2 years 8 months	2 years 4 months	8/12	2/12
Age when first seen	4 years 7 months	11/12	2 years 11 months	2 years 6 months	2 years 6 months	1 year 8 months
Fever	0	+	0	0	+	0
Passage of stones	+	0	0	0	+	0
Urinary infection	+	+	+	+	+	+
Hematuria	0	0	0	0	+	+
Abdominal mass	0	0	0	+	0	+
Hypertension	0	0	0	0	0	0
Anemia	0	+	+	0	+	+
Retardation of growth	+	+	+	+	0	+
Side affected	R	R	R	L	R	R
Stones visible on x-ray	+	+	+	0	0	+
Function as seen on x-ray	0	0	0	0	0	0
Contralateral kidney	Normal	Normal	Normal	Normal	Normal	Congenital hydronephrosis
Arteriography (hypovascularization)	?	?	?	?	+	+
Nephrectomy	+	+	+	+	+	
Cure	+	+	+	+	+	

other cases. The presenting symptoms include disturbances of micturition, discoloration of the urine, changes in general health, and stones discovered accidentally or causing retention of urine. The adult symptoms of fever and disturbances of general condition are rarely seen in children. The clinical picture is seldom sufficiently dramatic to indicate the need for hospitalization. For this reason, several years may elapse between the time the first symptoms became apparent and surgical treatment. Pyuria resistant to antibiotic treatment is a common feature. There may be retardation of growth, and an abdominal or loin mass may be palpable.

Laboratory Findings

There is nearly always hypochromic anemia and leukocytosis. The urine always contains pus, and the organism most commonly found is *Proteus*. There is a mild proteinuria related to the urinary infection. The blood levels of urea, electrolytes, calcium, phosphorus, alkaline phosphatase, proteins, and cholesterol are normal, and the urinary electrolytes, calcium, phosphorus, oxalic acid, amino acids, and reducing sugars are also normal.

Radiologic Signs

In every case, no dye was excreted by the affected kidney. In eight cases, opaque calculi could be seen on the affected side in the preliminary films. In two cases no calculi were seen, but one of these children had passed stones a short time previously.

The picture on the other side, in most cases, is normal, although in one case there was a congenital obstruction at the pelviuretenic junction.

Arteriography demonstrates hypovascularization of the involved kidney, and a renal scan shows both a lack of fixation of isotope on the involved side and compensatory hypertrophy of the healthy kidney.

Treatment

Nephrectomy was carried out in every case. The general prognosis is good. Many children reviewed some years after surgery have been found to be in good health, with no recurrence of their disease, and there is compensatory hypertrophy of the contralateral kidney.

Pathologic Anatomy

The macroscopic appearance is very suggestive. The pelvis and calyces are very dilated and filled with purulent material and stones (Figure 30). There is considerable atrophy of the cortex. A yellowish border appears around the calyceal cavities and there may be nodules of the same color in the nearby cortex.

On microscopic examination, necrotic zones with varying degrees of calcification are observed in the papillae, surrounded by an inflammatory granuloma consisting of lymphocytes, plasmocytes, polymorphonuclear cells, and most notably histiocytes filled with fat ("foam cells"), and giant cells. A band of inflammatory fibrous tissue separates this granulomatous zone from the cortex,

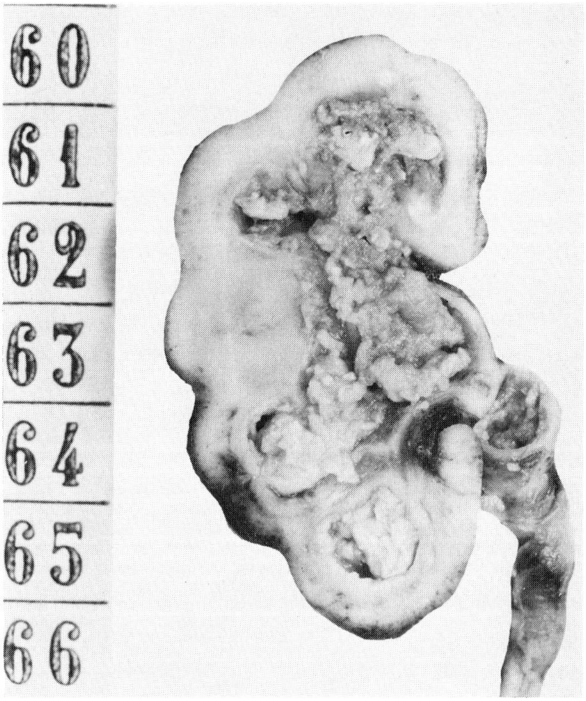

Figure 30. Xanthogranu-lomatous pyelonephritis: macro-scopic appearance. The calyces and pelvis are filled with puru-lent material and calculi.

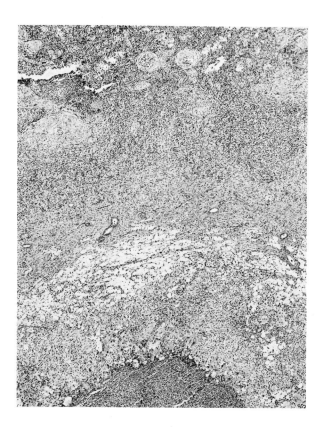

Figure 31. Xanthogranu-lomatous pyelonephritis. The cortex is atrophied by chronic pyelonephritis. Below the cortex is a fibrous zone and below this a granulomatous zone in which many foam cells and multinu-cleated cells can be seen. ×38.

which is atrophied by chronic pyelonephritis. Endarteritis and endophlebitis may occasionally be seen (Figure 31).

Localized Form

This form likewise is more rare in children than in adults, and we have seen only five cases. The children tend to be older at the time of diagnosis. The clinical history is relatively short, with fever, anemia, and pyuria. Intravenous urography reveals a space-occupying lesion at one pole of the kidney. No calculi were visible in any of the five cases. The treatment is nephrectomy, usually total because of the granulomatous involvement of the cortex and sometimes even of the perirenal fat.

Etiology

Many etiologic hypotheses have been put forward, including obstruction of the urinary tract, primary chronic suppuration in the kidney, unusually virulent organisms, antibiotic therapy, disorders of lipid metabolism, and venous disease.[8] Because of the particular topography of the disease, with involvement of all the papillae, we have suggested that the primary lesion may be papillary necrosis of ischemic origin. Calcification in the necrosis would be responsible for the stone formation. The xanthogranulomatous reaction and chronic pyelonephritis would then be secondary consequences of these phenomena.[9]

Conclusions

1. By definition pyelonephritis is a specific bacteriologic and anatomic entity. The term should be reserved strictly for lesions of the renal pelvis and interstitial tissue resulting from infection.

2. Urinary infection is very common in children. In the majority of cases, especially when there is no obstructive uropathy or associated renal malformation, this infection does not imply infection of the renal parenchyma.

3. When there is definite urinary infection, the classical clinical signs, disturbance of renal function, and abnormal urograms suggest acute pyelonephritis. However, these signs are not constant or may appear late, and they also are sometimes misleading, since they may be the result of some other condition. Greater diagnostic precision may be expected from analysis of the type of proteinuria and from studies of the antibodies against the bacteria responsible for the urinary infection. The prognosis is generally good.

4. The clinical, laboratory, urographic, and even histologic evidence may suggest chronic pyelonephritis, but the diagnosis should not be accepted without definite proof of infection. In such cases it is important to remember that there is a group of noninfectious interstitial nephropathies that are common in children.

5. Hypertension is rare in pyelonephritis. It usually is the result of segmental hypoplasia.

6. Despite the reservations we have expressed, recurrent urinary infection in children must not be neglected even if there is no sign of renal disease

and no abnormality in the urinary tract. Such cases should be treated as potential pyelonephritis.

REFERENCES

1. Andersen, H. J.: Clinical studies on the antibody response to *E. coli* O-antigens in infants and children with urinary tract infection, using a passive haemagglutination technique. Acta. Paediat. Scand. Suppl. *180*:1, 1968.
2. Aoki, S., Imamura, S., Aoki, M., and McCabe, W. R.: "Abacterial" and bacterial pyelonephritis. Immunofluorescent localization of bacterial antigen. New Eng. J. Med. *281*:1375, 1969.
3. Blank, E., and Girdany, B. R.: Prognosis with vesico-ureteral reflux. Pediatrics *48*:782, 1971.
4. Beeson, P. B.: What is chronic pyelonephritis? Symposium and discussion. *In* E. H. Kass: Progress in Pyelonephritis. Philadelphia, F. A. Davis, 1965, p. 367.
5. Bricker, N. S., Lubowtiz, H., and Rieselbach, R. E.: Renal function in chronic renal disease. Medicine *44*:263, 1965.
6. Brumfitt, W., and Percival, A.: Serum antibody response as an indication of renal involvement in patients with significant bacteriuria. *In* E. H. Kass: Progress in Pyelonephritis. Philadelphia, F. A. Davis, 1965, p. 118.
7. Brun, C., Raaschou, F., and Eriksen, K. R.: Simultaneous bacteriologic studies of renal biopsies and urine. *In* E. H. Kass: Progress in Pyelonephritis. Philadelphia, F. A. Davis, 1965, p. 461.
8. Chatelanat, F., Scopfer, P., and Mach, R.: Les pyélonéphrites xanthogranulomateuses. *In* "Actualités néphrologiques de l'Hôpital Necker. Paris, Flammarion, 1968, p. 263.
9. Habib, R., Lévy, M., and Royer, P.: La pyélonéphrite chronique xanthogranulomateuse chez l'enfant. Arch. franç. Pédiat. *25*:489, 1968.
10. Hanson, L. A., Holmgren, J., Jodal, U., and Winberg, J.: Precipitating antibodies to *E. coli* O-antigens: a suggested difference in the antibody response of infants and children with first and recurrent attacks of pyelonephritis. Acta. Paediat. Scand. *58*:506, 1969.
11. Hewstone, A. S., and Whitaker, J.: The correlation of ureteric urine bacteriology and homologous antibody titer in children with urinary infection. J. Pediat. *74*:540, 1969.
12. Kaufman, K. J.: Pyelonephritis. Round table. Ann. Radiol. *14*:217, 1971.
13. Kimmelstiel, P., Kim, O. J., Beres, J. A., and Wellmann, K.: Chronic pyelonephritis. Amer. J. Med. *30*:589, 1961.
14. Köllermann, M. W., and Ludwig, H.: Über den vesico-ureteralen Reflux beim normalen Kind in Saüglings—und Kleinkindalter. Z. Kinderheilk. *100*:185, 1967.
15. Lustik, B., Kniker, W. T., and Pryles, C. V.: Increased urinary glomerular basement membrane products in pyelonephritis. Pediat. Res. *4*:448, 1970.
16. Lackner, M., Wolfel, D., Banowsky, L., and Kornfeld, M.: Xanthogranulomatous pyelonephritis. J. Pediat. *75*:682, 1969.
17. Neter, E., Oberkircher, O. R., Rubin, M. I., Steinhart, J. M., and Krzeska, I.: Patterns of antibody response of children with infections of the urinary tract. Pediat. Res. *4*:500, 1970.
18. Neumann, C. G., and Pryles, C. V.: Pyelonephritis in infants and children. Amer. J. Dis. Child. *104*:215, 1962.
19. Scott, J. E., and Stansfeld, J. M.: Ureteric reflux and kidney scarring in children. Arch. Dis. Child. *43*:468, 1968.
20. Vasquez, J., and Herranz, G.: Pielonefritis xanthogranulomatosa. Rev. Med. Univ. Navarra *9*:127, 1965.
21. Williams, A. L., and Fowler, R.: Renal biopsy in recurrent urinary tract infection. Findings in children. Amer. J. Dis. Child. *105*:617, 1963.
22. Winberg, J.: Renal function studies in infants and children with acute, nonobstructive urinary tract infection. Acta Paediat. *48*:577, 1959.

Chapter Three

RENAL COMPLICATIONS
OF URINARY TRACT
MALFORMATIONS

The clinical incidence of urinary tract malformations is 0.6 to 5.4 per thousand, and the incidence at autopsy is 7 to 9.3 per thousand. The condition accounts for 4.5 cases in every thousand children admitted to a general pediatric department, and it is probably responsible for 50 per cent of cases of chronic renal failure.[21] Urinary tract malformation is very rarely familial,[22] but it is found in association with certain chromosome aberrations such as Turner's syndrome and abnormalities of chromosomes 13 and 18. The condition is often associated with congenital anorectal abnormalities, spina bifida, agenesis of the sacrum, aplasia of the abdominal muscles, congenital disorders of the heart, and a single umbilical artery. Boys are affected much more often than girls, and such disorders may be responsible for oligoamnios or, more rarely, hydramnios.

The renal complications are initially disorders of tubular function, especially defective concentrating ability, and later uremia.[1, 5, 7, 13, 14, 17, 19, 20, 25–27] The factors responsible for the renal complications are multiple, and the mechanism is only partly understood. The three principal factors are mechanical obstruction with increased pressure in the urinary tract, bacterial infection with secondary pyelonephritis, and the presence of dysplastic elements in the kidney. Although the concept of a reduced nephron population partly explains the defect in renal function, the type of renal insufficiency depends on other abnormalities.

The two important problems in theory and practice are the nature of the anatomic lesions in the kidney and the possibility of functional recovery after surgical correction of the uropathy.

Symptomatology

Mode of Onset

Attention may be drawn to the urinary tract by the presence of pyuria, polyuria, polydipsia, loin pain, or a renal mass. Disorders of micturition should be sought routinely in the newborn child; these include a defective urinary stream suggesting urethral valve in a boy or a neurogenic bladder; a continuous leak of urine indicating an ectopic ureter in girls; and a palpable, distended bladder. Hematuria or isolated proteinuria may be the result of obstructive uropathy, but hypertension is rare. In many cases, the signs are not very specific; there may be attacks of fever leading to a search for urinary infection or defective urinary concentration, abdominal pain, gastrointestinal disorders such as constipation or false diarrhea, general malaise, or failure to thrive.

Clinical Signs

Polyuria is virtually constant and may be as severe as in diabetes insipidus. Hypertension is rare but may occur under various circumstances. In the terminal stage of renal failure, hypertension is not specific and is a very poor prognostic sign. Hypertension may complicate acute renal failure resulting from urinary retention. At an early stage, and when there is good renal function, hypertension may be caused by high intrarenal pressure causing excessive secretion of renin. In such cases, the blood pressure returns to normal when the obstruction is relieved. In our experience, hypertension is more often the result of segmental hypoplasia in the kidney above the obstruction (see page 14). The growth defect is variable. It may be early and marked, or late and slight. Deficiency in growth is related to the degree of renal failure. Anemia is common and usually results from infection, with blocking of incorporation of iron into the red cells. Anemia with erythroblastopenia supervenes at the stage of advanced renal failure. In some cases of obstructive uropathy, there may be polycythemia. Bone disorders are variable and do not differ from those seen in the nephropathies (see page 395). Acidosis is generally latent, but it may become clinically important in attacks of acute infection or dietetic errors. Abnormal salt loss is nearly always latent and becomes clinically manifest only with excessive restriction of sodium intake or in attacks of intercurrent infection with diarrhea and vomiting. Signs of excessive salt loss include anorexia, nausea, vomiting, fatigability, and intention tremor. Failure to recognize a salt-losing syndrome may be very serious — even fatal — producing a clinical picture of collapse and extracellular dehydration, with a moist tongue. Stone is a common complication of obstructive uropathy (see page 195).

Renal Function[1, 7, 13, 19, 20, 25–27]

Obstructive malformations of the urinary tract primarily affect the tubular functions, and this cannot be explained merely on the basis of reduction of the nephron population. This fact, well known both in adults and experimentally, has also been demonstrated in children. There is nearly always a defect in concentrating ability, and this disorder can exist with normal glomerular filtration. For a given level of glomerular filtration, the defect in concentrating power is greater than that which occurs with reduction in the nephron population (Figure 32). This defective concentration may in effect produce a diabetes insipidus. We have recently been able to study function separately in each kidney.[17] This is a valuable model because both kidneys have the same environment.[6] In every case, the defect in concentrating power is greater in the damaged kidney or, if both kidneys are involved, in the more seriously affected of the two kidneys. We have even seen unilateral diabetes insipidus. There may also be defects in renal acidification function. The urinary pH does not drop sufficiently with an ammonium chloride load. Hydrogen ion excretion may be diminished both absolutely and when corrected per nephron unit —

that is to say, for normal glomerular filtration rate. These findings are confirmed in separate renal function studies. There may be unilateral inability to
lower pH (see Figure 36) and unilateral diminution in hydrogen ion excretion
per nephron unit. The renal ability to conserve sodium is not usually affected.[7, 19]
It is true that separate function studies show that the fraction of filtered sodium
excreted after five days of sodium restriction is greater on the more involved
side, but this does not lead to a clinically obvious salt-losing syndrome so long
as the glomerular filtration rate is above 25 ml./min./1.73 m.[2] In this regard,
the renal disorder in obstructive uropathy does not differ from that seen
when there is reduction in the nephron population. In the majority of cases,
there are no defects in the renal excretion of potassium, calcium, or phosphorus
other than those that appear when glomerular filtration is very poor.

Glomerular filtration may be normal or diminished to a varying degree.
At this stage of obstruction, it does not appear to be representative of the
number of residual nephrons because the diminished glomerular filtration
rate is partly functional. The filtration fraction and the ratio of glomerular
filtration to TmPAH are variable. The studies of this type which have been done
are insufficient to give an exact opinion on the significance of these two parameters. Experimentally, they are found to be decreased in acute obstruction
and elevated in chronic obstruction.[5, 7, 17]

In most cases, proteinuria is moderate—less than 1 g. per day. It rises

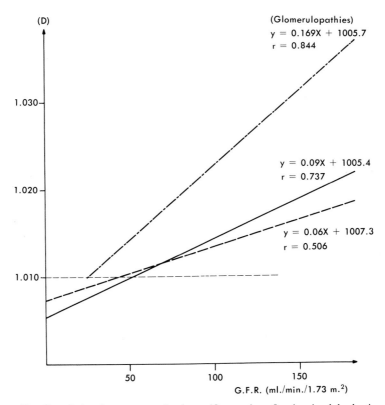

Figure 32. Correlation between maximal specific gravity of urine in dehydration (D) and
endogenous creatinine clearance (G.F.R.).

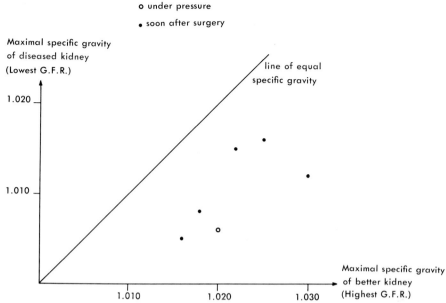

Figure 33. Comparison of maximal specific gravity of separate urines from each kidney in obstructive uropathy.

sharply when the glomerular filtration rate drops below 40 ml./min./1.73 m.² Hence, proteinuria has a definite value as an indicator of the degree of renal damage and of the number of nephrons remaining.

Defective concentrating ability is almost constant and is the first disorder to appear. It may exist without any deficiency in the ability of the kidney to regulate acid-base balance and without any diminution in glomerular filtration. The second abnormality to appear, which is never found in the absence of a defective concentrating ability, is defective power of acidification. Thus, a study of urine concentrating ability is the best test of kidney damage secondary to malformation of the urinary tract.[7, 19]

Renal damage may be unilateral and often is asymmetrical, and it may therefore be essential to perform separate renal function studies. The fixation of ¹⁹⁷Hg correlates well with glomerular filtration rate and gives a good idea of the function of each kidney (Figure 34).

Radiologic Studies[3, 7, 13, 16]

Radiologic studies establish the diagnosis of urinary tract malformation and give a rough idea of the degree of renal damage. In addition, they provide valuable information about ureteral contractility.

Hydronephrosis. In this condition, there is distention of the renal pelvis and calyces. The calyceal dilatation may be massive. True hydronephrosis must be differentiated from *megacalycosis* and from the condition that we call *megapelvis.*

In *megacalycosis,* the calyces are voluminous, with a flat base and decreased distance between calyx and cortex but a careful examination of the entire urinary tract, especially of the pelviureteric junction, reveals no malformation. The

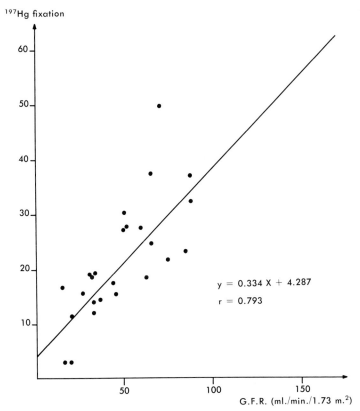

Figure 34. Relationship between glomerular filtration (G.F.R.) and fixation of [197]Hg.

renal pelvis is not dilated, its lower border remains concave, and it empties from its lowest point. The dynamics of filling and emptying are normal and synchronous with the opposite side.

In *megapelvis*, the renal pelvis is voluminous, and its inner border forms a straight line. At the outer part of the pelvis, the calyces are attached by very short stems, or stems may even be absent. However, the calyces remain concave, with the normal configuration of the papilla being preserved. Although the pelvis is very large, its lower border also remains concave, and it empties from its lowest point. Urography with induced diuresis does not show defective emptying of the pelvis, but the distinction from true hydronephrosis may be difficult in cases in which this minor abnormality is associated with malformation of the urinary tract on the other side.

Dunbar and Nogrady[9] have described the sign of the calyceal crescent. In the early films (during the first 20 minutes), linear shadows of high density appear in crescent form, more or less regularly arranged in the inner part of the renal parenchyma, whose limits are outlined by a nephrogram. These crescents are due to contrast material in the tubules and they are found when there is high intrapelvic pressure. This sign is specific for hydronephrosis and distinguishes it from multicystic kidney and in particular from nephroblastoma. When this sign is observed, it is an indication to take further films up to 24 hours if necessary, which will show that the kidney is in fact functioning and will reveal the obstructive uropathy.

Intravenous Urography. This has sometimes been suggested as a test of renal function, but it is of little value in obstructive uropathy.[3, 16] Delay in appearance of the contrast medium depends not only on glomerular filtration but also on the intrapelvic pressure.

An important criterion is the assessment of the amount of remaining renal parenchyma,[19] but this may be difficult. It is based on the measurement— which is approximate at best—of various parameters: the height of the calyces (C), the height of the kidney (K), and the theoretical height of kidney (TK), which is calculated by Hodson's formula[15]: TK = $0.057 \times X$ (height of patient in centimeters) + 2.646. Various ratios can be calculated. $\dfrac{C}{K}$ is normally 0.5, and any increase is related to the degree of hydronephrosis. $\dfrac{K-C}{K}$, whose value normally is 0.5, gives an approximate idea of the height of remaining renal parenchyma. The relationship of $\dfrac{K-C}{K}$ to $\dfrac{TK}{2}$ can be used as an index of the development of the remaining parenchyma in relation to normal kidney growth, but it must be remembered that these are measurements of projected images.

Ureteral Contractility. The radiologic examination should also assess ureteral contractility.[24] Precise information on this point is essential before making any decision about reimplanting the ureters into the bladder. Anti-reflux surgery causes increased pressure in the terminal ureter during bladder filling, and if the force of ureteral contraction is not able to overcome this pressure, the net result of the surgery will be ureteric dilatation and increase in the damage to the kidney. The ureteral contractility is assessed by cineradiography during intravenous urography or, better, by serial films taken with an image intensifier. If the child had previously undergone reimplantation of the ureters, the ureters should be studied with the bladder empty. The ureters can also be studied under various other conditions: during osmotic diuresis; with high perfusion flows in cases of cutaneous ureterostomy; and under the influence of various drugs that may affect ureteral peristalsis. Ureteric pressures may also be measured directly at the time of surgery.

Course

The rate of progression of renal damage varies enormously from case to case, even in the same type of obstructive lesion, depending on such things as secondary infection and surgical intervention (often including multiple surgery). Renal function may improve or stabilize, or it may deteriorate either gradually or in steps. Those cases that go on to terminal renal failure may benefit from a dialysis-transplantation program.

It is obvious that for better understanding of the various possibilities, two types of investigations are valuable—studies of the anatomic lesions in the kidney and studies of the possibilities of recovery after surgical intervention.

ANATOMIC ABNORMALITIES OF THE KIDNEY AND URINARY TRACT

Ureteric Lesions

The ureters are dilated and elongated to a varying degree and their walls are thickened by muscular hypertrophy. There are varying degrees of associated edema of the mucosa. Infection increases the edema and causes progressive fibrosis. Infection can also cause ureteral atony by a purely toxic effect. There may be stenosis of the lower end of the ureter and the ureteric orifice may be ectopic or located in a diverticulum. If no such abnormality exists, there is idiopathic megaureter, always associated with reflux. Therefore, the ureter may be obstructed, infected, or congenitally malformed. The quality of ureteral contraction depends on the severity and duration of all these factors.

Lesions of the Renal Parenchyma

The lesions of the kidney are multiple, and these are often difficult to interpret in nephrectomy or autopsy specimens. Renal biopsy gives only a small part of the picture.[4, 7, 11, 12, 23] There are three types of lesions. The first result from urinary obstruction and include reduction of the pelvic mucosa to a single cell layer, flattened papillae, dilated collecting tubules, and collapse and atrophy of the loops of Henle, with flattening of their lining. The lesions in the second group are caused by bacterial pyelonephritis secondary to the urinary infection; they may be acute, subacute, or chronic, and may be diffuse or localized, perhaps to one pole. The third group consists of the congenital abnormalities of the kidney associated with urinary tract malformation, most often a renal dysplasia of the type described by Ericsson and Ivemark[11, 12] (see Table 28). Adjoining the dysplastic zones is a very thin cortex containing only vessels and a few rare fetal or fibrous glomeruli, an appearance to which we have given the name *"cortical hypoplasia"*[7] (Figure 35). Much more rarely, the congenital anomaly is a segmental hypoplasia (see page 14). The vessels are generally normal except in segmental hypoplasia.

Table 28. Abnormalities of the Kidney in Urinary Tract Malformation (Nephrectomy and Autopsy Specimens)*

Type	Number of Cases	Interstitial Nephritis	Dysplasia	Segmental Hypoplasia	Vascular Lesions	Glomerulo-nephritis	Other
Congenital hydronephrosis	6	3	1	1	1	0	2
Megaureter	10	8	5	0	1	0	1
Ureteral duplication	10	6	8	0	2	2	0
Small kidney with vesicoureteral reflux	4	2	2	2	2	0	0
Ureteral hypoplasia	2	1	2	0	0	0	0
Obstruction of ureter	12	9	11	2	4	1	0
Total	44	29	29	5	10	3	3

*Many anomalies may coincide in the same kidney.

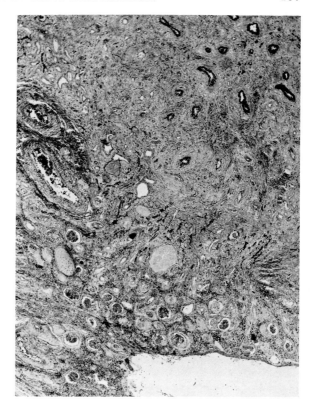

Figure 35. Cortical hypoplasia with medullary dysplasia in a boy with posterior urethral valves. ×35.

We have studied the type of lesion found in 100 cases of urinary tract malformations (56 biopsy specimens, 34 kidneys removed surgically, and 10 autopsy specimens). Table 28 summarizes some of the findings in whole kidneys and indicates the incidence of the various types of lesion and their distributions in the various types of urinary tract malformation. Table 29 gives the corresponding findings from renal biopsy specimens. Table 30 analyzes the lesions found in cases associated with hypertension; it will be noted that segmental hypoplasia was found in five of the eight cases of permanent hypertension.

Table 29. Abnormalities of the Kidney in Urinary Tract Malformation (Biopsies)

Type	Number of Cases	Normal Kidney	Interstitial Nephritis	Interstitial Fibrosis	Dysplasia	Segmental Hypoplasia	Vascular Lesions	Other
Congenital hydronephrosis	29	19	5	4	0	0	0	1
Megaureter	14	4	6	1	0	1	1	1
Ureteral duplication	1	1	0	0	0	0	0	0
Isolated vesicoureteral reflux	4	2	2	0	0	0	0	0
Vesicoureteral reflux with small kidney	5	1	1	0	2	1	0	0
Ureteral obstruction	3	0	2	0	1	0	0	0
Total	56	27	16	5	3	2	1	2

Table 30.   Abnormalities of Kidney in Cases of Urinary Tract Malformation with Hypertension*

Lesion	Transient Hypertension (6 cases)	Permanent Hypertension (8 cases)
Normal kidney	1	1
Interstitial nephritis	3	3
Interstitial fibrosis	1	0
Dysplasia	1	1
Segmental hypoplasia	0	5
Lesions of main vessels	0	0
Others	1	0

*Many lesions may coincide in the same case.

FUNCTIONAL RECOVERY AFTER SURGERY[13, 19, 20]

Many authors have reported that the concentrating power, the renal acidification function, and glomerular filtration may improve,[5, 7, 17, 26, 27] but the overall figures are pessimistic.[7, 20] In experimental studies, the renal damage becomes irreversible after the obstruction has been present for a certain length of time, and the longer the duration of obstruction the more limited the capacity for recovery.

We have studied this problem by comparative analysis of the function of each kidney.[13, 19] In some special cases, the renal damage is very asymmetrical, with the total function of the two kidneys close to normal, so that it is possible to study the particular consequences of obstruction. We have shown that the capacity for concentration and acidification (in all its parameters) can return to normal in the absence of any change in glomerular filtration. Thus, the tubular disorder, which is characteristic of the phase of obstruction, can regress completely without any change in the number of residual nephrons. Nephron function, unbalanced during obstruction, may return to a balanced state (Figures 36, 37 and 38).

Improvement in glomerular filtration is also possible. This may occur in two stages. In the first stage, there is a rapid rise in the glomerular filtration rate, suggesting that the lowered filtration during obstruction is partly the result of hemodynamic disorders caused by the increased urinary pressure and is not, in the presence of obstruction, representative of the number of residual nephrons. In the second stage, there may be slow improvement, probably an expression of compensatory hypertrophy.

Whenever tubule recovery is incomplete—and especially when there is a persistent disorder of concentration—detailed study is imperative. If the defect in concentrating ability is serious and out of proportion to the degree of glomerular insufficiency, it suggests poor drainage or some failure of surgery. If the defect in concentration is proportional to the diminution in glomerular filtration, it may be simply the result of the reduction in nephron population.

Thus, the minimal prognosis for renal function depends on the number of nephrons irreversibly damaged or, conversely, on the number of residual neph-

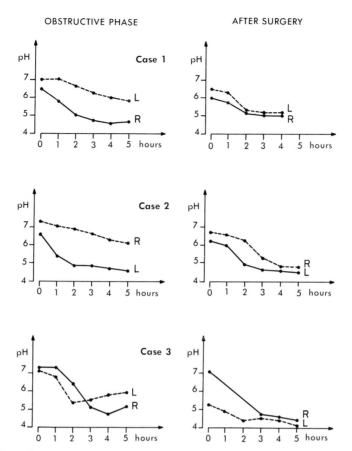

OBSTRUCTIVE PHASE · AFTER SURGERY

Case 1

Case 2

Case 3

Figure 36. Changes in urinary pH after NH₄Cl loading in the urine from the right (R) and left (L) kidneys before (left half of the figure) and after surgery (right half) in three cases of obstructive uropathy. Note the improvement in the damaged kidneys after surgery.

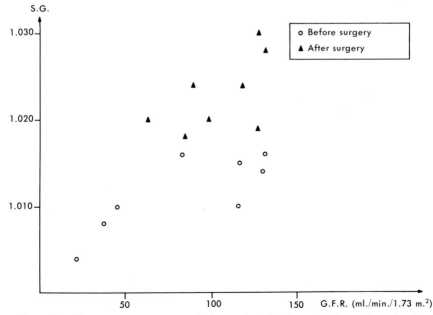

Figure 37. Homogenous recovery of glomerular filtration (G.F.R.) and maximal specific gravity of urine (S.G.) after surgical correction of urinary tract malformation.

169

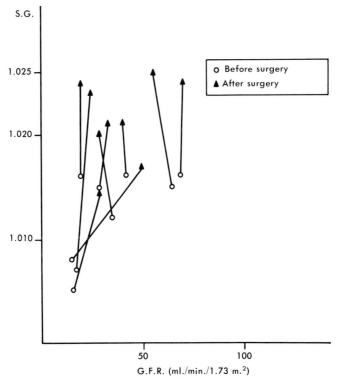

Figure 38. Separate renal function studies (separate ureterostomies). Relationship between glomerular filtration (G.F.R.) and maximal specific gravity of urine in dehydration (S.G.) before and after surgery.

rons. In practice, the situation may be assessed by measuring glomerular filtration some weeks after relief of the obstruction.

The results are influenced by various factors. In most cases, the urinary infection can be cured and recurrence prevented, except when the ureters have been diverted directly or indirectly onto the skin. Even in these situations, the infection can be greatly minimized. Minimal persistence of infection has not, in our experience, prevented recovery of renal function. The results of treatment are better with obstructive uropathy than with megaureter. This is probably a result of the difference in quality of ureteral contraction, which, as already noted, is such an important factor in determining the success of operations for reimplantation of the ureter into the bladder.

Cutaneous ureterostomy, combined with vigorous treatment of the urinary infection, improves or — at worst — stabilizes renal function, and sometimes good quality ureteral contractions may reappear.

In unilateral or predominantly unilateral uropathy, there is in general no improvement in glomerular filtration. It seems that the presence of the contralateral, healthy kidney inhibits compensatory hypertrophy in the diseased kidney, a fact that has been studied experimentally and confirmed in our own work. This concept must be taken into consideration in cases in which one kidney is healthy and the other very diseased, when a decision has to be made between nephrectomy and conservative surgery.

SPECIAL PROBLEMS

Decompression Syndrome[7, 8]

This disorder follows surgical relief of obstruction, ureterostomy, or even catheterization. It occurs not only with bilateral uropathy but also in unilateral cases, in which event the pediatrician may be taken off guard. It appears in the first few hours, the following day, or even several days after removal of the obstruction, and it develops progressively. The syndrome is characterized by obligatory polyuria, sometimes of a hyposthenuric type, with diminution of the TcH_2O associated with renal loss of sodium and potassium. The syndrome generally lasts for two or three days, but it may continue for a week or more. In severity, it seems to be proportional to the quality of renal function, the level of blood urea, and the degree of overhydration before surgery. The decompression syndrome is dangerous at the time it ccurs but does not, in the long run, carry a poor prognosis.

Problems of Uretero-Ileal Diversion

It is sometimes necessary to implant the ureters into an ileal loop (Bricker operation). This procedure may be complicated by stenosis and infection and also by renal lithiasis. The interposition of an ileal loop may also cause some metabolic disorders,[18] including an obligatory loss of bicarbonate, sodium, and chloride, the seriousness of which is directly related to the length of the ileal loop. These disorders are usually latent but may become evident with ill-advised sodium restriction, prolonged starvation, or intercurrent infection, presenting as an acidosis or especially a syndrome of sodium depletion. This may be a serious complication. In most cases, sodium bicarbonate supplementation is necessary. If the ammonium excretion on a normal diet is compared with that after an ammonium chloride load, it is found that the ammoniogenesis is often at its uppermost limit.

The presence of an ileal loop causes increased leukocyturia even when there is no infection. It also falsifies urine concentration tests, and so improvement in kidney function can be judged only by measuring glomerular filtration rate and ammonium excretion after an ammonium chloride load.

TREATMENT

Treatment of Infection

This has already been considered in detail (see page 138). Certain measures are peculiar to obstructive uropathy. Endoscopy must be restricted to the essential minimum. Retrograde ureteropyelography must be performed only immediately before surgery. Catheters are left in place for the shortest possible time. It is helpful in the prophylaxis of infection to use valved catheters to prevent reflux. Diversion to the skin surface should be made in the upper part of the abdomen where the stoma is easier to fit with a collecting device and less frequently contaminated. Finally, a high fluid intake favors both eradication and prophylaxis of infection.

Surgical Treatment

In every case of obstructive uropathy, the obstruction should be relieved as soon as possible. In cases of idiopathic megaureter, the prognosis is better with early surgery. There may, however, be irreversible renal damage. The indication for surgery depends on the renal concentrating ability.

In all abnormalities of the ureterovesical junction, of whatever type, surgical reimplantation of the ureter with an antireflux procedure should be undertaken only when ureteral contractility appears satisfactory.[19, 24] Hence, whenever renal damage is an indication for surgery and the ureter appears atonic, the only solution is cutaneous ureterostomy, however disagreeable this may be. Subsequent treatment depends on the return to normal of ureteral contractility. If ureteral contraction becomes satisfactory, continuity of the urinary tract may be reestablished. Conversely, if ureteral contraction remains poor, uretero-ileal diversion may preserve or even improve renal function.

In unilateral uropathy, a decision must be made between removing and attempting to preserve the damaged kidney. It is essential in the first instance to be certain that the contralateral kidney and its excretory tract are absolutely normal. It is then necessary to study the function of each kidney separately and also to determine the state of the ureter on the diseased side. Without doubt, if the ureter is atonic and there is serious damage to the kidney, with marked hypertrophy of the opposite kidney, there is little chance that the diseased kidney will recover normal function. Furthermore, it may be a source of infection. Unfortunately, the position is not always so clear-cut in practice.

Medical Treatment

When there is a considerable defect in concentration it is helpful to restrict the osmotic load in the diet, but this should not be done if there is any possibility that a salt-losing syndrome is present. In practice, there is no need to worry about the salt loss unless the glomerular filtration rate is less than 25 ml./min./1.73 m.^{2} Hyperchloremic acidosis is an indication for a diet with a low chloride content and for sodium bicarbonate supplementation. A corresponding amount of sodium must be withheld from the diet. In all cases, a high fluid intake spread evenly over the 24 hours is helpful, provided that there is a normal ability to dilute the urine.

Hypertension can be cured surgically only when it is the result of the high urinary pressure or of strictly unilateral segmental hypoplasia. In all other cases it must be treated medically (see page 411). The treatment of renal osteodystrophy is considered elsewhere (page 404).

The decompression syndrome can be prevented by careful measurement of the output of water, sodium, and potassium in the days following surgery. Each day, the losses of the preceding day must be replaced by giving the total amount multiplied by a factor between 1.2 and 1.7.

Patients with an ileal loop diversion may require a bicarbonate supplement. The need for this supplementation is best decided by studying the urinary ammonium output on a normal diet and following an ammonium chloride load.

CONCLUSION

It is obvious that prevention of kidney damage in cases of malformation of the urinary tract depends on early diagnosis; unfortunately, however, the diagnosis is often late. Special emphasis must be placed on the neonatal assessment of micturition and on the importance of searching for urinary tract and certain other malformations.

The renal disorder in this type of uropathy is not uniform, and diminished concentrating ability is the first sign of renal damage.

Renal function often improves after surgery. At the very least, a normal balance of renal function is restored in relation to the number of residual nephrons. Hence, the success of any surgery is judged by studies of concentrating ability and of the renal regulation of acid-base balance.

The ultimate prognosis depends on the number of residual nephrons. This may be difficult to establish, but in practice it seems that measuring the glomerular filtration rate some weeks after surgery and determining the renal fixation of ^{197}Hg give the closest approximations of this number, and so these are the best parameters for determining the likelihood of kidney recovery. The degree of proteinuria is also a very significant factor.

The problem of ureteral contractility lies at the core of all decisions about abnormalities of the ureterovesical junction. Unfortunately, we still lack satisfactory methods of measuring ureteral function.

Every decision about treatment and management in cases of urinary tract malformation requires the collaboration of pediatric nephrologists, surgeons, biochemists, and bacteriologists. It is probable that closer collaboration will eventually improve the outlook for these malformations, whose prognosis remains unsatisfactory at the present time.

REFERENCES

1. Barratt, T. M., and Chantler, C.: Obstructive uropathy in infants. Proc. Roy. Soc. Med. *63*: 1248, 1970.
2. Ten Bensel, R. W., and Peters, E. R.: Progressive hydronephrosis, hydroureters, and dilatation of the bladder in siblings with congenital nephrogenic diabetes insipidus. J. Pediat. 77:439, 1970.
3. Berg, U., Aperia, A., Broberger, O., Ekengren, K., and Ericsson, N. O.: Relationship between glomerular filtration rate and radiological appearance of the renal parenchyma in children. Acta Paediat. Scand. *59*:1, 1970.
4. Bernstein, J.: The morphogenesis of renal parenchyma maldevelopment (renal dysplasia). Pediat. Clin. N. Amer. *18*:395, 1971.
5. Bricker, N. S.: Obstructive nephropathy. *In* M. B. Strauss and L. G. Welt: Diseases of the Kidney. Boston, Little, Brown & Co., 1963, p. 72.
6. Bricker, N. S., Klahr, S., Lubowitz, H., and Rieselbach, R. E.: Renal function in chronic renal disease. Medicine *44*:263, 1965.
7. Chaptal, J., Mathieu, H., Jean, R., and Habib, R.: Le rein au cours des uropathies obstructives. *In* XXe Congrès Pédiat. Langue franç. (volume 1). Nancy, 1965. Paris, Expansion Scientifique Française, 1965, p. 229.
8. Chapman, A., Gay, M., and Legrain, M.: La levée d'obstacle de la voie excrétrice urinaire. Étude de la fonction rénale et de l'équilibre hydro-électrolytique. Nephron 7:258, 1970.
9. Dunbar, J. S., and Nogrady, M. B.: The calyceal crescent. A roentgenographic sign of obstructive hydronephrosis. Amer. J. Roentgenol. *110*:520, 1970.
10. Eknoyan, G., Suki, W. N., Martinez-Maldonado, M., and Anhalt, M. A.: Chronic hydronephrosis: observations on the mechanism of the defect in urine concentration. Proc. Soc. Exp. Biol. Med. *134*:634, 1970.
11. Ericsson, N. O., and Ivemark, B. I.: I. Renal dysplasia and pyelonephritis in infants and children. Arch. Path. *66*:255, 1958.
12. Ericsson, N. O., and Ivemark, B. I.: II. Primitive ductules and abnormal glomeruli. Arch. Path. *66*:264, 1958.
13. Gagnadoux, M. F.: Le retentissement fonctionnel rénal des uropathies obstructives de l'enfant. Thèse méd., Université Paris V, 1970, U.E.R. Necker-Enfants-Malades.

14. Gillenwater, J. Y., Westerfelt, F. B., Vaughan, E. D., Jr., and Carter, C. B.: Impaired renal function in unilateral hydronephrosis. *In* Proceedings of the Fourth International Congress of Nephrology. Basel, S. Karger, 1969, p. 160.
15. Hodson, C. J., Drewe, J. A., Karn, M. N., and King, A.: Renal size in normal children. A radiographic study during life. Arch. Dis. Child. *37*:616, 1962.
16. Ladefoged, J., and Pedersen, F.: Relationship between roentgenological size of the kidney and the kidney function. J. Urol. *99*:239, 1968.
17. Legrain, M., Bitker, M., and Kuss, R.: Obstructive nephropathy in adults. *In* Proceedings f the Third International Congress of Nephrology (Washington 1966). Basel, S. Karger, 1967, Vol. 2, p. 336.
18. Mathieu, H., Chedru, M. F., Chalchat, M. A., Guedeney, J., and Chatelain, C.: Ionic disturbances in urinary ileal diversion. Third meeting, European Society of Paediatric Nephrology, 1969, p. 14.
19. Mathieu, H., and Gagnadoux, M. F.: Possibilités de récupération des fonctions rénales après intervention dans les uropathies malformatives de l'enfant. *In* Journées parisiennes de Pédiatrie. Paris, Flammarion, 1971, 0. 41.
20. McCory, W. W., Shibuya, M., Leumann, E., and Karp, R.: Studies of renal function in children with chronic hydronephrosis. Pediat. Clin. N. Amer. *18*:445, 1971.
21. Neimann, N., Manciaux, M., and Rachmut, H.: Dépistage et diagnostic précoce des uropathies obstructives. *In* XXᵉ Congrès Pédiat. Langue franç. (Volume 1), Nancy, 1965. Paris, Expansion Scientifique Française, 1965, p. 5.
22. Royer, P , Frézal, J., Bois, E., and Feingold, J.: Les néphropathies héréditaires. Arch. franç. Pediat. *27*:293, 1970.
23. Rubenstein, M., Meyer, R., and Bernstein, J.: Congenital abnormalities of the urinary system. I. A post-mortem survey of developmental anomalies and acquired congenital lesions in a children's hospital. J. Pediat. *58*:356, 1961.
24. Williams, D. I.: The ureter, the urologist and the paediatrician. Proc. Roy. Soc. Med. *63*:595, 1970.
25. Winberg, J.: Renal function studies in infants and children with acute nonobstructive urinary tract infection. Acta Paediat. (Uppsala) *48*:577, 1959.
26. Winberg, J.: Renal function in water-losing syndrome due to lower urinary tract obstruction before and after treatment. Acta Paediat. (Uppsala) *48*:149, 1959.
27. Zetterstrom, R., Ericsson, N. O., and Winberg, J.: Separate renal function studies in predominantly unilateral hydronephrosis. Acta Paediat. (Uppsala) *47*:540, 1958.

Chapter Four

NONBACTERIAL
INTERSTITIAL NEPHRITIS

Nonbacterial interstitial nephritis is characterized by initial damage to the interstitial tissue, exclusive or predominant, caused by a local nonsuppurative process.[7, 11, 16] Thus, "it must be fundamentally distinguished from pyelonephritides, interstitial lesions provoked by the local action of bacteria."[16] Much of the credit for defining this condition should be given to Zollinger.[16]

ACUTE INTERSTITIAL NEPHRITIS

This condition used to be relatively common as a complication of scarlet fever or diphtheria. Though these diseases are no longer frequently encountered, there is a resurgence of interest in acute interstitial nephritis because it may be provoked by various drugs.[5, 14] The etiology can not always be determined.[4]

Pathologic Anatomy[4, 7, 16]

The kidneys are enlarged and appear inflamed. The cortex and the columns of Bertin are pale and the papillae congested. The pelvis and major vessels are normal. Microscopic examination discloses infiltration of the interstitial tissue, either diffuse or localized around veins or arteries, particularly obvious at the corticomedullary junction. There is often edema. The proportion of histiocytes, lymphocytes, and plasmocytes varies, with plasmocytes predominating in the early stages and lymphocytes later. The density of the infiltration is variable. In some types, there is a large number of eosinophils. The glomeruli remain intact and the tubules are preserved or may show changes in their epithelium.

There is no difficulty in diagnosis. In the newborn child a similar appearance may be produced by persisting local hematopoiesis. The limited character of the tubular lesions differentiates them from tubular disorders secondary to certain poisons, hemolysis, shock, or burns. There is also interstitial infiltration in rejected homotransplanted kidneys.

Clinical Features[4]

Acute interstitial nephritis in children is, in our experience, uncommon. Zollinger, in a 10 year period, found 107 cases in a total of 10,000 autopsies.

175

The clinical features may suggest a tubular disorder: proteinuria and leuko-cyturia without hematuria or pyuria, continued diuresis, absence of edema, marked diminution of concentrating ability, and hyperchloremic acidosis. More often, there are no specific features. In some varieties, macroscopic or microscopic hematuria is the rule. A significant number of cases present with anuria. Hypertension is rare. The clinical picture is completed by symptoms peculiar to the causal diseases.

The condition declines over several weeks once the cause has been re-moved, and complete cure is obtained. Certain anuric forms formerly were very dangerous (108 deaths in 147 cases in Zollinger's statistics[16]), but the prognosis for such cases is now better.[6]

Etiology

The main causes of acute interstitial nephritis are indicated in Table 31. Some etiologic factors merit a special comment.

Infectious Diseases

The interstitial nephritis is not the result of local proliferation of bacteria, and the mechanism of the disease is poorly understood. Possible factors are the effect of bacterial toxins[16] and antigen-antibody reactions.[6]

In acute interstitial nephritis occurring as a complication of scarlet fever or typhoid fever, the infiltration is predominantly perivascular, but in lepto-spirosis, the infiltration is diffuse and most marked at the corticomedullary junc-tion.[16] A case of acute interstitial nephritis was described recently as a compli-cation of infection with the beta hemolytic streptococcus.[6] As well as diffuse infiltration, there was tubular necrosis, with swelling of the cells and fragmenta-tion of the basement membrane observed on electron microscopy.

We have seen two cases of uncertain but probably infectious etiology

Table 31.   Causes of Acute Interstitial Nephritis

Infections	Streptococcus Scarlet fever Diphtheria Typhoid fever Leptospirosis Unidentified infection, with iridocyclitis
Antibiotics	Colistin Polymyxin B } Direct action Kanamycin Amphotericin
	Penicillin Methicillin } Allergy Sulfonamides
Various drugs	Phenindione Para-aminosalicylic acid Bismuth (thioglycolate) Phenylbutazone

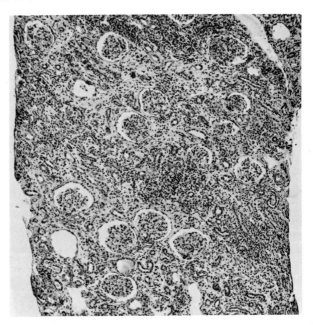

Figure 39. Renal biopsy from a case of acute interstitial nephritis with iridocyclitis. Note the intense round cell infiltration. This boy, aged 8 years, had proteinuria, leukocyturia, moderate renal insufficiency and bilateral iridocyclitis. He was treated with steroids and after four months he was permanently cured. Etiology could not be established.

in which diffuse infiltration of the kidney was associated with *iridocyclitis* that persisted for six months and disappeared completely (Figure 39).

Colistin[1, 5, 13]

Colistin has a direct toxic action on the kidney. The kidney is not usually damaged unless the daily dose is high, of the order of 10 million units/1.73 m.^{2}/day given intravenously. The toxic dose is lower in cases of renal insufficiency. The renal disorder is preceded by nausea, vomiting, and neurologic disorders, including paresthesia of the limbs and circumoral region, vertigo, ataxia, hypotonia and loss of tendon reflexes, and convulsions. There may be clouding of consciousness and behavior disturbances in the absence of any water or electrolyte imbalance. The renal insufficiency is progressive and often latent. Hence, it must be sought by routine estimation of blood urea and creatinine levels. The renal disorder generally resolves in a matter of weeks or months.

Some other antibiotics are nephrotoxic and can cause similar complications (Table 32). The renal toxicity of gentamycin is low and much less to be feared than its ototoxicity.

Penicillin and Methicillin[3]

Renal damage probably results from a combination of direct toxic action and allergy. It generally follows the administration of high doses, such as 20 to 60 million units of penicillin G per 1.73 m.^{2} per day or 20 to 24 g. of methicillin per 1.73 m.^{2} per day. Renal damage is much more common with methicillin than with penicillin G. After an interval, which varies from 8 to 44 days, the temperature rises and a morbilliform rash appears, with marked eosinophilia being present. Kidney involvement is revealed by a hematuria that is often

Table 32.   Renal Toxicity of Various Antibiotics

Medication	Toxic (T) or Allergic (A) Effect	Degree	Type of Lesion		
			Interstitial	Tubular	Calcareous Deposits
Gentamycin	T	±	?	+?	0
Colistin	T	+	+++	+	0
Kanamycin	T	+	+++		
Polymyxin B	T	+	Hyperemia with eosinophils	+	0
Bacitracin	T	+++	++	++	+
Amphotericin	T	+++	++	++	+++
Penicillin G	A, rare		+++	±	0
Methicillin	A, rare		+++	±	0
Sulfonamides	A or T, rare		+++ (A)	+ (T)	0
Tetracyclines (out-of-date)	T	++	0	++ (proximal)	0
Cephaloridine	T	+	0	++ (acute)	
Neomycin	T	+++	0	+++	0
Beta-lactamines					
Cephalothin					
Chloramphenicol	0	0	0	0	0
Streptomycin					
Oligosaccharides					
Cycline					

macroscopic, proteinuria, and a variable degree of disturbance of renal function. Circulating antibodies can sometimes be found by immunologic tests, and skin sensitivity tests may be positive. The situation returns to normal in a matter of weeks. Only one case has been recorded in which the anuria persisted, with a fatal outcome, and in that case penicillin therapy had been continued.

The interstitial infiltration of the kidney is diffuse. It consists of lymphocytes and eosinophils, but not plasmocytes. The glomeruli and vessels are normal. The tubules in the cortex may be damaged and even necrosed. Specific antibodies have been localized by immunofluorescent techniques in the zones of tubular necrosis and in the basement membranes of the tubules and the glomeruli.

The *sulfonamides* can produce a similar clinical picture quite apart from the anuric complications arising from their precipitation within the tubules.

Phenindione

This commonly used anticoagulant may affect the kidney in two ways, producing (1) a proteinuria with or without a nephrotic syndrome, and (2) chiefly, acute interstitial nephritis. This nephritis is allergic in type. It appears after a latent interval ranging from 11 days to 7 weeks. The renal disturbance is but one of a whole series of allergic manifestations that includes pyrexia, erythema of various types—sometimes bullous, sometimes purpuric—eosinophilia, hepatomegaly, occasionally with cholestatic jaundice. The onset is insidious, often with hematuria followed frequently by anuria. The mortality is high, in the region of 50 per cent. The interstitial infiltration is diffuse, consisting of lymphocytes and plasmocytes and also polynuclear cells, with a high proportion of eosinophils. The prognosis is improved by the use of steroids and symptomatic treatment of the renal insufficiency.

CHRONIC NONBACTERIAL INTERSTITIAL NEPHRITIS

This differs from chronic bacterial pyelonephritis by (1) the absence of urinary infection, (2) the fibrous rather than cellular nature of the interstitial lesions and the absence of polynuclear cells, abscesses, and pelvic infection, and (3) the presence of particular causes, whether genetic, geographic, toxic, or metabolic.

Excluded from this group are the cases of fibrocellular infiltration of the interstitial tissue that at various stages of their evolution may complicate different nephropathies, such as, for example, glomerular diseases, partial necrosis of the renal cortex, some nephrotic syndromes of young children (nephrotic syndrome with complex tubular insufficiency), uninfected hydronephrosis, Alport's syndrome, oligomeganephronia, and certain hereditary nephropathies, such as cystinosis and oxalosis.

Finally, it is important to emphasize the fundamental difference between chronic interstitial nephritis and segmental hypoplasia of the kidney, in which the interstitial infiltration consists of foci of tubular cells and includes very severe vascular lesions (see page 16).

Clinical Features

There is fatigue, polyuria, polydipsia, and moderate proteinuria of the mixed type, in which there is albuminuria and triple globulinuria.[15] Anemia presents early. Hypertension is rare in our experience. Glomerular filtration and para-aminohippuric acid clearance diminish late and together. The filtration fraction remains normal. For a long time, the principal disorder of renal function is defective concentration of urine and a tubular acidosis of the proximal type, with loss of bicarbonate. Urinary loss of sodium or potassium, or both, is also common, and there may be glycosuria or hypophosphatemia. The disease develops very slowly but inevitably progresses to chronic uremia.

The clinical picture may vary according to the cause.

Etiology

Chronic Interstitial Nephritis Caused by Analgesics

The most important cause of analgesic nephropathy is phenacetin. For a long time, the interstitial nephritis is reversible if the patient stops taking phenacetin. Complications include hemolytic anemia and papillary necrosis. Because of the doses and length of time necessary to produce an analgesic nephropathy, this type is unlikely to occur in children. The same can be said for chronic fluoride, beryllium, and cadmium poisoning.[1]

Chronic Interstitial Nephritis of Metabolic Origin

This is seen as a complication of potassium depletion, hypercalcemia, and hyperuricemia.[2]

Potassium Depletion.   Both in experimental animals and in man, potassium depletion causes vacuolization in the tubules and, in the long run, an interstitial nephropathy that may not be reversible.[2, 8] Conditions that are accompanied by potassium depletion in children include distal tubular acidosis, cystinosis, and idiopathic De Toni-Debré-Fanconi syndrome. This potassium depletion is probably responsible for some of the chemical and anatomic features of these conditions. It is above all in Bartter's syndrome (see page 58) that this situation is accentuated in childhood. In addition to the hypertrophy of the juxtaglomerular apparatus and the vacuolization of the proximal tubule, some patients may develop a variable degree of interstitial fibrosis leading to serious uremia. A role for potassium depletion in the development of this situation is possible but has not been proved.

Hypercalcemia and Hypercalciuria.   When these conditions, regardless of their cause, are present for a long time, they can produce chronic interstitial nephritis often accompanied by nephrocalcinosis that can be identified on x-ray films or in renal biopsy specimens (see page 184).

We have often found foci of chronic interstitial nephritis in cases of idiopathic hypercalciuria, but the significance of this finding is not obvious (see page 65).

Hyperuricemic Nephropathy.[12]   In addition to the renal complications of uric acid lithiasis, with or without infection, there is also a hyperuricemic nephropathy.

Hyperuricemia is rarer in childhood than in adult life, gout being quite exceptional. Possible causes include physiologic hyperuricemia of the newborn, rapid cell destruction during treatment for leukemia and malignant tumors, terminal renal failure, and organic acidoses (ketosis and lactic, propionic, and methylmalonic acidoses) that block the tubular secretion of uric acid.

Various renal disorders may be induced by hyperuricemia, including medullary urate infarcts in the newborn; tubular blockage by crystals and a tubulo-interstitial reaction with acute renal failure in periods of rapid cell destruction; and chronic interstitial nephropathy with crystals of uric acid in the renal parenchyma. These findings have been noted in type 1 glycogenosis with lactic acidosis, and we have seen a similar picture in methylmalonic acidemia. Chronic hyperuricemic tubulo-interstitial nephropathy is an important localization of hereditary hyperuricemia with sex-linked recessive transmission (syndrome of Lesch-Nyhan). In one of our cases, pitressin-resistant polyuria was the first symptom (see page 78) (Figure 40).

Hyperuricemic nephropathy is prevented and treated by allopurinol (Zyloric), a xanthine oxidase inhibitor, given in doses of 200 to 400 mg./1.73 m.[2]/day.

In hyperuricemia secondary to chronic renal failure, the lesions of hyperuricemic nephropathy may be superimposed on those of the causal kidney

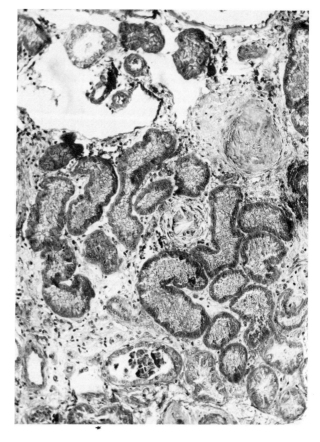

Figure 40. Hyperuricemic chronic interstitial nephritis in a boy of 14 years with the Lesch-Nyhan syndrome. The renal disorder presented the clinical picture of a vasopressin-resistant diabetes insipidus. Note, in addition to the intersitial fibrosis, the presence of a uric acid crystal in the center of the preparation.

disease. This secondary hyperuricemia is a constant feature of terminal uremia in children and is little affected by maintenance dialysis (see page 378).

Primary Chronic Interstitial Nephritis

Hereditary Chronic Interstitial Nephritis.   The oculo-cerebro-renal syndrome of Lowe may progress to chronic interstitial nephritis after a lengthy period.[9] Nevertheless, the most characteristic type of hereditary chronic interstitial nephritis is nephronophthisis with or without tapetoretinal degeneration (see page 42).

Balkan Nephropathy.[10]   This is a peculiar endemic nephropathy that occurs in certain districts of Bulgaria, Rumania, and Yugoslavia and in some wooded regions of Canada and Scandinavia. The disease may be found in children, adolescents, and adults. It has not been possible so far to detect specific genetic or environmental etiologic factors, but persons who emigrate from the regions in which the disease is endemic are not affected. The lesion consists of a tubulo-interstitial nephropathy going on to total sclerosis and atrophy of the kidneys. The principal symptoms are polyuria and polydipsia without hypertension. The condition progresses to chronic uremia without going through any stage of the nephrotic syndrome.

Sporadic Chronic Interstitial Nephritis.   Cases of this type may be seen in children. The various causes already mentioned should be sought for and excluded. The majority are cases of nephronophthisis that appear isolated because there are few children in the family or because the chances for this condition to appear (hereditary distribution) are slight (see page 44).

CONCLUSIONS

Acute and chronic nonbacterial interstitial nephropathy must be distinguished clearly from bacterial pyelonephritis. Clinical and laboratory features, etiology, and treatment are entirely different. The current interest in these conditions is focused on the role of certain drugs, metabolic disorders, and genetic and geographic factors that are still poorly understood.

REFERENCES

1. Amiel, C.: Néphrites interstitielles toxiques. Rev. Prat. (Paris) *16*:2233, 1966.
2. Ardaillou, R.: Les néphrites interstitielles d'origine métabolique. Rev. Prat. (Paris) *16*:2247, 1966.
3. Baldwin, D. S., Levine, B. B., McCluskey, R. T., and Gallo, G. G.: Renal failure after interstitial nephritis due to penicillin and methicillin. New Eng. J. Med. *279*:1245, 1968.
4. Chazan, J. A., Garella, S., and Esparza, A.: Acute interstitial nephritis. A distinct clinicopathological entity? Nephron *9*:10, 1972.
5. Fillastre, J. P., Morel-Maroger, L., Mignon, F., and Mery, J. P.: Néphropathies aiguës médicamenteuses. *In* Actualités néphrologiques de l'Hôpital Necker. Paris, Flammarion, 1969, p. 155.
6. Knepshied, J. H., Carstens, P. H. B., and Gentile, D. E.: Recovery from renal failure due to acute diffuse interstitial nephritis. Pediatrics *43*:533, 1969.
7. Morel-Maroger, L., and Verger, D.: Anatomie pathologique des néphrites interstitielles. Rev. Prat. (Paris) *16*:2143, 1966.
8. Muehrcke, R. C., and McMillan, J. C.: The relationship of "chronic pyelonephritis" to chronic potassium deficiency. Ann. Intern. Med. *59*:427, 1963.
9. Ores, R. O.: Renal changes in oculo-cerebro-renal syndrome of Lowe. Arch. Pathol. *89*:221, 1970.
10. Popov, N. G.: La néphropathie endémique des Balkans. Rev. Prat. (Paris) *16*:2247, 1966.
11. Richet, G.: Place des néphrites interstitielles parmi les affections rénales. Rev. Prat. (Paris) *16*:2139, 1966.
12. Royer, P.: L'hyperuricémie héréditaire précoce avec troubles neurologiques et rénaux. *In* Actualités néphrologiques de l'Hôpital Necker. Paris, Flammarion, 1968, p. 301.
13. Schreiner, G. E., and Maher, J. F.: Toxic nephropathy. Amer. J. Med. *38*:409, 1965.
14. Simenhoff, M. K., Guild, W. R., and Dammin, G. J.: Acute diffuse interstitial nephritis. Review of the literature and case report. Amer. J. Med. *44*:618, 1968.
15. Traeger, J., Revillard, J. P., and Manuel, Y.: La protéinurie des néphrites interstitielles. Rev. Prat. (Paris) *16*:2183, 1966.
16. Zollinger, H. U.: Interstitial nephritis. *In* F. P. Mostofi and D. E. Smith, eds.: The Kidney. Baltimore, Williams & Wilkins, 1966, p. 269.

Chapter Five

NEPHROCALCINOSIS AND THE KIDNEY IN HYPERCALCEMIA

Nephrocalcinosis signifies an orderly deposition of calcium salts in the renal parenchyma. Depending on the intensity of the deposition, the condition may be obvious on radiologic examination (so-called "radiologic nephrocalcinosis") or on histologic examination of biopsy or autopsy specimens (so-called "histologic nephrocalcinosis"). Calcareous deposits visible on microscopy are found in 15 to 20 per cent of autopsies in adults.[16] They were also found in 60 of 1475 autopsies (57 of these patients under the age of 2 years) that we performed in children,[20] an incidence of 8 per cent. Radiologic nephrocalcinosis is rare. Incidences of 7 in 1418[14] and 27 in 9000[1] have been reported. Wenzl and his colleagues[22] found six cases, compared with 77 cases of lithiasis, in a period of 25 years at the Mayo Clinic. We have seen 31 cases in 15 years (Table 33).

Table 33. Severe Nephrocalcinosis in Childhood
(Personal Series, 1955–1970)

	Nephrocalcinosis Detected	
Cause	Radiologically	Histologically
Bilateral cortical necrosis	0	2
Xanthogranulomatous pyelonephritis	0	6
Oxalosis	7	4
Distal tubular acidosis (gradient type)	10	4
Vitamin D poisoning	4	6
Hypercalcemia with elfin facies	1	4
Idiopathic hypercalciuria	2	2
Hypophosphatasia	1	1
Precocious metaphyseal dysostosis	1	?
Thyroid deficiency	1	4
Familial hypercholesterolemia	1	1
Calcifying arterial disease	0	1
Immobilization (paraplegia)	1	?
Cause unknown	2	3
Total	31	38

Nephrocalcinosis may at times complicate various diseases of infants and children. The mechanism of the abnormal deposition has been clarified by experimental work, including electron microscopy[2, 4, 7] and microanalysis by electron probe.[2, 7]

Clinical Features

In most cases, nephrocalcinosis is clinically silent. There may be symptoms of urinary lithiasis or of renal insufficiency. Diagnosis depends on radiology and on histologic study of renal biopsy specimens.

Radiology

A plain film with no other preparation than gastric insufflation may provide a picture varying from small specks to large opacities outlining the papillae or even diffuse opacity of the entire kidney parenchyma. The calcifications may be located in the papillae, in the medulla, in the corticomedullary region, or in the cortex. There may be associated lithiasis or arterial calcification (Figure 41).

Renal Biopsy

We prefer semi-open biopsy to avoid taking too deep a fragment. There are three important points to be noted: Bouin's solution should not be used as a fixative because it may dissolve the calcium deposits; the hardness of the deposits creates difficulties in cutting fragments embedded in paraffin; and, lastly, special precautions are necessary in making preparations for electron microscopy to avoid detachment of the deposits.

The nature of the deposits may be shown by Von Kossa's stain for phosphates, by polarized light demonstrating the birefractive calcium oxalate crystals, and by microanalysis by electron probe.

Localization of the deposits is variable, and one particular segment of the

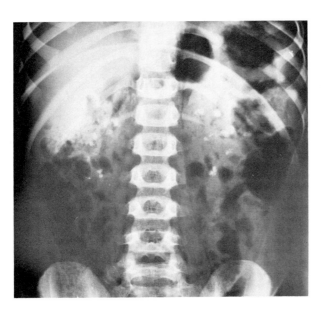

Figure 41. Plain x-ray film of the abdomen in a child suffering from oxalosis. Dense opacities of nephrocalcinosis can be seen in each renal area, as well as several calculi.

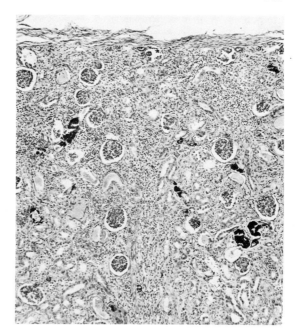

Figure 42. Nephrocalcinosis in a child with idiopathic hypercalcemia and elfin facies. Very dense calcium deposits can be seen, and there is also an intense interstitial reaction.

nephrons or the interstitial tissue may be affected. Even the localization within the cells may vary; the calcific deposits may be in the basement membrane or within the cell cytoplasm or in the tubular lumen. The exact significance of these different distributions in human pathology is not yet known. The nephrocalcinosis of chronic tubular acidosis is localized to the medulla, having a radial disposition, whereas in hypercalcemia and vitamin D intoxication the nephrocalcinosis is diffuse, with no special pattern. The renal arterioles may be calcified, which seems to be a particular hallmark of vitamin D poisoning. The adjacent renal parenchyma may be healthy or affected to a varying degree by interstitial nephritis (Figure 42).

Evolution

When there is a permanent cause for the nephrocalcinosis, the deposits tend to increase in both extent and intensity. When the cause can be removed or compensated for by treatment, the nephrocalcinosis may stabilize or even regress. This has been noted in cases of parathyroid adenoma, vitamin D poisoning, and prolonged immobilization.

In both men and animals, the calcific deposits in the renal parenchyma are responsible for urinary calculus formation on deposits detached from the papilla and for the development of chronic sclerosing interstitial nephritis leading ultimately to renal failure and hypertension (see page 179, *Chronic Nonbacterial Interstitial Nephritis*).

Etiology

Intense diffuse progressive nephrocalcinosis presents an important practical problem because of the risk of serious and progressive renal insufficiency. The causes in children are summarized in Table 34.

Table 34.   Causes of Nephrocalcinosis in Children

1. *Nephrocalcinosis secondary to kidney disease:*
   Medullary sponge kidney.
   Cortical necrosis, either partial or maintained on hemodialysis.
   Xanthogranulomatous pyelonephritis.
   Various other conditions.

2. *Oxalosis* (hyperoxaluria of types I and II).

3. *Disordered acid-base balance with alkaline urine:*
   Distal tubular acidosis.
   Bartter's syndrome.
   Overload of alkali.

4. *Hypercalcemia and/or hypercalciuria:*
   Immobilization.
   Vitamin D excess.
   Idiopathic hypercalcemia.
   Idiopathic hypercalciuria.
   Hyperparathyroidism.
   Hypothyroidism.
   Hyperthyroidism.
   Hypophosphatasia.
   Precocious metaphyseal dysostosis.
   "Blue diaper" syndrome.

5. *Calcification of renal vessels:*
   Calcifying arterial disease.
   Severe familial hypercholesterolemia.

Many of these causes are considered in other sections of the book, including renal cortical necrosis (page 23); precalyceal canalicular ectasia (page 24); xanthogranulomatous pyelonephritis (page 155); oxalosis (page 65); distal tubular acidosis (page 70); and idiopathic hypercalciuria (page 65).

Intrarenal calcification residing in fact in the walls of the arteries and arterioles may be found in the calcifying arteriopathy of infants and in severe cases of familial hypercholesterolemia (cutaneotendinous xanthomatosis). In three of our cases of nephrocalcinosis, there was no obvious cause; one was a case of familial nephrocalcinosis with pigmented retinitis, the second was a case of hypertension with nephrocalcinosis, and the third was a rapidly fatal nephrotic syndrome with intratubular precipitation of calcium.

Special emphasis should be laid on the *renal disorders associated with hypercalcemia.*[5, 6]

Hypercalcemia causes a functional nephropathy with lowering of glomerular filtration, of renal plasma flow, and of the TmPAH. Three tubular abnormalities are common—increased urinary output of sodium and potassium, defective tubular reabsorption of water with pitressin-resistant polyuria, and an increased urinary excretion of hydrogen ions with aciduria and metabolic alkalosis or sometimes, conversely, a disorder of ammoniogenesis. In hyperparathyroidism, the specific action of parathormone causes defective bicarbonate reabsorption and acidosis despite the hypercalcemia. These disorders can be reversed until there is diffuse nephrocalcinosis with interstitial nephritis. Many causes of hypercalcemia are therefore factors in nephrocalcinosis.

Vitamin D Intoxication

This may occur in children as a result of therapeutic mistakes or as a complication of the use of high doses of vitamin D in the treatment of chronic hypoparathyroidism or idiopathic vitamin-resistant rickets.[13, 15, 21] The compounds concerned include cholecalciferol, ergocalciferol, and dihydrotachysterol. The current practice of using 25-hydroxycholecalciferol (and possibly dihydroxylated derivatives in the near future) may run the risk of producing hypercalcemia and nephrocalcinosis because of the suppression of the normal regulation of the activation of vitamin D.

The clinical picture includes renal, alimentary, neurologic, and psychic disorders, and failure to grow. X-ray studies reveal increased density of the metaphyses and sometimes demineralization of the diaphyses. The urinary calcium output may rise before the blood calcium level rises. Soft tissue calcification may develop around the joints, in various viscera, in the arteries, and in subcutaneous tissue. In the cornea, there is calcific band keratopathy, which is capable of regression if the excessive intake of vitamin D is stopped.

The nephrocalcinosis is usually microscopic and rarely visible on x-ray films. In experimental pathology, the calcium deposits are found initially in the basement membrane of not only the proximal tubules, as in calcium overload situations, but also the medullary and distal tubules.[7] Bowman's capsule may also be calcified. The deposits consist of a collection of small rounded granules containing calcium and phosphorus in well-defined proportions, very similar to those found in microcrystals of hydroxyapatite. There are associated cell lesions[19] and calcareous deposits in the intima of the arterioles. These deposits may extend to involve all the arteries and even such large vessels as the aorta.

The pathophysiology of these lesions presents difficult problems. In the rat, the calcifications are not dependent on the hypercalcemia but on the vitamin D itself.[6, 10] This constantly produces a disorder of cell function with defective oxidative phosphorylation in the mitochondria and diminished uptake of calcium.[19] There are also degenerative lesions of the arterial walls.[6] These lesions apparently precede the mineral deposition.[19] The increased urinary calcium output is a better indicator of excessive intake of the vitamin than is the rise in plasma calcium.[11]

The prognosis in vitamin D intoxication is probably favorable if the condition is recognized in time. Most of the disorders can regress even when there are discrete foci of nephrocalcinosis. Death may occur in the acute phase from dehydration or vascular disorder.[6] The long-term prognosis should perhaps be guarded if there is serious renal involvement, hypertension, or any vascular disorder (Table 35).

The treatment is above all preventive. Excessive vitamin D dosage must be avoided; in most cases, 1000 I.U. per day is quite enough. In cases of vitamin-resistant rickets and hypoparathyroidism, the therapeutic doses should be lowered when the urinary calcium reaches 4 mg./kg./day or the blood calcium rises above 10.5 mg. per 100 ml.[11]

Once intoxication occurs, treatment includes stopping administration of the vitamin, instituting a low calcium diet, and the administration of cortisone. With very severe hypercalcemia, it is important to prevent dehydration. It may be helpful to use intravenous chelating agents or thyrocalcitonin in doses of 10 to 25 M.R.C. units/m.[2]

Table 35.   Serial Study of Two Cases of Vitamin D Poisoning

Dates*	Age (months)	Height (cm.)	Weight (kg.)	Blood Pressure (mm. Hg)	Serum Calcium (mg./100 ml.)	Urinary Calcium (mg./kg./day)	Glomerular Filtration Rate (ml./min./1.73 m.²)
September 1970	18	71	7.440	95/50	10.8	5.5	75
June 1971	26	83	11.700	105/50	10.4	2.7	105

*This patient is a boy born March 17, 1970, who had acute vitamin D poisoning with moderate histologic nephrocalcinosis. The principal effect is on tubular function, with defective concentration, inadequate lowering of urine pH, and defective excretion of ammonia. A cure was obtained in a matter of months.

Dates†	Age (months)	Height (cm.)	Weight (kg.)	Blood Pressure (mm. Hg)	Blood Calcium (mg./100 ml.)	Urinary Calcium (mg./kg./day)	Glomerular Filtration Rate (ml./min./1.73 m.²)
September 1971	23	75	7.100	160/100	11.5	20	41
February 1972	28	78	8.650	120/60	10.2	3	60

†This patient is a girl born September 28, 1969, who had prolonged vitamin D poisoning with severe histologic nephrocalcinosis. This child was studied two months after stopping administration of vitamin D. There is persistent hypercalcemia and moderate hypertension, and the renal damage affects all functions. The rise in cholesterol and lipid levels should also be noted. There was little improvement in a period of five months.

Idiopathic Hypercalcemia with Special Facies[6]

This syndrome appears soon after birth and presents with alimentary and renal disorders, defective growth, a cardiac murmur, hypertension, disorders of psychomotor development, and hypotonia. The facial appearance is very striking. The forehead is wide, and its central part protrudes. Commonly there is epicanthus with a convergent squint. The bridge of the nose is flattened, and there is hypoplasia of the lower jaw with prominence of the upper lip and drooping cheeks. The ears are large, prominent, and placed low on the skull. There are also dental abnormalities. There are often complex vascular abnormalities, including supravalvular aortic stenosis, stenosis of the pulmonary arteries, and more or less extensive hypoplasia of the aorta, with stenosis of various arteries, such as the renal and mesenteric arteries.

The blood pressure is often raised. The reasons for this are complex and include hypercalcemic nephropathy, aortic stenosis, renal artery stenosis, and sometimes even associated segmental hypoplasia of the kidneys. There is always mental disorder, with a very low IQ, inability to learn, and apathy or sometimes agitation during hypercalcemic phases. The serum calcium level may vary from 11.0 to 16.5 mg. per 100 ml. and may vary by as much as 2 or 3 mg. per 100 ml. in the course of a single day. The urinary calcium output is elevated. The intestinal coefficient of absorption of calcium is raised. The bones are dense and osteosclerotic, with a thick cortex and a succession of opaque metaphyseal bands. The centers of ossification in the epiphyses have a cockade ap-

Table 35.   Serial Study of Two Cases of Vitamin D Poisoning — *Continued*

| Urine Osmolarity in Dehydration (mOsm./kg.) | *Urine Studies with Short Course of NH₄Cl* | | | |
	Lowest Urine pH	Titratable Acidity	NH₄ (μEq./min./1.73 m.²)	H⁺
436	5.8	45	63	106
967	4.9	43	116	159

| Urine Osmolarity in Dehydration (mOsm./kg.) | *Urine Tests with Ammonium Chloride Loading* | | | | | |
	Lowest Urine pH	Titratable Acidity	NH₄	H⁺ (μEq./min./1.73 m.²)	Cholesterol (mg. per 100 ml.)	Lipids (mg. per 100 ml.)
429	4.9	19	30	49	440	1210
490	5.2	18	40	58	240	600

pearance, with a very dense center. The clinical features of the renal disorder are those found in any hypercalcemia. Discrete nephrocalcinosis is often visible radiologically, with a distribution similar to that found in vitamin D poisoning. There may also be calcareous deposits in other tissues.

With time, the disorders of calcium metabolism and the skeletal abnormalities regress, but the prognosis is poor because of the dysmorphia, the neurologic disorder and mental retardation, the cardiac malformations and hypertension, and the renal impairment.

It is of some nosologic interest that a similar syndrome has been described by Williams and Beuren, in which there is the same type of dysmorphia and cardiac and vascular malformations, but there is no disorder of calcium metabolism and no nephrocalcinosis.

The disease sets in during intrauterine life, and the exact stage can often be determined by the type of cardiovascular malformation. Vitamin D poisoning in pregnant rabbits reproduces the same pattern of cardiovascular malformation. The condition has been found several times in monozygous twins and triplets, but as yet it is impossible to say if the condition is hereditary or a result of some embryopathy.

It has been suggested that the disease results from disordered vitamin D metabolism or more generally from disordered sterol metabolism, but there is a good deal of evidence against this hypothesis.

The treatment is the same as in vitamin D intoxication. Thyroid extract has been used, with a favorable effect on the general condition and bone lesions, but without improvement in the hypercalcemia. The action of thyrocalcitonin is variable; we have used it successfully, in association with a low-calcium diet, to lower the blood calcium in some of our patients.

Primary Hyperparathyroidism[6]

This condition is rare in children, and parathyroid adenoma is seldom found before the age of 8 years. When it does occur, the clinical picture differs in no way from that seen in adults.

A more special problem is presented by hyperparathyroidism of the newborn owing to diffuse clear-cell hyperplasia of all the parathyroid glands. This disease is probably hereditary, of the autosomal recessive type. The infant exhibits severe dehydration and gross hypercalcemia. Sometimes the disease does not present until later in infancy. The prognosis is poor.

Nephrocalcinosis is common, and experimental studies[2, 4] have shown that the calcium is deposited in the cell cytoplasm, in the tubular lumen, and in the basement membranes. The intracytoplasmic deposits are in the form of needles. They are independent of intracellular organelles, although they are associated with mitochondrial lesions. The calcific deposits contain calcium, phosphorus, magnesium, and oxygen, and the intratubular deposits also contain sulfur. The deposits in the basement membranes are dense and rounded and contain only phosphorus and calcium. Often the main deposits are in the proximal tubules. Identical lesions have been seen in a patient with a parathyroid adenoma.[2] The physiopathology is determined by the hypercalciuria, the hyperphosphaturia, and the mobilization of mucopolysaccharides by the parathyroid hormone.

Nephrocalcinosis Owing to Immobilization

This formerly was common but today is rare because prophylaxis is better. Immobilization, for whatever reason, provokes considerable osteolysis and consequent hypercalcemia, hypercalciuria, and ultimately nephrocalcinosis of the same type as that seen with calcium overloads. In our experience, sodium phosphate is more likely to be effective in reducing the urinary calcium level than is calcitonin.

Thyroid Deficiency Nephrocalcinosis[18]

Both macroscopic and microscopic nephrocalcinosis has been seen in thyroid deficiency states in children, both before and after treatment.

There are marked associated abnormalities of phosphorus and calcium metabolism, including hypercalcemia, hypercalciuria (in some cases), osteosclerosis, and increased absorption of calcium from the gut. The fundamental disorder is probably slowing of bone metabolism with diminished accretion and especially osteolysis. Thus, the hypothyroid patient has little defense against stimulus to hypercalcemia, such as increased dietary intake of calcium or vitamin D, calcium perfusion, or parathormone injection. In such circumstances, both the blood and urinary calcium levels rise considerably. Conversely, ethylenediamine tetraacetic acid (EDTA) is poorly tolerated and produces prolonged hypocalcemia, which may prove dangerous. The absence of thyroxine is more important than the absence of thyrocalcitonin in these situations.

Prevention of nephrocalcinosis depends on early diagnosis, although it may exist in the first months of life. When osteosclerosis is present, treatment with thyroid extract must be carried out cautiously and the dose varied according to the urinary calcium output. There are reports of nephrocalcinosis being brought on by treatment.

Various Other Causes

In children, hypercalcemia and hypercalciuria may occur as a complication of leukemia and of the bone metastases of neuroblastomas. There is rarely time for nephrocalcinosis to develop.

Some hereditary bone disorders may be accompanied by hypercalcemia, hypercalciuria, and even nephrocalcinosis. These include hypophosphatasia, precocious metaphyseal dysostosis, and the "blue diaper" disease with indicanuria.

The recent introduction of high doses of orthophosphate in treatment of hypercalcemia and hypercalciuria raises the possibility that patients so treated may subsequently develop nephrocalcinosis. Experimentally, a phosphate overload provokes nephrocalcinosis[7, 12] with crystalline deposits containing calcium and phosphorus in specific proportions occurring in the cytoplasm of the tubular cells. It has been suggested that phosphate therapy may have been responsible for some cases of human nephrocalcinosis.[3] There is no doubt that phosphate therapy must not be introduced without careful consideration and proper monitoring of the renal status.

Conclusions

Nephrocalcinosis is rare in children. The causes have been clearly established. Because the future course of nephrocalcinosis in children is uncertain, it is probably important to emphasize practical rules of preventing this disorder. Prevention depends above all on early diagnosis of the underlying disorder.

In idiopathic distal tubular renal acidosis the corrected dose of bicarbonate is not that which restores the blood pH to normal but that which reduces the hypercalciuria.

In treatment or prophylaxis of rickets, not more than 5 to 10 mg. of vitamin D should be given in any one year.

Whenever large doses of vitamin D are indicated, the urinary calcium output must be monitored. Administration of the vitamin must be discontinued if the urinary calcium output rises above 4 mg./kg./day.

If a child must be immobilized, it is dangerous to prescribe calcium and vitamin D. The best way to prevent decalcification and the risks of nephrocalcinosis is to ensure normal bone metabolism by early mobilization, and, if necessary, by the use of a mechanical turning device.

It is essential to avoid the intemperate intake of calcium, phosphates, and alkalis.

If the diagnosis is late, the treatment of congenital myxedema, or cretinism, must be monitored by regular estimations of blood and urine calcium.

REFERENCES

1. Antoine, B., Provenzal, O., and Watchi, J. M.: Néphrocalcinoses. Rev. Prat. (Paris) *16*:4067, 1966.

2. Berry, J. P.: Néphrocalcinose expérimentale par injection de parathormone. Etude au micro-analyseur à sonde électronique. Nephron, 7:97, 1970.
3. Breur, R. I., and Le Bauer, J.: Caution in the use of phosphates in the treatment of severe hypercalcemia. J. Clin. Endocr. 27:695, 1967.
4. Caulfield, J. B., and Schrag, P. E.: Electron microscopy study of renal calcification. Amer. J. Path. 44:365, 1964.
5. Epstein, F. H.: Calcium and the kidney. Amer. J. Med. 45:700, 1968.
6. Fourman, P., and Royer, P.: Calcium et tissue osseux. Paris, Flammarion, 1970.
7. Galle, P.: Les néphrocalcinoses: nouvelles données d'ultra-structure et de microanalyse. In Actualités Néphrologiques de l'Hôpital Necker. Paris, Flammarion, 1967, p. 303.
8. Györy, A. Z., Edward, K. D. G., Robinson, J., and Palmer, A. A.: The relative importance of urinary pH and urinary content of citrate, magnesium and calcium in the production of nephrocalcinosis by diet and acetazolamide in the rat. Clin. Sci. 39:605, 1970.
9. Harrison, A. R., and Ghose, R. R.: Nephrocalcinosis. Proc. Roy. Soc. Med. 56:925, 1963.
10. Mathieu, H., Cuisinier-Gleizes, P., Habib, R., Dulac, H., Lacoste, M., Gyrard, E., and Royer, P.: Action toxique de la vitamine D sans hypercalcémie chez le rat parathyroïdectomisé. I. Étude des lésions anatomiques. Path. Biol. 12:674, 1964.
11. Mathieu, H., Cuisinier-Gleizes, P., Dulac, H., Gyrard, E., Hérouard, S., and Royer, P.: Action toxique de la vitamine D sans hypercalcémie chez le rat parathyroïdectomisé. II. Action sur la calciurie. Valeur séméiologique de l'hypercalciurie. Path. Biol. 12:688, 1964.
12. Meyer, D. L., and Forbes, R. M.: Effects of thyroïd hormone and phosphorus loading on renal calcification and mineral metabolism of the rat. J. Nutr. 93:361, 1967.
13. Moncrieff, M. W., and Chance, G. M.: Nephrotoxic effect of vitamin D therapy in vitamin D refractory rickets. Arch. Dis. Child. 44:571, 1969.
14. Mortensen, J. D., and Emmett, J. L.: Nephrocalcinosis: a collective and clinicopathologic study. J. Urol. (Baltimore) 71:398, 1954.
15. Paunier, L., Kooh, S. W., Conen, P. E., Gibson, A. A. M., and Fraser, D.: Renal function and histology after long term vitamin D therapy of vitamin D refractory rickets. J. Pediat. 73:833, 1968.
16. Pyrah, L. N.: The calcium-containing stone. Proc. Roy. Soc. Med. 51:183, 1958.
17. Royer, P.: Les néphrocalcinoses de l'enfant. In Modern problems in Paediatrics. Vol. 5. Basel, Karger, 1960, p. 359.
18. Royer, P., Mathieu, H., and Balsan, S.: Troubles du métabolisme calcique dans l'insuffisance thyroïdienne de l'enfant. Ann. Endocr. 29:610, 1968.
19. Scarpelli, D. G.: Experimental nephrocalcinosis. A biochemical and morphologic study. Lab. Invest. 14:123, 1965.
20. Shanks, R. A., and MacDonald, A. M.: Nephrocalcinosis infantum. Arch. Dis. Child. 34:115, 1959.
21. Stickler, G. B., Jowsey, J., and Bianco, A. T.: Possible detrimental effects of large doses of vitamin D in familial hypophosphatemic vitamin D resistant rickets. J. Pediat. 79:68, 1971.
22. Wenzl, J. E., Burke, E. C., Stickler, G. B., and Utz, D. C.: Nephrolithiasis and nephrocalcinosis in children. Pediatrics 41:57, 1968.

Chapter Six

URINARY LITHIASIS

Urinary stones in infants and children are an important cause of urinary infection and of progressive deterioration in kidney function. The causes and mechanisms of calculus production are still very imperfectly understood. The calculi consist of a crystalline fraction and a protein matrix that represents between 2.5 and 10 per cent of the weight of the stone. The crystalline fraction consists of calcium phosphate, calcium oxalate, or magnesium ammonium phosphate, more rarely of uric acid or cystine, and extremely rarely of xanthine or glycine. The incidence of urinary lithiasis in infants and children varies from one part of the world to another and in different periods of time. Consequently, it is customary to distinguish between endemic and sporadic urinary lithiasis.

ENDEMIC URINARY LITHIASIS[6, 21, 22]

Endemic urinary lithiasis still exists in many countries in the Middle East, in the Far East, and in Africa. There is evidence that it once existed in western Europe and gradually disappeared toward the beginning of the twentieth century. If often affects infants, especially boys. The endemic form is characterized by the high percentage of bladder calculi, the predominance of calcium urate and oxalate in the constitution of the stones, and its predilection for the children of the poorer classes of society. Many factors—ethnic, nutritional, climatic, and parasitic—have been blamed, but the true etiology is far from clear. However, the condition tends to disappear as the socioeconomic status rises.

SPORADIC URINARY LITHIASIS

The sporadic type is observed mainly in Europe and North America. The calculi are found principally in the upper urinary tract.

Incidence[2, 4, 9, 10, 12, 16, 17, 19]

The published statistics are summarized in Table 36. Urinary lithiasis is not very rare in children; it has been found in 1.11 per cent of cases at autopsy.[27] Thirty per cent of cases occur before the age of 2 years and 50 per cent before the age of 4 years. Stones may even be found in the neonatal period.

Table 36. Etiology of Urinary Lithiasis in Children

| | Known Causes | | | | |
Authors	Abnormalities of the Urinary Tract	Metabolic	Total	Cause Unknown	Total
Myers[16]	25	9 (+5)	39	46 (54 per cent)	85
Houllemare[12]	25	18	43	37 (46 per cent)	80
Royer (1962)	Excluded	22	22	13 (37 per cent)	35
Wenzl et al.[25]	37	13	50	27 (35 per cent)	77
Willnow[27]	15	—	—	—	—
Bruezière et al.[4]	(25 per cent)	(25 per cent)	(50 per cent)	(50 per cent)	105
Prandi[17]	44	28	72	128 (64 per cent)	200

Another peculiarity of infantile lithiasis is that it is bilateral in one third of cases, whereas it is unilateral in 90 per cent of cases in older children. The condition is more common in boys than in girls. Boys are affected in 80 to 85 per cent of cases before the age of 2 years, but 60 to 65 per cent of patients over the age of 4 years are males, and only 55 per cent of adult patients are males. The figures are the same for lithiasis secondary to ureteropelvic obstruction. There is no explanation for the male preponderance (Table 37). Table 38 summarizes the causes of lithiasis in infants in our own experience.

Clinical Features

Stones may be passed in the urine or discovered in the diapers. There may be pyuria, hematuria, pain, abdominal distention and vomiting, disorders of micturition and retention of urine, and even anuria. The course and prognosis depend on the cause, on the treatment, and on secondary disorders in the kidneys; there may be definitive cure, recurrence, or even chronic uremia and death.

Table 37. Incidence of Urinary Lithiasis in Children
According to Age and Sex

| | Age | | Sex | |
Authors	Per Cent Under 2 Years	Per Cent Over 2 Years	Male (Per Cent)	Female (Per Cent)
Houllemare[12]	41	59	72	28
Wenzl et al.[25]	—	—	65	35
Willnow[27] (autopsies)	80 (<1 year)	—	50	50
Bruezière et al.[4]	33	67	75	25
Prandi[17]	—	—	78	22
Royer	40	60	72	28
Myers[16]	29	71	61	39

Table 38. Lithiasis in Children Under the Age of 30 Months
(Personal Series, 1968)

Causes	Sex		Progress			
	Male	Female	Currently Cured	Recurrence	Death	Status Unknown
Obstructive uropathy (33 per cent)	10	1	1	3	0	7
Metabolic stone (18 per cent)						
Cystinuria-lysinuria	2	2	1	1	1	1
Xanthinuria	1	—	1	—	—	—
Distal tubular acidosis	—	1	—	1	—	—
Xanthogranulomatous pyelonephritis (12 per cent)	3	1	4	—	—	—
Nonrecurrent phosphocalcific lithiasis with mental retardation (12 per cent)	3	1	3	—	1	—
Cause unknown (25 per cent)	6	2	3	2	—	3
Total (33 cases)	25 (75 per cent)	8 (25 per cent)	13 (40 per cent)	7 (20 per cent)	2 (6 per cent)	11 (34 per cent)

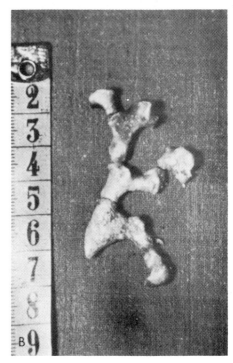

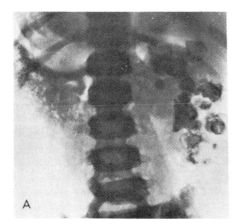

Figure 43. Idiopathic staghorn calculus in a boy aged 8 years. *A*, Plain x-ray before surgery. *B*, The stones removed at surgery. Bivalving the kidney enabled all the stones to be removed, with an excellent result.

If urinary lithiasis is suspected, the investigations should include a plain radiograph of the abdomen, intravenous urography, measurement of both the urinary output and the blood concentration of calcium, magnesium, oxalic acid, and uric acid, and chromatographic studies of urinary amino acids. It should be noted that nearly all calculi are radiopaque except xanthine and sometimes uric acid stones. If any calculi are recovered, they should be analyzed chemically and by crystallography. The study is completed by searching for urinary infection and by performing renal function studies (Figure 43).

Etiology

Two main groups of causes can be distinguished, and the relative importance of these varies depending on the source of the case material in the different centers. These types are (1) the lithiases associated with malformation in the urinary tract or kidney, and (2) the lithiases of metabolic origin. A cause has been found in 36 to 64 per cent of cases in different statistics.

Lithiases Associated with Urinary Tract Malformation[9, 10, 12, 17, 19, 27]

Lithiasis is associated with malformation of the urinary tract in about 25 per cent of cases. Every kind of abnormality of the urinary tract may be complicated by calculus formation, but the most important is obstruction of the pelviureteric junction. In most cases, the calculi consist of calcium phosphate and magnesium ammonium phosphate. It seems that both stasis and urinary infection (which raises the pH if the infection results from a urea-splitting organism such as *Proteus*) predispose to lithiasis. It is not clear why the complication is relatively rare or why it occurs more often in boys: it is found in 3 per cent of cases of pelviureteric obstruction in girls but in 17 per cent in boys.

The connection between lithiasis and malformation is not always obvious. In some cases, the malformation is clearly primary, but in other cases may be responsible for the stenosis by causing inflammation and progressive sclerosis. Whether it is primary or secondary, the stenosis must be treated surgically. The role of reflux is difficult to interpret, and it may disappear after treatment of the lithiasis.[1]

Sometimes, instead of the usual calculi there are the so-called "matrix stones," and these may even occur, though more rarely, without any urinary tract malformation.[4] They usually present with urinary infection and may be evident on a plain x-ray film by reason of a narrow rim of calcification at the periphery or even in the center of the matrix. On intravenous urography these matrix stones appear as a filling defect. The mode of formation of matrix stones is not known, but they may destroy the kidney.

Lithiasis may also occur as a complication of urinary diversion to a segment of gut and in certain conditions such as medullary sponge kidney (see page 24), megacalycosis, horseshoe kidney, renal dysplasia, and especially xanthogranulomatous pyelonephritis (see page 155).

Metabolic Lithiases

These account for about one fourth of the cases of lithiasis. They require extensive investigation because the cause must be found and treatment instituted in order to prevent recurrence. The most common cause is hypercalciuria, which accounts for about half of the cases. The remaining half comprises urinary lithiasis owing to a disorder of urate or oxalate metabolism or of tubular transfer of amino acids.

Calcium Stones.[7] This group includes calculi consisting of calcium oxalate or calcium phosphate, or both, accompanied by hypercalciuria (see page 65). This definition excludes cases in which the stones contain calcium (90 per cent of stones) but in which hypercalciuria does not occur. Also excluded from this group are the lithiases with hyperoxaluria which are symptomatic of an oxalosis that may be accompanied by hypercalciuria.[15]

This group accounts for some 10 per cent of stones in children and about half of the cases of metabolic lithiasis. The stones are frankly radiopaque. They are often single, more rarely multiple. They may be associated with nephrocalcinosis that may be obvious at the outset and must in any case be sought for routinely (see page 183).

Cystine Stones.[5] These account for between 1 and 5 per cent of cases of lithiasis. They are the most common form of calculus caused by abnormal tubular transfer. Cystine stones most often result from defective tubular reabsorption of cystine, arginine, lysine, and ornithine (classical cystinuria or cystinuria-lysinuria). There is another hereditary disorder in which isolated cystinuria occurs (hypercystinuria). Cystinuria-lysinuria is a hereditary disease, and two varieties have been described: one is an autosomal recessive condition in which the heterozygous subjects are healthy; the other form is an incompletely recessive condition. The heterozygous subjects eliminate more cystine in the urine than normal subjects, and the urinary cystine levels may vary from close to normal to levels identical to those found in homozygous victims of the disease. There are other clinical differences between the two types. In the recessive form, the clearance of cystine is greater than the clearance of arginine. Intestinal transfer of cystine and of basic amino acids is affected in a parallel manner. The plasma cystine level is lowered. In the incompletely recessive form, the cystine clearance is greater than the inulin clearance and the arginine clearance is greater than the lysine clearance. The disorder of intestinal transfer may be identical to the first type or the cystine clearance may be relatively unaffected. In the latter variety, the plasma cystine level is not lowered.

The diagnosis of cystine lithiasis is relatively easy. The calculi are generally large, multiple, molded to the outline of the calyces and pelvis, and radiopaque. Macroscopically they are soft, yellowish, waxy, and malleable. The cystine can be identified chemically and by x-ray diffraction. Its crystals have a hexagonal form.

Urinary examination reveals an excessive output of cystine. Brand's test gives a red-magenta color that is not specific and is in fact positive for any sulfhydryl compounds. Sullivan's test is more sensitive and gives a specific red color. Two-dimensional paper chromatography reveals the high urinary output of cystine and basic amino acids, and, when applied to the patient's relatives as well, will reveal the type of transmission. Normal persons excrete 0.01 to 0.02 g. of cystine in the urine in 24 hours, whereas sufferers from cystine lithiasis excrete between 0.5 and 1 g. in 24 hours.

Treatment includes several special measures. Cystine is only weakly soluble, and even less so at an acid pH. The urine should be rendered alkaline and kept at a pH of 7 or above as much as possible. To this end, sodium bicarbonate is prescribed in progressive doses of 2 to 5 g./day, the dose is fractionated throughout the day, and the pH is checked at each micturition with special test papers until it remains permanently at 7 or above. With this treatment alone, recurrence of lithiasis can be prevented in many cases.

It has been suggested that the dietary intake of cystine and of methionine should be restricted, but this is very difficult to achieve when there must, at the same time, be an adequate intake of protein and of methionine, an essential amino acid. Restriction of sulfur containing amino acids does reduce the intake of hydrogen ions and so raises the pH of the urine.

D-Penicillamine is a very active drug.[5, 14] It reacts with cystine to form a compound that is more soluble and less easily crystallized. It also reduces the urinary output of cystine by combining with its precursors to form cysteine-penicillamine and penicillamine disulfide. The dosage necessary is of the order of 1 to 2 g./1.73 m.^{2}/24 hours. This treatment can produce excellent results in preventing recurrence and even in achieving the dissolution of large calculi, but it is fraught with numerous complications. The problems include sensitivity reactions similar to those seen with penicillin, but more frequent and often very serious, nephrotoxicity and possibly a nephrotic syndrome, and also granulocytopenia and lymphocytopenia. The patient must be observed very closely and the drug must be withdrawn, despite its remarkable efficacy, as soon as any complications appear.

Table 39. Changes in Blood Uric Acid Levels in Childhood (mg./100 ml.)*

Age	0 to 48 hours	48 hours to 10 days	10 days to 2 years	2 to 6 years	over 6 years
Maximal value	9.0	8.4	4.2	5.7	5.0
Mean	6.79	4.65	2.36	4.06	4.10
Minimal value	5.2	3.9	1.6	2.8	3.2

*After Castelle and colleagues.

Uric Acid Stones.[11] Uric acid calculi are much less common in children than in adults. They are only slightly radiopaque. Three varieties may be distinguished: lithiasis with hyperuricemia, lithiasis with hyperuricosuria without hyperuricemia, and an idiopathic uric acid lithiasis that possibly may be hereditary.

The normal blood uric acid level is of the order of 3 to 4 mg. per 100 ml. in children (Table 39). Hyperuricemia may result from many causes, but the most common is the use of cytotoxic drugs for certain malignant conditions.

The hereditary hyperuricemia of Lesch-Nyhan is a rare disease in which there is hyperuricemia, chronic encephalopathy, a tendency to self-mutilation, macrocytic anemia, and a gouty type of interstitial nephritis with or without lithiasis. It is a result of lack of hypoxanthine-guanine-phosphoribosyl-transferase. Gout with urinary lithiasis has very occasionally been noted in type 1 glycogenoses with a deficit of glucose phosphatase. Primary gout is very rare in children.

Hyperuricosuria without hyperuricemia is seen mainly during treatment with drugs that block the tubular reabsorption of uric acid, such as probenecid. Such drugs are rarely used in children. The condition can also result from a very high intake of protein and purine. An isolated primary disorder of the tubular reabsorption of uric acid has also been recorded.

Idiopathic uric acid lithiasis without hyperuricemia or hyperuricosuria is common in adults but rare in children. De Vries has, however, described an autosomal recessive familial form with early and recurrent calculus formation. This disease may be linked to a defect in renal ammoniogenesis leading to increased excretion of free hydrogen ions with permanent lowering of urinary pH that will encourage the precipitation of uric acid even if there is no increase in the amount excreted.

Treatment includes several measures. As in cystinuria, alkalinization of the urine prevents recurrence and may even lead to dissolution of the stones. If there is associated hyperuricemia, allopurinol (Zyloric) should be prescribed. This drug blocks xanthine oxidase and diminishes the plasma and urinary levels of uric acid. It is g ven in doses of 200 to 400 mg./1.73 m.^{2}/day. It prevents recurrence and may even encourage dissolution of calculi. It is usually well tolerated apart from occasional allergic skin reactions.

Oxalic Stones.[15, 26] Oxalic calculi are not uncommon in children; they may be large, and are radiopaque, regular in outline, and bristle with tiny spikes. They are particularly likely to cause hematuria. These calculi may occur as a complication of primary hyperoxaluria or oxalosis, or there may be idiopathic oxalic lithiasis unassociated with either hyperoxaluria or hypercalciuria. Oxalate is also the anionic substance involved in hereditary glycinuria and hypercalciurias.

More than 100 cases of familial oxalosis have been described since 1925. Oxalate is deposited in all the tissues, particularly in the kidney, and there are hyperoxaluria, nephrocalcinosis, and massive kidney stones. There are two biochemical types, and the prognosis is poor because of the early onset of renal failure (see page 107).

In some cases of oxalate lithiasis without hypercalciuria or hyperoxaluria, the calcium-magnesium ratio in the urine may be increased because of diminished magnesium excretion. In such cases, recurrence may be prevented by an oral supplement of magnesium.

Xanthine Stones.[20] These are very rare. Only some 40 cases have been described, and two of these patients were brothers. They result from lack of xanthine oxidase, the enzyme responsible for the transformation of hypoxanthine and xanthine into uric acid. It was feared that the treatment of hyperuricemia with allopurinol, a drug that inhibits xanthine oxidase, might lead to formation of xanthine stones, but in fact only one such case has been reported. Xanthine calculi are radiolucent unless they are of a mixed nature—for example, combined with calcium oxalate. They are yellowish-brown and friable and consist of crystals with tapering ends. Xanthine may be identified by its staining reactions; murexide gives an orange-red color. Spectrophotometry and electrophoresis are more specific. The urinary xanthine content is elevated, being above 15 mg./1.73 m.²/day. The uric acid levels in blood and urine are low. There is no specific treatment, but it is advisable to make the urine alkaline. Allopurinol diminishes the excretion of xanthine while raising the excretion of hypoxanthine, which is much more soluble.

Hereditary Glycinuria.[24]   In 1957, De Vries and his colleagues described a stone-producing condition characterized by hyperglycinuria with no increase in plasma glycine levels, which apparently is linked to defective tubular reabsorption of glycine. Transmission is probably dominant. The calculi are of calcium oxalate but contain 0.5 per cent glycine. Diagnosis depends on chromatography of the urinary amino acids. There is no known specific treatment.

Lithiasis of Unknown Origin.   In most cases there are large calcium phosphate or magnesium ammonium phosphate stones. These stones have little tendency to recur. The prognosis is good if there is no serious renal damage. The pathogenesis, however, is not clear. Because of the biochemical composition of the stones, there is a tendency to incriminate a preceding urinary infection, especially with urea-splitting organisms. It is also possible that such stones might be initiated during temporary states of pathologic crystallization owing to severe dehydration.

Included in this group of calcium phosphate stones of unknown origin in infants is a curious syndrome described by us in which there is urinary lithiasis, psychomotor retardation, and hip malformation[18] (Table 40). The calcium phosphate calculi are very numerous and usually bilateral, and at first sight the prognosis would appear to be poor. There is retardation of growth and psychomotor development: this may be moderate but can be obvious from the earliest months. The hip disorder can simulate osteochondritis, a condition that is rare at this age. There are no biochemical or histologic renal disorders. Despite appearances, the prognosis is good, with recovery of the hip disease,

Table 40. Multiple Phosphocalcific Lithiasis in Early Childhood
with Mental Retardation and Hip Disorders

Case	Sex	Age at Diagnosis	Presenting Symptoms	Phospho-calcific Lithiasis	Growth (in S.D.)	Mental Retardation	Hips	Progress
1	F	20 months	Anuria	Multiple bilateral	+1 S.D.	+	Fragmentation	Surgical death
2	M	3 months	Pyuria	Multiple bilateral	−1 S.D.	+	Abnormal	Cure
3	M	3 months	Pyuria	Multiple bilateral	−1 S.D.	+	Normal	Cure
4	M	5 months	Pyuria	Multiple bilateral	−1 S.D.	+	Fragmentation	Cure

improvement of the mental state, and absence of recurrence after removal of the calculi.

LITHOGENESIS

The prophylactic treatment of urinary lithiasis depends on the specific elements in each type of stone and on the analysis of the general causes of calculus formation.[13, 23]

Normal urine is a better solvent than water. It contains various substances in apparent supersaturation and in an unstable physicochemical state. The factors concerned in precipitation of calculi are urinary flow, the volume of water, the ionic strength, the pH, the presence of substances affecting solubility, and the existence of a nucleus of crystallization.

The urinary flow plays an important part, and there is no doubt that urinary stasis predisposes to stone formation. The amount of urinary water affects the concentration of the particular substance involved; there seems to be little doubt that calculi are more easily precipitated from the concentrated urine during the night. In infants, the urine may become very concentrated because of abnormal extrarenal losses of water, owing, for example, to a high ambient temperature or to diarrhea. The ionic concentration is significant, and solubility is improved by an increase in the content of sodium, chloride, sulfate, and also urea. The pH is a fundamental factor. Calcium phosphate and magnesium ammonium phosphates are less soluble at a pH above 6. Uric acid is more soluble at a pH above 6 and cystine is more soluble at a pH above 7. Infection with a urea-splitting organism, such as *Proteus*, raises the pH of the urine and predisposes to precipitation of magnesium ammonium phosphate. Any possible nucleus of crystallization, such as a foreign body, an indwelling catheter, or even a mass of bacteria, may encourage precipitation. Emphasis has also been placed on the lithiasis-inhibiting role of magnesium (over and above its contribution to ionic strength), of citrate, of pyrophosphates, and of peptide inhibitors, some of which have been isolated.

The organic protein matrix plays an essential part in stone formation.[3] In fact, calculi consist of an aggregate of organic or inorganic crystals in an organic matrix that accounts on average for 2.5 per cent of the weight of the calculus. The matrix is the nucleus on which the stone forms by epitaxy and successive deposition. According to this hypothesis, a calculus is fundamentally a matrix that is secondarily mineralized. The origin of the matrix is unknown. This hypothesis is not universally accepted. Vermeulen's experiments[23] have shown that in animals the crystallization is the initial phenomenon and occurs in the region of the papilla in which the concentration is highest. According to this hypothesis, the protein matrix plays only a secondary role, providing cohesion for the stone and preventing its dissolution during periods when the urine is no longer supersaturated. Stasis prolongs the time available for crystallization and serves to retain the developing calculus thus formed. In fact, the degree of supersaturation of urine necessary to initiate lithiasis is much greater than that necessary for calculi to grow. It may be conceived that, at some particular moment, certain unusual conditions pertain — such as those owing to dehydration, for example — which provoke the genesis of a calculus. The stone continues to grow even though the physicochemical condition of the urine returns to normal. The specific initiating factor may never be identified. This attempt to explain idiopathic lithiasis is interesting although as yet hypothetical.

Attempts are being made to treat lithiasis by controlling crystallization in the urine with the use of inhibitors, such as the magnesium ion and especially pyrophosphates.

Treatment

Surgery

In the great majority of cases, surgery is necessary. The object is to remove all calculi and to preserve the kidney. The difficulties and risks vary with the site and size of the stones. Cystotomy, ureterotomy and pyelotomy are simple operations. On the other hand, some operations, such as nephrolithotomy, extended pyelolithotomy associated with nephrolithotomy, and particularly major nephrolithotomy, all of which involve extensive bisection of the kidney, carry a significant risk. This latter type of operation is generally indicated for large calculi impacted in the renal pelvis and extending out into the calyces. In these conditions, complete removal of the stones may not be possible without destructive surgery. In some cases, partial nephrectomy may be necessary. Lastly, in cases of pyonephrosis in which the opposite kidney is healthy, even the entire kidney may have to be removed.

The indications for surgical treatment depend on the chances of spontaneous passage, the unilateral or bilateral nature of the stones, the probable difficulties of the surgery, the renal damage caused by the lithiasis, the danger involved in not operating, and finally the risks of major recurrence in cases of metabolic stone disease and of soft calculi. Any surgery may be contraindicated by the degree of renal failure.

When an operation is to be performed, a certain number of precautions are indicated. If the stone is in the ureter, its position must be verified radiographically immediately before operation to be sure that it has not moved. In cases of staghorn calculus, it is helpful to get precise information about its extensions by preoperative nephrotomography. During surgery, it is essential to verify the complete removal of all stones with the aid of contact x-ray films. Catgut suture material should be fine and all knots should be tied on the exterior. Catheters should be left in place for the shortest possible time. Silastic catheters are softer, better tolerated, and less prone to produce infective complications. There should be a high urinary output. When soft or matrix stones are removed, it is wise to leave in a nephrostomy tube for lavage with proteolytic enzymes, because stones of this type tend to recur early.

The results of surgery are variable. Despite every precaution there may be residual calculi or recurrence. Reoperation is sometimes necessary and may present surgical difficulties. However, it is very important to treat any obstruction in the urinary tract, whether this is primary or secondary.

Medical Treatment

Apart from the special needs of particular varieties of lithiasis, there is one medical treatment that should be applied in common to all types of calculi, whether submitted to surgery or not. The essentials of this therapy are rigorous treatment of infection and a high fluid intake.

Treatment of any infection is very important because the infection may predispose to further calculus formation and may aggravate any existing renal damage (see page 138).

The increased fluid intake is designed to keep the urine specific gravity below 1.010 permanently. The purpose is to avoid conditions favorable to the precipitation of calculi and possibly even create conditions that favor their dissolution. The extra water intake required is of the order of 2 liters/m.^{2}/day. The fluid intake should be divided equally over the 24 hours and should include a portion at the time of going to bed and one in the middle of the night. Even more fluid may be needed in the presence of fever, high ambient temperature, or fluid lost from the alimentary tract.

Some prophylactic measures are effective. Paraplegic patients and patients in extensive plaster casts require active and passive mobilization, using a mechanical bed if necessary; the administration of orthophosphates may also be indicated, with dosage monitored by observations of urinary calcium level. In cystinuria-lysinuria, alkalis should be prescribed. This treatment may be given prophylactically to relatives of patients with lithiasis who have not yet developed calculi themselves. In more general terms, preventative treatment includes an immediate rehydration of patients with acute diarrhea and the avoidance of excessive intake of calcium or vitamin D.

CONCLUSION

Whenever a stone is discovered, a patient search must be undertaken in the hope of uncovering a specific metabolic cause. However carefully conducted, this search will prove vain in a large number of cases, and the explanation for this annoying fact may be found in certain experimental studies. It has been shown that once the nucleus of a calculus has been formed it continues to grow even when urine returns to normal. It is even possible that the initial episode of stone formation might have occurred during intra-uterine life.

Decisions about surgical intervention may be difficult, and in cases of large calculi, the operation itself may present considerable problems. Surgery may fail if any stone is left behind.

Emphasis must be placed on the prevention of lithiasis and the importance of a carefully supervised regimen with a high fluid intake.

REFERENCES

1. Auvert, J.: Calcul de rein et reflux vésico-urétéral chez l'enfant. Disparition du reflux après ablation du calcul. J. Urol. Nephrol. *71*:482, 1965,
2. Beane, H. C., Magoss, I. V., Staubitz, W. J., and Jewett, T. C., Jr.: Urolithiasis in childhood. J. Urol. *97*:537, 1967.
3. Boyce, W. C.: Organic matrix of human urinary concretions. Amer. J. Med. *45*:673, 1968.
4. Bruezière, J., Lasfargues, G., Gallet, J. P., and Boulesteix, J.: Les coagulums uroprotidiques chez l'enfant. Vie Méd. *23*:3013, 1969.
5. Crawhall, J. C., and Watts, R. N. E.: Cystinuria. Amer. J. Med. *45*:736, 1968.
6. Eckstein, H. B.: Endemic urinary lithiasis in Turkish children. Arch. Dis. Child. *36*:137, 1961.
7. Epstein, F. H.: Calcium and the kidney. Amer. J. Med. *45*:700, 1968.
8. Fleisch, H., Bisaz, S., and Care, A. D.: Effect of orthophosphate on urinary pyrophosphate excretion and the prevention of urolithiasis. Lancet, *1*:1065, 1964.
9. Gallet, J. P : La lithiase urinaire du nourrisson. Vie Méd. *23*:2967, 1969.
10. Gallet, J. P : La lithiase urinaire de l'enfant. Vie Méd. *23*:2977, 1969.
11. Gutman, A. B., and Yu, T. F.: Uric acid nephrolithiasis. Amer. J. Med. *45*:756, 1968.
12. Houllemare, L.: La lithiase urinaire de l'enfant. *In* Actualités Pédiatriques (M. Lelong), 4th series. Paris, Doin, 1962, p. 117.
13. Howard, J. E., and Thomas, W. C., Jr.: Control of crystallization in urine. Amer. J. Med. *45*: 693, 1968.
14. McDonald, J. E., and Henneman, P H.: Stone dissolution in vivo and control of cystinuria with D-penicillamine. New Eng. J. Med. *273*:578, 1965.
15. Mathieu, H., Gagnadoux, M. F., Mongour, P , Czernichow, P., Volter, F., and Kaplan, M.: Oxalose familiale, étude de 2 cas—essai de traitement. Soc. Méd. Hop. Paris *119*:719, 1968.
16. Myers, W. A. A.: Urolithiasis in childhood. Arch. Dis. Child. *30*:165, 1955; and *32*:48, 1957.
17. Prandi, D.: Lithiase rénale de l'enfant. Thèse Méd. Paris, 1968 (no. 713 [dactylographie]).
18. Royer, P., and David, L.: La lithiase urinaire phosphocalcique multiple et non récidivante du nourrisson avec retard psychomoteur et anomalies des hanches. Arch. franç. Pédiat. *26*: 607, 1969.
19. Royer, P., and Lévy, M.: La lithiase urinaire des nourrissons. *In* Acquisitions médicales récentes: Journées médicales annuelles de Broussais-la-Charité. Paris, Expansion Scientifique Française, 1969, p. 51.
20. Seegmiller, J. E.: Xanthine stone formation. Amer. J. Med. *45*:780, 1968.
21. Thomson, J. O.: Urinary calculus at the Canton hospital, Canton, China, based upon 3,500 operations. Surg. Gynec. Obstet. *32*:44, 1921.
22. Valyasevi, A., and Van Reen, R.: Pediatric bladder stone disease; current status of research. J. Pediat. *72*:546, 1968.
23. Vermeulen, C. W., and Lyon, E. S.: Mechanisms of genesis and growth of calculi. Amer. J. Med. *45*:684, 1968.
24. de Vries, A., Kochwa, S., Lazebnik, J., Frank, M., and Djaldetti, M.: Glycinuria, a hereditary disorder, associated with nephrolithiasis. Amer. J. Med. *23*:408, 1957.
25. Wenzl, J. E., Burke, E. C., Stickler, G. B., and Utz, D. C.: Nephrolithiasis and nephrocalcinosis in children. Pediatrics *41*:57, 1968.
26. Williams, H. E., and Smith, L. H., Jr.: Disorders of oxalate metabolism. Amer. J. Med. *45*: 715, 1968.
27. Willnow, U.: Nephrolithiasis. Deutsch. Med. Wschr. *92*:1668, 1967.

PART
III

Glomerulopathies

RENÉE HABIB

INTRODUCTION

Glomerular pathology in children is very important because of its incidence and the many problems of its course and treatment. Glomerular disorders in children have a reputation for being benign, but a recent study of our own material shows that 26 per cent of the cases of chronic renal failure in children result from glomerular nephropathy.

Four parameters may be used to define a glomerular disorder – the mechanism, the histology, the clinical and biochemical features, and the etiology. In most glomerular nephropathies, the mechanism is still obscure, but there is a great deal of evidence that some are of immunologic origin. This subject is considered in Chapter 1 of Part III.

Renal biopsy has made it possible to accumulate considerable morphologic data. The various histologic findings are now well codified; each one may be associated with a variable clinical picture, but each has a specific course. This new and fundamental information about the natural history of glomerular disease and the consequent therapeutic concepts are set out in Chapter 2.

The clinical and biochemical features of the various diseases have been the longest known, but the introduction of renal biopsy revealed that each of the known syndromes corresponded to various different histopathologic lesions, demonstrating that the clinical picture alone is a poor guide to prognosis. The major syndromes of glomerular nephropathy are studied in Chapter 3.

The causes of glomerular disease are known to some extent. The important role of certain types of hemolytic streptococcus has been known for a long time. Some glomerulopathies appear to be no more than particular localizations of systemic disease. More than half of glomerular nephropathies are idiopathic. Discovery of the cause is important for prognosis and treatment only in those systemic diseases in which extrarenal factors play an important part. The renal manifestations of systemic disease are considered in Chapter 4.

THE MECHANISM OF
GLOMERULONEPHRITIS*

There is experimental, clinical, laboratory, and histologic evidence that most glomerulopathies are of immunologic origin. Two immunologic mechanisms that can give rise to glomerulonephritis are known. The first is production of antibodies that can react with the subject's own glomerular basement membrane. The second is the production of antibodies that can react with endogenous or exogenous nonglomerular antigens, with the formation of circulating antigen-antibody complexes that are secondarily fixed on the glomerular basement membrane.

EXPERIMENTAL EVIDENCE

Glomerulonephritis Produced by Antibodies Against Basement Membrane

The "hetero-immune" glomerulonephritis of Masugi is produced by injecting into a rat the serum of a rabbit or duck previously immunized by crushed rat kidney. It has been shown that the antibodies concerned are directed essentially against the antigens on the basement membrane of the rat. A similar glomerulonephritis can be produced in animals immunized with antigens of heterologous basement membrane. The evidence for the role of anti-basement membrane antibody is very strong. The glomerulonephritis can be transmitted by injecting serum from a nephritic animal to a healthy animal of the same species and the transmission is just as effective if the immunized animal has had both kidneys removed.

Histologically, there is endocapillary and extracapillary proliferation and an influx of neutrophil polymorphonuclear cells. These phenomena are associated with a fall in the level of serum complement. This type of glomerulonephritis has a characteristic appearance on electron microscopy or immunofluorescent study: there is a uniform linear deposit on the endothelial aspect of the basement membrane. Immunofluorescence study shows that this deposit consists of antibodies and complement.

The relationship between these experimental models and human glomerulonephritis is not evident. Glomerulonephritis resulting from anti-basement membrane antibodies can appear in man under different conditions.

---

*This chapter was written in collaboration with C. Loirat.

207

Endogenous antigens of glomerular or other origin, normally inaccessible to the immune system, may be liberated in certain circumstances. Glomerulonephritis can be produced by injecting rabbits with normal autologous or homologous urine; certain normal urinary glycoproteins possess antigens in common with the basement membrane and provoke the appearance of anti-basement membrane antibodies. Antibodies against aorta, lung, or placenta can also produce glomerulonephritis owing to the antigenic relationship of many organs.

Certain exogenous antigens may also have antigenic similarity with basement membrane. For example, there is a cross reaction between the parietal antigen of the hemolytic streptoccocus and the anti-basement membrane antibodies. The deposits found in man in acute poststreptococcal glomerulonephritis are not, however, of the type characteristic of the glomerulonephritis resulting from anti-basement membrane antibody. The possibility remains that certain cases of glomerulonephritis from anti-basement membrane antibody are of streptococcal origin.

Glomerulonephritis Caused by Deposition of Antigen-Antibody Complexes

Experimental Serum Disease

A glomerulonephritis can be produced in animals by the injection of a nonglomerular, heterologous protein. The disease presents after an interval of 10 days, during which the antibodies are formed. It is acute and curable, with endocapillary proliferation and a transient fall in the level of serum complement if only one injection of heteroprotein is given. The disease becomes chronic with repeated injections of antigen in such quantity that there is a slight excess of antigen, permitting the formation of soluble antigen-antibody complexes that have most chance of becoming fixed on the vascular walls.

This type of glomerulonephritis is characterized by the presence of granular deposits in clumps on the epithelial aspect of the basement membrane. Immunofluorescence shows that they consist of antibodies, antigen, and complement.

There are experimental situations in which antibodies initially directed against exogenous antigens combine equally well with autologous antigens. For example, Heyman's glomerulonephritis is produced by injecting rats with antigens obtained from the brush border of human proximal convoluted tubules. The corresponding antibodies combine with the injected antigen and also with the immunologically similar antigens of the host present in the circulation. In the same way, injection of heterologous thyroglobulin into a rabbit causes the formation of antibodies that react with the thyroglobulin of the host to form complexes that cause kidney disease.

Spontaneous nephritis in animals is associated in most cases with deposits of immune complexes. It often appears to be the result of a chronic viral infection, with deposition of complexes made up of the infecting agent, the corresponding antibodies, and complement. This is the case, for example, in the glomerulonephritis found in mice chronically infected either by the virus of lymphocytic choriomeningitis or by coxsackie B virus, or in mink affected by Aleutian disease. Viral infection may also play a role in the glomerulonephritis of hybrid NZB/W mice (see page 211).

MECHANISM OF FORMATION OF RENAL LESIONS
IN GLOMERULONEPHRITIS

There is still a great deal to be learned about how glomerular lesions are produced by the deposition of immune complexes or of anti-basement membrane antibodies.

The Role of Complement

A certain number of reactions that are known to play an important part in the genesis of glomerular lesions (for example, the liberation of histamine with increased permeability of glomerular capillaries and attraction of polymorphonuclear cells) depend on the activation of complement. The role of complement is well proved in the experimental Masugi glomerulonephritis, in which the lesions are very much less severe if there has been a previous depletion of complement or polymorphonuclear cells.

The fall in the level of serum complement and the presence of deposits of complement in the glomeruli seen in certain cases of human glomerulonephritis, like those in experimental glomerulonephritis, are evidence that complement also plays an important part in the genesis of the glomerular lesions in man.

The Role of Immunoglobulins

There is good evidence that the antibodies fixing complement are those that induce the most significant glomerular lesions. It is known that the ability to fix complement varies with the type of immunoglobulin. Five types of immunoglobulin are known in man — IgG, IgM, IgA, IgD, and IgE. Complement is fixed only by antibodies composed of IgM and certain IgG antibodies. Human IgG is divided into four subgroups, IgG_1, IgG_2, IgG_3, and IgG_4, of which only IgG_1 and IgG_3 fix complement. The type of immunoglobulin entering into the constitution of anti-basement membrane antibodies, or the antibodies forming part of an antigen-antibody complex, may thus be one of the elements determining the type and extent of the glomerular lesions.

The Role of Coagulation Phenomena[23]

In Masugi glomerulonephritis, there is always a deposit of fibrin and of fibrinogen derivatives between the epithelial cells and in the mesangium. The pathogenic role of these coagulation phenomena is underlined by the effectiveness of heparin therapy, which prevents not only deposition of fibrin and its derivatives but also the formation of epithelial crescents and glomerular sclerosis. Similar observations have been made in certain glomerulonephritides resulting from deposition of immune complexes, in particular in the glomerulonephritides of NZB mice.

Immunofluorescent studies show that there are also deposits of fibrinogen derivatives in the glomeruli in certain cases of human glomerulonephritis. These deposits are present in variable amounts in the intercapillary cells (probably as a result of phagocytosis), proliferating in acute endocapillary proliferative glomerulonephritis. The deposits are constantly found in malignant glomerulonephritis in the epithelial crescents and in the zones of glomerular sclerosis. They are found also in the glomerulonephritis of lupus, along the epithelial surface of the basement membrane, in amounts that vary with the nature of the lesions. Fibrin degradation products are commonly found in the blood or urine in various types of glomerulonephritis. These deposits are constantly found at a very early stage in the glomerular lesions of rheumatoid purpura.

The good results of early heparin therapy in human malignant glomerulonephritis are, if confirmed, an additional argument in favor of the important role of coagulation phenomena in the genesis of the glomerular lesions.[9]

The role of *delayed hypersensitivity* reactions in human glomerulonephritis remains largely hypothetical.

HUMAN GLOMERULONEPHRITIS

It is not possible at the present time to propose a mechanism for every histologic type of human glomerulonephritis. The experimental glomerulonephritides never reproduce exactly the histologic lesions of glomerulonephritis in man. The comparison between the experimental models and human glomerulonephritis relies essentially on the evidence of immunofluorescent studies, but this is by no means conclusive in all cases.

Poststreptococcal Glomerulonephritis with Endocapillary Proliferation

There is still considerable mystery about the mechanisms by which *Streptococcus* produces a nephropathy. The hypothesis that it is an immune process, with deposition of antigen-antibody complexes, rests on several arguments. The interval between the streptococcal infection and the onset of renal symptoms can be compared with that noted in serum disease. In addition, there is a transient diminution in the level of complement (total hemolytic complement or $C'3$ fraction [B_1C-B_1A]). The most important evidence is histologic: the endocapillary proliferation with polymorphonuclear infiltration and especially the presence of granular deposits in humps on the epithelial aspect of the basement membrane, shown on immunofluorescence to consist of IgG and $C'3$. These features are common to both acute glomerulonephritis and the serum disease.

The presence of streptococcal antigen in these deposits, reported by Andres and his colleagues,[1] has not been confirmed by other authors. On the other hand, it has been possible to isolate from the serum of subjects with acute glomerulonephritis an IgG that fixes on the glomeruli of other subjects with acute glomerulonephritis. This activity is inhibited by previous absorption of serum with a preparation of streptococcal cell membrane.[22] It might thus be thought that the streptococcal antigen fixes on the basement membrane and that the antibodies made by the host fix secondarily at the same site. The IgG included in the deposits has not, however, been isolated, nor has its possible antistreptococcal action been studied.

The antigenic relationship between the streptococcal cell membrane and certain antigens of the basement membrane has been emphasized.[15]

Linear deposition of IgG might be expected, but a glomerulonephritis with granular deposition has been produced in monkeys by the injection of rabbit antistreptococcal membrane antibodies, which might suggest that the antigenic components of the basement membrane that are immunologically related to the streptococcal antigens are not distributed in a uniform manner.[16]

Lupus Glomerulonephritis

This is a well-known example of glomerular disease associated with the deposition of immune complexes.

The fact that there is diminution in the level of total complement and of many of its constituents, which varies with the activity of the disease, is a strong argument in favor of an immune process.

On immunofluorescence, granular deposits are seen. Their topography varies, as does the histologic type of lupus glomerulonephritis. The deposits consist of immunoglobulins, mainly IgG, but also IgA, IgM, and C′3. By elution, it has been shown that these immunoglobulins are antinuclear antibodies with particular anti-DNA activity. DNA has also been found in these deposits.[10] It thus seems well established that immune complexes, at least DNA–anti-DNA, are responsible for the renal disorder of systemic lupus erythematosus. The variability of the histologic lesions and the exact cause of the disease remain to be explained. In this regard, a viral etiology is often suggested.

One of the arguments in favor of this hypothesis is the similarity between the human disease and the disease found in mice of the NZB and hybrid NZB/W strains. The mouse disease is characterized by a Coombs positive hemolytic anemia, by the presence of LE cells in the circulating blood, and by glomerulonephritis in 98 per cent of cases. As in human lupus glomerulonephritis, the immunoglobulins present in the glomeruli are anti-DNA antibodies. It is thus very probable that here also the glomerulonephritis is linked to the deposition of DNA–anti-DNA complexes. The NZB and NZB/W mice have a genetic predisposition to produce anti-DNA antibodies in abnormally large amounts, expecially when infested by various viruses. It may be that there is a similar basis for the human disease.

In patients with systemic lupus erythematosus, anti-DNA antibodies have been found that react more strongly with double-chain RNA of viral type than with the monocatenary RNA of mammalian type.[20]

Tubular formations of viral appearance have been demonstrated in the endothelial cells.[18] The presence of measles antigen[21] has been disputed.[19]

Glomerulonephritis with Anti-Basement Membrane Antibodies

This condition is rare in man. Goodpasture's syndrome is the prototype, but it is exceptional in children. The same linear deposit of IgG and C′3 is found on the glomerular basement membranes and on the walls of the pulmonary alveoli. A single antibody would seem to be responsible for both the kidney and the lung lesions.

Other Types of Glomerulonephritis

The mechanism of *other types* of glomerulonephritis is even less well elucidated.

Extramembranous glomerulonephritis is often compared with the chronic serum disease because of the presence of granular deposits on the epithelial aspect of the basement membrane, which are composed mainly of IgG and sometimes C'3 or C'4.[4]

In *membranoproliferative glomerulonephritis*, granular deposits of IgG, IgM, and C'3 may be found on the walls of the glomerular capillaries (membrano-proliferative glomerulonephritis with intermembrano-endothelial deposits) or there may be deposits consisting exclusively of C'3 in irregular humps along the walls and especially in the mesangial axes (membranoproliferative glomeru-lonephritis with dense deposits). It is in the latter type of membranoproliferative glomerulonephritis that the serum level of C'3 is most constantly very low.[12] The mechanism of this abnormality is uncertain. Some authors have demon-strated diminished synthesis of C'3, others a diminished half-life and still others a C'3 inhibitor. It must be emphasized that the C'3 level does not parallel the clinical evolution of the nephropathy. The level of C'3 may become normal at a stage when the nephropathy is progressive,[24] or it may be very low at a time when all signs of nephropathy have regressed.[17] The fact that C'3 levels return to normal after bilateral nephrectomy is an argument in favor of the role of the kidney in this abnormality, but this return to normal is not absolutely constant.[7] The reproduction of the disease in a grafted kidney, especially in identical twins who receive no immunodepressive therapy, is an-other argument in favor of an immune process.

The evidence from immunofluorescent studies in *endocapillary and extra-capillary glomerulonephritis* is still confused. Anti-basement membrane antibodies may be involved.[11]

The segmental and focal glomerulonephritides of rheumatoid purpura are charac-terized on immunofluorescence by granular deposits of IgG, IgA, and C'3 and of fibrinogen in the mesangial axes. This suggests the existence of antigen-antibody complexes, but it has yet to be explained why they are found only in the intercapillary axes. This localization is observed when the complexes are insoluble, as occurs when the amounts of antigen and antibody are equivalent. Here again the causative antigen is unknown, and the immune nature of the condition remains hypothetical.

The problem of glomerulonephritides characterized by *membranous de-posits* of IgA, IgG, and C'3 is no clearer. An argument in favor of the immune nature of this nephropathy is the rapid reproduction of the disease in a kidney graft in those rare cases that have gone on to renal failure and been submitted to transplantation.[3]

The presence of IgM and C'3 in the lesions of *segmental and focal hyalinoses* does not seem in any way specific or related to an immune process. In the neph-rotic syndrome with *minimal glomerular lesions*, the constant sensitivity of the disease to steroids and to immunosuppressive agents and the occurrence of cases clearly linked to allergic phenomena[25] are arguments that can be ad-vanced in favor of an immune process. But evidence against this hypothesis is the absence of any deposit of immunoglobulins or C'3.[4] The discovery of IgE deposits along the walls of the glomerular capillaries[6] has yet to be confirmed.

CONCLUSION

Histologic and immunofluorescent studies provide evidence for certain comparisons between experimental and human glomerulonephritis and suggest that immune phenomena may be responsible for some cases of the disease in man. However, the prime mover of the supposed immune phenomenon, in particular the nature of the responsible antigen, remains unknown. There is also an almost complete lack of any explanation of how the presence of an anti-basement membrane antibody or of antigen-antibody complexes causes histologic lesions of variable type and severity.

Recent work, in particular on the activation of the complement system and properdine, gives promise of very rapid developments in this field. By way of example, some recent discoveries may be summarized.

1. It is certain that the coagulation process is involved in the pathogenesis of nephritis associated with anti-basement membrane antibodies, but this process does not appear to play a significant part in the development of nephritis associated with circulating immune complexes, such as the nephritis of serum sickness.[2]

2. Antibodies against glomerular and tubular basement membrane have been found in certain patients presenting with focal or proliferative endocapillary and extracapillary glomerulonephritis and also in cases of periarteritis nodosa. Abnormal rosette tests or leukocyte migration tests have also been found in these patients. These abnormalities would seem, however, to be secondary to the renal disease rather than implicated in its pathogenesis.[14]

3. A more sophisticated understanding of the activation of complement may presage interesting developments. The circulating immune complexes act on the classic activation pathway: C1, C4, and C2 react to elaborate C3-convertase, which catalyzes the activation of C3 and factors C5 to C9. The components of C1 (C1q, C1r, and C1s), have been purified. However, an alternative pathway of terminal activation of the complement system is known, comprising factor A, factor B or C3 proactivator, and properdine. Many new discoveries have followed. Deposits of properdine have been found in the glomeruli, but only in diffuse endocapillary proliferative glomerulonephritis, membranoproliferative glomerulonephritis, and lupus. Factors C3, C4, and B are decreased in lupus, but only C3 is diminished in membranoproliferative glomerulonephritis.[8] We have, however, recently found elective lowering of C4 in certain cases of membranoproliferative glomerulonephritis. Lastly, particular kidney disorders have been found in cases of hereditary deficiency of the subcomponents of C1, notably C1r.[5]

REFERENCES

1. Andres, G. A., Accini, C., Hsu, K. C., Zabriskie, J. B., and Seegal, B. C.: Electron microscopic studies of human glomerulonephritis with ferritin conjugated antibody. J. Exp. Med. *123*:399, 1966.
2. Baliah, T., and Drummond, K. N.: The effect of anticoagulation on serum sickness nephritis in rabbits. Proc. Soc. Exp. Biol. Med. *140*:329, 1972.
3. Berger, J.: IgA deposits in renal disease. Transplant. Proc. *1*:939, 1969.
4. Berger, J., Yaneva, H., and Hinglais, N.: Immunofluorescence des glomérulonéphrites. *In* Actualités néphrologiques de l'Hôpital Necker. Paris, Flammarion, 1971, p. 17.
5. Day, N. K., Geiger, H., Stroud, R., De Bracco, M., Mancado, B., Windhorst, D., and Good, R. A.: C1r deficiency. J. Clin. Invest. *51*:1102, 1972.
6. Gerber, M. A., and Paronetto, F.: IgE in glomeruli of patients with nephrotic syndrome. Lancet *1*:1097, 1971.
7. Pickering, R. J., Herdman, R. C., Michael, A. F., Vernier, R. L., Fish, A. J., Gewurz, H., and

Good, R. A.: Chronic glomerulonephritis associated with low serum complement activity (chronic hypocomplementemic glomerulonephritis). Medicine *49*:207, 1970.

8. Hunsicker, L. G., Ruddy, S., Carpenter, C. B., Schur, P. H., Merrill, J. P., Müller-Eberhard, H. J., and Austen, K. F.: Metabolism of third complement component (C3) in nephritis. New Eng. J. Med. *287*:835, 1972.

9. Kincaid-Smith, P., Saker, B. M., and Fairley, K. F.: Anticoagulants in "irreversible" acute renal failure. Lancet *2*:1360, 1968.

10. Koffler, D., Schur, P. H., and Kunket, H. G.: Immunological studies concerning the nephritis of systemic lupus erythematosus. J. Exp. Med. *126*:607, 1967.

11. Lerner, R. A., Glossock, R. J., and Dipon, F. J.: The role of antiglomerular basement membrane antibody in the pathogenesis of human glomerulonephritis. J. Exp. Med. *126*:989, 1967.

12. Levy, M., Loirat, C., and Habib, R.: Idiopathic membranoproliferative glomerulonephritis in children, correlations between light, electron and immunofluorescent microscopic appearances and serum C3 and C4 levels. Biomedicine *19*:447, 1973.

13. Lewis, E. J., and Couser, W. G.: The immunological basis of human renal disease. Ped. Clin. N. Amer. *18*:467, 1971.

14. Mathieu, P., Dardenne, M., and Bach, J. F.: Detection of humoral and cell mediated immunity to kidney basement membranes in human renal disease. Amer. J. Med. *53*:185, 1972.

15. Markowitz, A. S., and Lange, C. F.: Streptococcal related glomerulonephritis. I. Isolation, immunochemistry of soluble fractions from type 12 nephritogenic streptocci and human glomeruli. J. Immunol. *92*:565, 1964.

16. Markowitz, A. S.: Streptococcal-related glomerulonephritis in the Rhesus monkey. Transplant. Proc. *1*.985, 1969.

17. Northway, J. D., McAdams, A. J., Forristal, J., and West, C. D.: A "silent" phase of hypocomplementemic persistent nephritis detected by reduced serum B_1C globulin levels. J. Pediat. *74*:28, 1969.

18. Norton, W. L.: Endothelial inclusions in active lesions of systemic lupus erythematosus. J. Lab. Clin. Med. *74*:369, 1969.

19. Pincus, T., Blacklow, N., Grimey, P., and Bellanty, J.: Glomerular microtubules of systemic lupus erythematosus. Lancet *2*:1057, 1970.

20. Schur, P. H., and Monroe, M.: Antibodies to ribonucleic acid in systemic lupus erythematosus. Proc. Nat. Acad. Sci. *63*:1108, 1969.

21. Tannenbaum, M., Hsu, K. C., Buda, J., Grant, J. P., Lattes, C., and Lattimer, J. K.: Electron microscopic virus-like material in systemic lupus erythematosus: with preliminary immunologic observations on presence of measles antigen. J. Urol. *105*:615, 1971.

22. Treser, G., Senar, M., McVicar, M., Franklin, M., Ty, A., Sagel, I., and Lange, K.: Antigenic streptococcal components in acute glomerulonephritis. Science *163*:676, 1969.

23. Vassali, P., and McCluskey, R. T.: Rôle des protéines de coagulation dans les affections glomérulaires d'origine immunologique. *In* Actualités néphrologiques de l'Hôpital Necker. Paris, Flammarion, 1971, p. 55.

24. West, C. D., and McAdams, A. J.: Serum B_1C globulin levels in persistent glomerulonephritis with low serum complement: variability unrelated to clinical course. Nephron *7*:193, 1970.

25. Wittig, H. J., and Goldman, A. S.: Nephrotic syndrome associated with inhaled allergens. Lancet *1*:542, 1970.

For additional recent information, see:

a. Peltier, A.: Le système complémentaire. Path. Biol. *20*:1013, 1972.

Chapter Two

HISTOLOGIC CLASSIFICATION AND CLINICOHISTOLOGIC CORRELATIONS OF GLOMERULAR LESIONS*

The progress achieved during the past 15 years in the understanding of glomerular disease has been made possible by the routine practice of renal biopsy, by improvements in light and electron microscopy, and more recently by the application of the technique of immunofluorescence.

All glomerular nephropathies present with the sudden appearance or chance discovery of proteinuria that may or may not be accompanied by a nephrotic syndrome and may or may not be associated with hematuria. An additional feature in one third of cases is early renal insufficiency, or, in 20 per cent of cases, hypertension.

The clinical pattern is the same, with variations in the frequency and severity of individual features, whatever the histologic type of the glomerular disease. This means that the clinical presentation is of little help in evaluating the prognosis. Even identification of the etiology does not help to orient the physician because a specific etiology may be associated with many different histologic findings and variable clinical patterns.[10, 19, 20]

The importance of histologic study resides in the fact that the appearance of the lesions will indicate the natural history and prognosis of a glomerular nephropathy. The classification we propose is based on the study of 1368 patients with a clinical diagnosis of glomerular disease in which we have studied renal biopsies. In practice, four main groups can be distinguished (Table 41).

1. The glomeruli are normal or present minimal glomerular lesions.

2. The glomeruli present specific lesions—in other words, the lesions indicate the causal disease.

3. The glomeruli present nonspecific lesions that do not point with certainty to a precise diagnosis or to a correlation with a particular clinical pattern. The lesions do, on the other hand, indicate the prognosis and this in itself is sufficient justification for the renal biopsy. It is in this group that precise classification is of fundamental importance.

---

*This chapter was written in collaboration with C. Kleinknecht and M. C. Gubler.

Table 41. Classification of Glomerular Nephropathy (1368 Cases)

I. GLOMERULAR NEPHROPATHIES ASSOCIATED WITH MINIMAL GLOMERULAR LESIONS (586 CASES)	
Pure idiopathic nephrotic syndrome	317
Idiopathic nephrotic syndrome with hematuria	110
Idiopathic "proteinuria-hematuria" syndrome	82
Isolated proteinuria	55
Isolated hematuria	22
II. GLOMERULAR NEPHROPATHIES ASSOCIATED WITH SPECIFIC GLOMERULAR LESIONS (142 CASES)	
Thrombotic microangiopathy	110
Amyloidosis	9
Diabetic glomerulosclerosis	2
Malarial "membranous" glomerulonephritis	21
Lupus nephritis (with hematoxylin bodies)	0
III. GLOMERULAR NEPHROPATHIES ASSOCIATED WITH NONSPECIFIC GLOMERULAR LESIONS (607 CASES)	
A. *Diffuse glomerular lesions*	
1. Nonproliferative	
Extramembranous glomerulonephritis	50
"Membranous" glomerulonephritis	10
Infantile mesangial sclerosis	10
2. Proliferative	
Pure endocapillary glomerulonephritis	86
Endocapillary and extracapillary glomerulonephritis (with focal crescents)	121
Endocapillary and extracapillary glomerulonephritis (with diffuse crescents)	27
Membranoproliferative and lobular glomerulonephritis	106
B. *Focal glomerular lesions*	
1. Segmental and focal glomerulonephritis	99
2. Focal glomerular sclerosis	
Segmental hyalinization	74
Global fibrosis	24
IV. UNCLASSIFIABLE GLOMERULAR LESIONS (33 CASES)	
Alport's syndrome	6
Focal "membranoproliferative" glomerulonephritis	4
Extramembranous glomerulonephritis with mesangial proliferation	4
Lesions too advanced for classification	19

4. The glomerular lesions are so disorganized or advanced that no classification is possible.

MINIMAL GLOMERULAR LESIONS

In 586 cases we found no significant lesion in the glomeruli. Most of these were idiopathic nephrotic syndromes, either pure (317 cases) or accompanied by hematuria (110 cases), which was usually microscopic and transient. In 82 cases the patient presented with "proteinuria with hematuria," one or the other being predominant. In this group, especially in cases of recurrent macroscopic hematuria, immunofluorescence studies have on some occasions revealed mesangial deposits of IgA and IgG (14 cases).

In 55 cases, permanent, isolated, idiopathic proteinuria had been discovered. In 22 cases, there was isolated hematuria. The discovery of minimal glomerular lesions has a negative significance but is no guarantee of a favorable prognosis.

SPECIFIC GLOMERULAR LESIONS

These are by far the least common, being found in fewer than 10 per cent of cases of glomerular disease in children. We include in this group: (1) thrombotic microangiopathy, the histologic picture underlying the hemolytic uremic syndrome (110 cases); (2) amyloidosis (9 cases); (3) diabetic glomerulosclerosis of the Kimmelstiel-Wilson type, very rare in children (2 cases); (4) malarial membranous glomerulonephritis, a lesion that we have seen in 21 black African children from the Ivory Coast suffering from a steroid-resistant nephrotic syndrome; and (5) lupus nephritis, for which the diagnosis can be made with certainty only if there are hematoxylin bodies in the lumina of the glomerular capillaries.

Thrombotic Microangiopathy

Glomerular lesions are associated with lesions of the arterioles and rarely of the larger caliber renal arteries. The glomerular lesion is characterized by thickening of the walls of the glomerular capillaries without endocapillary hypercellularity. This thickening results from swelling of the intermembrano-endothelial zone, which takes on a tufted, finely fibrillary appearance. The basement membrane is intact. There may be subendothelial fibrinoid deposits and fibrin thrombi in the lumina of the capillaries. Glomerular lesions of varying age and appearance may be found in the same preparation, suggesting the possibility of successive attacks on the glomeruli.

The vascular lesions involve principally the preglomerular arterioles and sometimes the interlobular arteries. There is most often swelling of the subendothelial zone that may involve the muscle wall, and sometimes fibrinoid necrosis. The lumen of the vessels is partly obstructed by a fibrin thrombus that is usually adherent to the necrotic wall. There is no perivascular granuloma.

The basic lesion is identical in both fatal and curable cases. In the curable cases, the glomerular lesions are less diffuse, the fibrinoid intracapillary thrombi are less common, and the arteriolar lesions are much less frequent. With immunofluorescence, there is no fixation of anti-IgG, anti-IgA, anti-IgM, anti-B_1C, or antialbumin sera. We have, on the other hand, noted fixation of antifibrinogen sera in five cases,[18] and other authors have reported the same finding in two cases.[37] This fixation occurs in the intracapillary and intra-arteriolar thrombosis and also in the walls of the glomerular capillaries and on the arteriolar walls.

Electron microscopy[11, 18, 37] reveals a very particular appearance: hypertrophy and cytoplasmic ramifications of the endothelial cell, whose phagocytic activity is increased; a deposit under the lamina densa of irregular disposition and density; abundant platelets in the lumina of the capillaries, with zones of intimate contact between these platelets and the sublaminar regions where the deposit is elaborated. The red blood cells have a particular morphology; their contours are polyhedral, with rectilinear borders. This is probably the ultrastructural equivalent of the anisocytosis found in the peripheral blood. There are also particles suggestive of viral nucleotides.[11, 18]

Amyloidosis

Amyloidosis (Figure 44) is easily diagnosed. The characteristic infiltration in the mesangium and the walls of the glomerular capillaries and in the base-

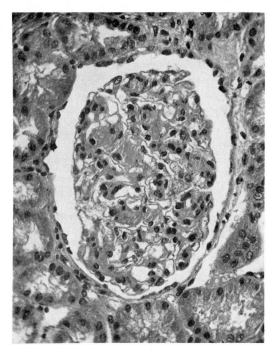

Figure 44. Renal amyloidosis. The entire mesangium and all the glomerular capillary walls are infiltrated by an amorphous substance that has the staining characteristics of amyloid. ×410.

ment membranes of the tubules and the arterioles by blobs of an eosinophilic, acellular substance, metachromatic to crystal violet and staining with Congo red, cannot be confused with any other lesion.[16] Of our nine patients, three had primary amyloidosis, three had familial Mediterranean fever, and in three the disease was secondary to chronic rheumatoid arthritis.

Diabetic Glomerulosclerosis of the Kimmelstiel-Wilson Type[25]

This is very rare in children, and we have never seen a case in a patient below the age of 15 years. The characteristic nodular lesions are formed at the periphery of the glomerulus and follow the contours of a capillary loop. The capillary loop surrounding a small nodule generally is dilated, whereas the lumen of the loops surrounding large nodules usually is obliterated. The nodules are hyaline, with a lamellar structure. They vary in number and size within the same glomerulus. Variable numbers of glomeruli in the renal parenchyma present the characteristic nodular lesions.

Malarial "Membranous" Glomerulonephritis[23, 31] (Figure 45)

We have found this particular lesion in 21 African children from the Ivory Coast suffering from a steroid-resistant nephrotic syndrome. The characteristic feature is a gross anomaly of the walls of the glomerular capillaries, which are thickened in an irregular fashion, twisted, and have a double contour. There are no extramembranous deposits and no endocapillary proliferation, but in the very occasional capillary loop there is a voluminous inter-membrano-endothelial fibrinoid deposit. In the majority of cases, in addition

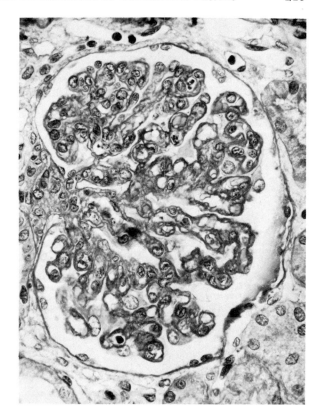

Figure 45. Malarial "membranous" glomerulonephritis. There is diffuse thickening and a double contour appearance of the walls of the glomerular capillaries, but there is no mesangial proliferation. ×350.

to these parietal lesions, there are focal and segmental lesions produced by coalescence of several capillary loops.

Lupus Nephritis with Hematoxylin Bodies

The diagnosis of lupus nephritis cannot be made in the absence of hematoxylin bodies. The hematoxylin bodies of Gross are specific, but they are very rare (we have never seen them in children). They are rounded or ovoid structures, about the size of a nucleus or larger, stained purple or lavender by hematoxylin, Feulgen positive, and located in the lumen of the glomerular capillaries, generally in zones of endocapillary proliferation. Wire-loop lesions (or intermembrano-endothelial deposits) produce thickening of some of the capillary walls, but these and the karyorrhexis emphasized by some authors seem less specific.

NONSPECIFIC GLOMERULAR LESIONS

These are the most common, being found in about half of all cases of glomerular nephropathy. They merit detailed consideration, and the etiology and clinical and laboratory features of each type of lesion will be discussed here.

The nonspecific glomerular lesions may be *diffuse* (that is to say, they involve all the observed glomeruli), or *focal* (meaning that only some glomeruli are involved, whereas others are normal).

Diffuse Glomerulonephritis

Two principal types may be seen, those with and those without proliferation of the mesangial cells.

Nonproliferative Glomerulonephritis

Extramembranous Glomerulonephritis.   This type of glomerulonephropathy was originally described as a specific lesion of the adult nephrotic syndrome. Many recent publications have been devoted to this entity.[2, 3, 8, 9, 12–14, 17, 21, 33, 34] Most authors report observations in children, at the same time emphasizing the great rarity of the condition in childhood.[10, 34, 40] This has not been our experience, however; this group has accounted for some 10 per cent of all nonspecific glomerular nephropathies we have seen.[19, 20, 35]

HISTOLOGY.   On light microscopy, the glomerular lesion is characterized by regular and diffuse thickening of the capillary walls with no associated endocapillary proliferation (Figure 46). As shown by trichrome stains, this thickening results from the presence of a more or less continuous fibrinoid or hyaline deposit on the epithelial aspect of the basement membrane, between the lamina densa and the epithelial covering. One of the most precise elements of histologic diagnosis is that, in the majority of cases, silver stains reveal characteristic spikes on the membrane or wall, provided that the lesions are neither very early nor very late (Figure 47).

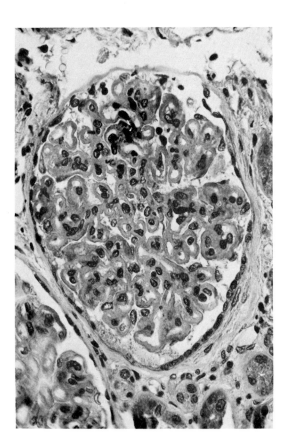

Figure 46. Extramembranous glomerulonephritis. Note the regular and diffuse thickening of all the glomerular capillary walls and also the absence of mesangial proliferation. ×500.

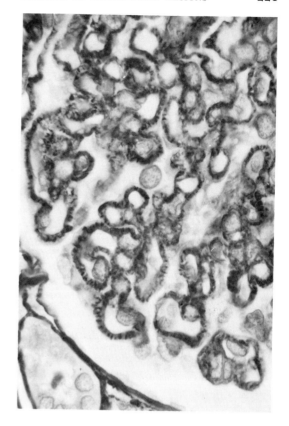

Figure 47. Extramembranous glomerulonephritis. With this stain, the basement membrane has a very characteristic hatched appearance. Silver stain, ×1190.

Examination with the electron microscope confirms the presence of an abnormal subepithelial deposit in confluent masses. The lamina densa is sometimes intact, sometimes thinned, and often completely fused with the deposit. Silver staining is necessary to localize the deposit in relation to the lamina densa. This stain also reveals the perpendicular spikes on the lamina densa separating the abnormal deposits from one another. In advanced cases, the spikes may completely surround the deposits, giving a twisted appearance to the wall (Figure 48).

In every case in which immunofluorescent studies of renal biopsy material have been possible, diffuse granular fixation of anti-IgG and anti-B_1C sera has been found along all the walls of the glomerular capillaries.

CLINICAL FEATURES.   Our series of 50 cases includes children of all ages, including the first year of life (8 months and 10 months). Two thirds of the children were boys. In 60 per cent of cases, the nephropathy developed without any definite antecedent or associated disorder. In the remaining cases, various etiologic circumstances were noted. Nine patients had had an infective episode, two had a giant urticaria, six had multiple joint pains and fever, and three were African children with sickle cell anemia.

There was no laboratory evidence of systemic lupus erythematosus in the 35 patients studied. In 27 children, the nephropathy was discovered by chance on examination of urine. In 19 children, the onset was marked by edema and in four others by macroscopic hematuria.

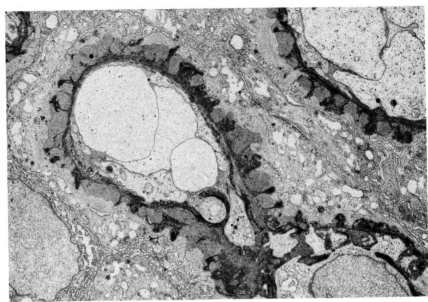

Figure 48. Electron micrograph of extramembranous glomerulonephritis. The large deposits on the epithelial aspect of the basement membrane are separated from one another by spicules of varying shape and size, lying perpendicular to the lamina densa, and argentaffins like the lamina densa. Silver stain, ×5700.

Proteinuria, sometimes selective, sometimes not very selective, was present in all patients, varying in degree from patient to patient and even in the same patient from day to day. In 44 cases, there was an associated nephrotic syndrome. A nephrotic syndrome was present from the onset in 31 children but appeared at a later stage in the other 13 patients. The nephrotic syndrome persisted throughout the period of observation in 11 children, while in the other 33 it was transient and disappeared, in the majority of cases, in a few months. Six patients did not have a nephrotic syndrome at any stage. Hematuria was noted at some stage in all but two patients, but it was macroscopic in only 11.

Hypertension was noted at onset in only three patients, and two of these had transient elevation of blood urea nitrogen. Complement (C'3) levels were always normal.

The various treatments used (prednisone and immunodepressive agents) did not seem effective (Table 42). In all, 34 patients received steroids. We have seen remissions in six patients so treated but the remission occurred between three and seven months after starting treatment. Immunodepressive agents were used in 21 patients and of these four had remissions eight to 12 months after beginning treatment. In 10 patients, combined treatment with prednisone and immunodepressive agents was associated with four remissions after three to 16 months of treatment. On the other hand, 19 patients who received no treatment also had complete remissions (five of these had never been treated and in the other 14 treatment had been stopped for more than six months).

In our experience, the evolution may follow one of two patterns.

In the first of these, 26 children had one or more remissions (Figure 49). In 17 of the 26 there was complete remission after one disease episode of varying duration. In the nine other cases, the remissions lasted from two months to five years and were followed by one or more relapses, more often consisting

Table 42. Response of Extramembranous Glomerulonephritis to Different Treatments

Treatment		Number of Cases	Response		
			Remission	Amelioration	Failure
First treatment (less than six months)	Steroids	24	5	4	15
	Immunodepressive drugs	6	2	3	1
	Steroids and immunodepressive drugs	3	0	1	2
	No treatment	17	5	0	12
Subsequent treatment	Steroids	10	1	3	6
	Immunodepressive drugs	15	2	1	12
	Steroids and immunodepressive drugs	7	4	2	1
	No treatment	20	14	1	5

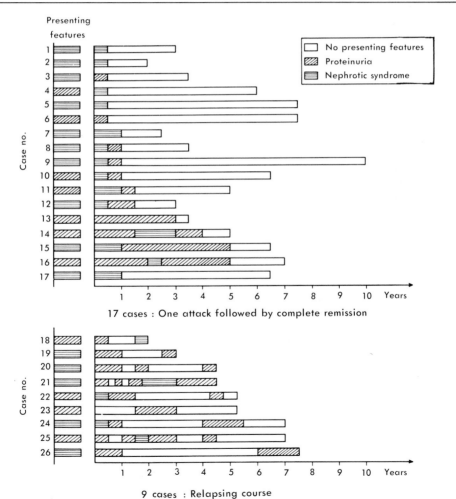

Figure 49. Glomerulonephritis with extramembranous deposits. Course with remissions in 26 cases.

223

of a moderate proteinuria than a nephrotic syndrome. In both groups, when the nephrotic syndrome was present at the outset, it has generally been mild and transient and never lasted more than one year. We have never seen an unfavorable outcome in this type.

In the second pattern, the nephropathy progressed without remission in 24 patients (Figure 50). In 12 patients, the nephrotic syndrome was absent or transient, and in the remaining 12, the nephrotic syndrome was permanent. Only in this group have we seen an unfavorable outcome. Five patients developed chronic renal failure at intervals of 18 months to five years after the onset of the disease. Two of these children are dead, one after three and a half years and the other after eight years. In the latter, the nephrotic syndrome began at the age of 10 months, and there were signs or tubular insufficiency, with glycosuria, hyperchloremic acidosis, and a salt-losing syndrome preceding the onset of global renal failure, which appeared 18 months after the first signs of disease. It thus seems that a permanent nephrotic syndrome carries a very poor prognosis.

The present situation after a follow-up of one to 10 years (four years on

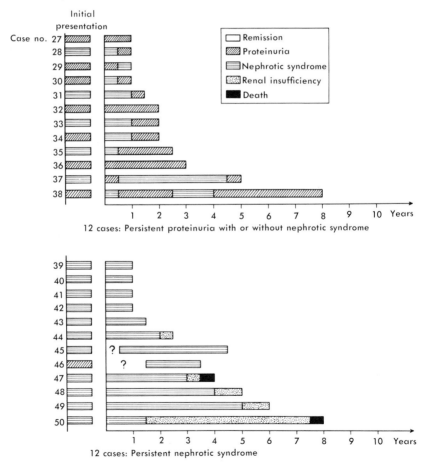

Figure 50. Glomerulonephritis with extramembranous deposits. Course without remission in 24 cases.

average) is as follows: two patients are dead or on maintenance dialysis, three have renal insufficiency, nine have a persistent nephrotic syndrome, 15 have moderate proteinuria, and 21 are in complete remission. Some of these remissions are recent, and so the possibility of relapse remains. However, in eight of the children, the remission has lasted for more than three years and may signify permanent cure.

"Membranous" Glomerulonephritis. We have isolated this group of 10 cases because of the special histologic appearance. The glomerular lesions are characterized by regular and diffuse thickening of the capillary walls in the absence of any mesangial proliferation. No deposits can be seen on the epithelial aspect of the basement membrane, and silver staining shows a twisted appearance of walls and the absence of spikes. It is possible that this appearance may represent only a particular evolutionary stage of extramembranous glomerulonephritis, as suggested by the work of Bariéty and associates.[3] This would seem to be confirmed by the similarity of the clinical features, including the same predominance in males, the same age at onset (four cases before the age of 2 years, including two at the age of 6 months), the same idiopathic nature of the nephropathy, the same symptomatology (seven nephrotic syndromes with hematuria, three proteinuria with hematuria), and the same type of evolution of the nephropathy (except for one patient who died after two years).

Diffuse Mesangial Sclerosis (10 Cases) (See Page 267). This has not to our knowledge been described previously. It is very interesting because of the early onset of the nephropathy (during the first year of life) and because of the familial character in many cases.[21, 27] There is simultaneous involvement of all the glomeruli. There is no mesangial proliferation, but fine argentaffin fibrils invade the mesangium, leading to retractile sclerosis of the tuft. The epithelial cells surround the tuft like a crown. The 10 patients in our series with this type of lesion all presented with an idiopathic nephrotic syndrome, and this was accompanied by microscopic hematuria in three cases. The prognosis is very poor. Nine of the 10 are dead, all having died before the age of three years.

Proliferative Glomerulonephritis

Mesangial or Pure Endocapillary Proliferative Glomerulonephritis (86 Cases). The characteristic feature of this condition is a varying degree of proliferation of the mesangial or endocapillary cells and hypertrophy of the intercapillary tissue without any thickening of the walls of the glomerular capillaries (Figure 51). This type of lesion is found principally in two circumstances of totally different significance—authentic cases of curable acute glomerulonephritis (with or without nephrotic syndrome), and certain cases of idiopathic nephrotic syndrome that are usually steroid-resistant.

In the early stage of acute glomerulonephritis, in addition to the mesangial proliferation, there are polymorphonuclear cells in the lumen of the glomerular capillaries and humps (small, widely spaced fibrinoid deposits) on the epithelial aspect of the basement membrane. On immunofluorescence, the humps appear to consist of IgG and B_1C and form a line of granular deposits along the walls of the glomerular capillaries. However, in the phase of resolution, these proliferated cells concentrate in the intercapillary axes, the humps disappear, immunofluorescence is negative, and only here and there is the diagnosis in-

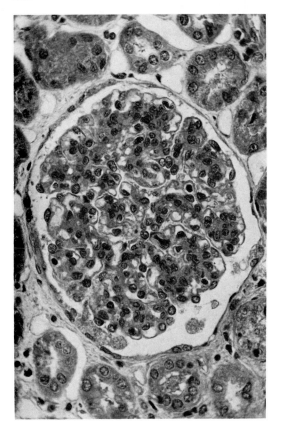

Figure 51. Diffuse endocapillary
glomerulonephritis in a patient with glomerulonephritis of acute onset following infection. Note the intense mesangial proliferation and the integrity of
the walls of the glomerular capillaries.
×410.

dicated by the hypercellularity, which is more marked in acute glomerulonephritis than in the cases of idiopathic nephrotic syndrome.

Of the 86 cases presenting this type of glomerular change, the nephropathy appeared in six during the course of a systemic disease. Fifty-five of the
cases were authentic acute glomerulonephritis, of which 51 developed after an
episode of sore throat, whose streptococcal origin was proved in only half of the
cases. All presented with proteinuria and hematuria that was usually macroscopic. Sixteen of the patients had, in addition, a fall in serum protein level,
with a mild, transient nephrotic syndrome. In two thirds of the cases of acute
glomerulonephritis a rise in the blood urea or hypertension or both occurred
in the initial stage of the disease. All these patients recovered completely at
intervals varying from three to 13 months.

The 25 other patients presented with a frank idiopathic nephrotic syndrome, either pure (four cases) or accompanied by hematuria that was usually
microscopic (21 cases). In five of these patients, a second renal biopsy revealed
disappearance of the mesangial proliferation and the appearance of segmental
and focal hyalinization. Unlike the acute glomerulonephritis group, the disease
pursued a chronic course in the patients presenting with a nephrotic syndrome
and mesangial proliferation; the condition was usually steroid-resistant, and
four of these patients died between one and a half and four years after the onset.
One other patient has reached the stage of chronic renal failure. Clearly it is
essential to distinguish between these two histologic entities.

Proliferative Endocapillary Glomerulonephritis with Focal Epithelial Crescents (121 Cases).   The characteristic histologic feature of this group is the association of diffuse endocapillary proliferation in all the glomeruli, with epithelial or extracapillary proliferation of varying degree and extent, but never involving more than 80 per cent of the glomeruli (Figure 52). We have found that diffuse extracapillary proliferation involving all the glomeruli has a very sinister significance,[19] and hence this group is considered in a special chapter. This type of glomerular nephropathy can be found in many etiologic circumstances, but there is usually a definite cause (only 15 cases were idiopathic). This disease is most often identified in the context of a systemic disease (62 cases), but it may be found also in glomerulonephritis of acute onset occurring after infection, which perhaps is rather more severe than the average (54 cases).

In more than half the cases, the clinical picture is that of a nephrotic syndrome with hematuria, but the hematuria is usually transient and rarely gross. In the other cases, one finds the classical picture of acute glomerulonephritis with proteinuria, hematuria that is often macroscopic, elevation of the blood urea nitrogen level, or hypertension. The prognosis in this type of glomerular disorder is a function of the number of glomeruli involved in the extracapillary proliferation. Death has rarely been seen in this group, and then only in cases of systemic disease. One third of the patients have recovered, apparently completely. The remaining patients retain some evidence of nonprogressive nephropathy over many years, generally a proteinuria.

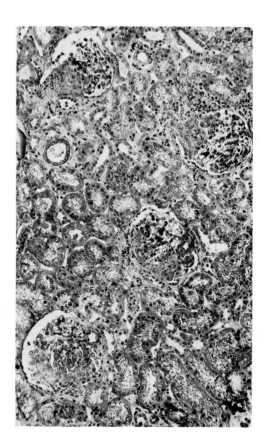

Figure 52. Endocapillary and extracapillary proliferative glomerulonephritis with focal crescents. There is diffuse mesangial proliferation in all the glomeruli, but in some of the glomeruli there is in addition an extracapillary proliferation producing fusion of the most affected parts of the tuft with Bowman's capsule. ×115.

Endocapillary Glomerulonephritis with diffuse Epithelial Crescents[27]
(see page 282).   There are 27 patients in this group, and the histologic characteristic is the presence, in 80 to 100 per cent of glomeruli observed, of voluminous epithelial or fibroepithelial crescents, sometimes containing fibrin, encircling
a glomerular tuft that itself is grossly abnormal, in which the lesions can be
difficult to analyze (Figure 53). In eight cases it was apparent that these epithelial
crescents were superimposed on a typical membranoproliferative glomerulonephritis. These eight patients are specially considered with the group of membranoproliferative glomerulonephritis. In the other cases, a mixture of endocapillary proliferation, in places varying from loop to loop, of mesangial
sclerosis and of deposits in the walls makes any classification impossible. In one
of these cases, we were able to identify by immunofluorescence techniques
linear deposits of IgG and B_1C on the walls, and the presence of circulating
anti-basement membrane antibody was reminiscent of Goodpasture's syndrome,
even though there was no evidence of associated lung disease.

Most often, this type of glomerular nephropathy develops in the context of
a systemic disease. In some patients, the disorder presents as acute postinfective
glomerulonephritis. In a few cases no cause can be found. All the patients with
this type of nephropathy have one point in common, the severity of the disease.
They have, for the most part, a nephrotic syndrome with hematuria appearing
concomitantly or secondarily, and the most notable feature is early renal insufficiency that may be accompanied by oliguria or even anuria. Sometimes the

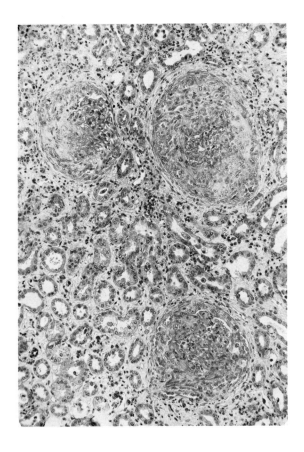

Figure 53. Endocapillary and
extracapillary proliferative glomerulonephritis with diffuse crescents.
Huge   circumferential   epithelial
crescents occupy Bowman's space
in all the glomeruli. ×110.

renal failure develops gradually, but, in either case, it progresses inevitably to death. All the patients in this group died within 20 months, with the exception of two in whom the course of the disease was more prolonged (2 years 10 months and 3 years 7 months).

Membranoproliferative Glomerulonephritis (106 Cases). The incidence of membranoproliferative glomerulonephritis is high in children, accounting for 20 percent of nonspecific glomerulonephritides.[19] The isolation of this variety within the group of prolonged glomerulonephritis is fairly recent and resulted from the practice of renal biopsy.[17, 20] Many names have been given to this variety, including mixed membranous and proliferative glomerulonephritis,[1] parieto-proliferative glomerulonephritis,[4] and mesangiocapillary glomerulonephritis.[10]

Immunofluorescence in these cases has revealed deposits of immunoglobulin and complement in the walls of the glomerular capillaries.[29] Gotoff and his colleagues[15] and West and associates[39] have found significant and permanent lowering of the C'3 fraction of serum complement, and they term this variety "hypocomplementemic persistent glomerulonephritis." There have been several recent studies of this type of nephropathy.[2, 7, 24, 30, 38]

Our description of the natural history of the disease is based on a clinical study of 98 cases of idiopathic membranoproliferative glomerulonephritis. Similar lesions may be found in systemic diseases. Among such on our service have been three cases of lupus, two cases of rheumatoid purpura, two cases of periarteritis nodosa, and one case of unidentified systemic disease. One additional patient with "shunt nephritis" (see page 322) presented typical membranoproliferative lesions.

HISTOPATHOLOGY. The membranoproliferative glomerulonephritides are defined by the association of endocapillary proliferation with hypertrophy of the mesangial substance and a diffuse but often irregular thickening of the walls of the glomerular capillaries. Light microscopy, confirmed by ultrathin sections and by electron microscopy, reveals, depending on the type of thickening, two different varieties.

1. *Membranoproliferative glomerulonephritis with intermembranoendothelial deposits or a "double contour" appearance of the walls of the glomerular capillaries (Figures 54 and 58).* The double contour appearance is the result of infiltration of both cellular and fibrillary elements of the mesangium between the basement membrane of the capillary and the endothelium, leading to progressive narrowing of the lumen of the glomerular capillaries. We have seen 69 cases.

2. *Membranoproliferative glomerulonephritis with dense basement membrane deposits.*[5] In these cases, the lamina densa, infiltrated by a very chromophilic deposit, takes on a quite characteristic ribbon appearance. We have seen 29 cases (Figures 55 and 59).

Whatever the nature of the parietal deposit, three forms of membranoproliferative glomerulonephritis can be described.

Most often (59 cases), the parietal lesions (whether of the "double contour" or "dense deposits" types) and the proliferative lesions are isolated (pure membranoproliferative glomerulonephritis) (Figures 54 and 55).

Sometimes (26 cases) there is in addition an accumulation of membranoid substance expanding the intercapillary axes and giving the tuft a lobulated appearance. This is what is called lobular glomerulonephritis (Figures 56 and 57).

Lastly, in 13 cases, in addition to the membranoproliferative lesions of the

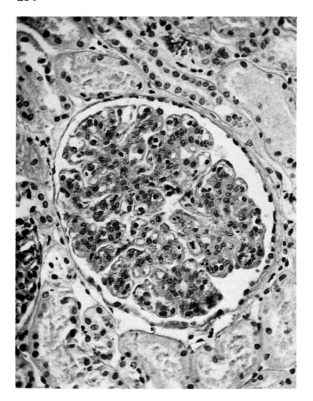

Figure 54. Membranoproliferative glomerulonephritis with subendothelial deposits and a double-contour appearance of the walls of the glomerular capillaries. ×285.

Figure 55. Membranoproliferative glomerulonephritis with dense deposits in the basement membranes. The appearance is comparable to that of Figure 54, the only difference being the nature of the deposit thickening the walls of the glomerular capillaries. ×290.

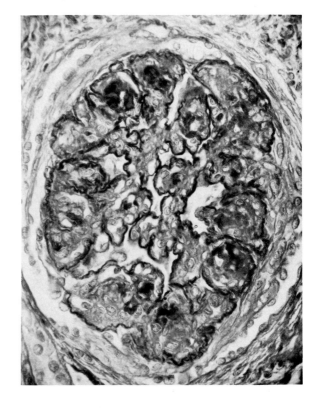

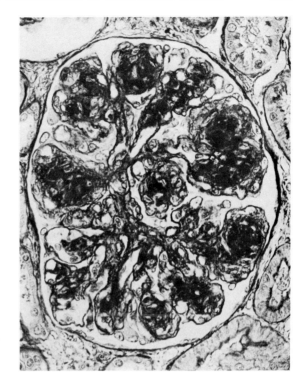

Figure 56. Lobular glomerulonephritis with subendothelial deposits. The accentuation of the mesangial tissue produces lobulation of the tuft. ×350.

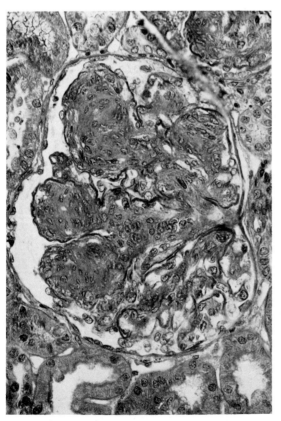

Figure 57. Lobular glomerulonephritis with dense deposits in the basement membranes. ×500.

tuft, there was extracapillary proliferation of variable extent (involving between 30 and 100 per cent of glomeruli), leading to the formation of epithelial or fibroepithelial crescents filling the space between the capsule and glomerular tuft.

We studied 20 cases by immunofluorescence and the results differed according to the type of thickening of the wall. In the 15 cases in which light microscopy had revealed intermembrano-endothelial deposits or double contours, there were two different findings. In 12 cases, for which most of the biopsies were taken early, a constant finding was endomembranous fixation of anti-IgG sera varying in intensity from one capillary loop to another, and an inconstant and lesser fixation of anti-IgM sera. Anti-C′3 sera were also fixed and in three cases this fixation was very intense, diffused through all of the capillary walls and with both parietal and mesangial localization, whereas there was only slight fixation of anti-immunoglobulin sera. In these three cases, biopsies were taken late, 2 years 4 months, 4 years, and 4 years 6 months after the onset of the disease.

In the five cases in which light microscopy had revealed dense deposits in the basement membranes, we found slight and irregular fixation of anti-IgG and anti-IgM sera on the walls of the glomerular capillaries, but the fixation of anti-C′3 serum was variable. In three cases the anti-C′3 serum was fixed in the mesangium and in very small amounts on the capillary walls, whereas in the other two cases it was fixed diffusely and intensely exclusively on the walls of the glomerular capillaries.

We have never found significant changes in the lesions on repeated biopsy, whatever the time interval between the biopsies. We have observed an increase in the amount of the deposits or a diminished intensity of cellularity, but we have never seen membranoproliferative glomerulonephritis become lobular or vice versa.

CLINICAL FEATURES. This type of nephropathy affects girls more often than boys (57 girls and 41 boys) and, in 80 cases, it developed after the age of 8 years. We have never seen it before the age of 2 years. In 42 children, the nephropathy was discovered following an upper respiratory tract infection or a sore throat whose streptococcal nature was proved only in 10 patients by a rise in the antistreptolysin titer. In 56 other cases, no etiologic factor could be discovered. It should be recorded, however, that two of these children presented a partial lipodystrophy of the Barraquer-Simons type.

The presenting feature was edema of varying degree in 38 cases and macroscopic hematuria in 19 cases. In the remaining 41 patients, proteinuria was discovered by routine examination of the urine prior to a vaccination or after a febrile sore thorat. In one third of the cases, acute glomerulonephritis was diagnosed because of the sudden onset, following a sore throat, of hematuria, proteinuria, renal insufficiency, or hypertension.

The urinary protein is rarely more than 250 mg./kg./24 hours at the onset of the disease, and in more than half of the cases it is less than 100 mg./kg./24 hours. In the cases in which this was studied, the proteinuria was found to be only moderately or slightly selective. Serum proteins were measured in 74 patients and were found to be normal in 16; only in eight patients were they grossly lowered. The serum lipids were measured in 68 cases and were found to be very high in only three but normal in 36 cases. Edema was absent in more than half of the cases, but even when present, it is slight.

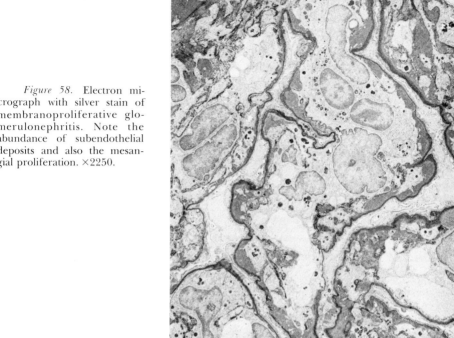

Figure 58. Electron micrograph with silver stain of membranoproliferative glomerulonephritis. Note the abundance of subendothelial deposits and also the mesangial proliferation. ×2250.

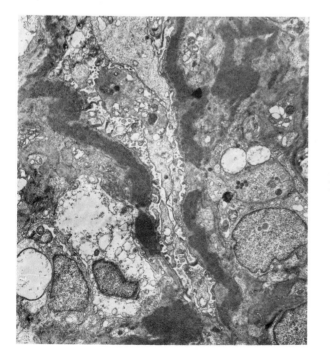

Figure 59. Electron micrograph of membranoproliferative glomerulonephritis with dense deposits in the basement membranes. ×3400.

These patients have been followed for periods varying from one and a half to 18 years (five and a half years on average), and during this period most developed a nephrotic syndrome. Usually this nephrotic syndrome is mild and may even be purely a laboratory finding. Serous effusions were found in only five patients. The nephrotic syndrome was permanent in 23 patients; it appeared late but then became permanent in 19. It was intermittent or transient in 40 patients, and 16 patients did not present a nephrotic syndrome at any stage.

Hematuria is virtually constant. Only in three patients was it not present at any stage. In the first year of the disease, macroscopic hematuria was noted in 35 patients. In one patient, the hematuria did not become macroscopic until the second year of the disease. This hematuria persists over the years, but has a tendency to diminish spontaneously with time. The macroscopic hematuria frequently seen during the first year becomes rare at a later stage and this observation may give some guidance in dating the onset of the disease.

A blood urea level between 60 and 200 mg. per 100 ml. was noted at the onset of the disease in 31 patients, proving regressive in 24 of them.

There was hypertension at onset in 21 patients, but the blood pressure returned to normal in all but three (two of these died very soon afterward and one remained hypertensive after 10 years).

In half of the cases, the rise in blood urea level and the hypertension are associated in the same patient. There was profound anemia (red cell count between 2 and 3.2 million per cubic millimeter) at onset in 19 patients and 11 of these had a lobular glomerulonephritis. In most cases, this anemia is independent of any chronic renal failure.

The C′3 fraction of complement was measured by the immunodiffusion technique in 24 patients on one or more occasions. The C′3 level was low or extremely low in 17 cases. In five patients, it remained low. In eight patients, the C′3 level rose subsequently with or without immunodepressive treatment. Only one measurement was made in four of the patients. The complement level was normal in the seven other cases. In two of these, it was repeatedly found to be normal, and in the five other patients, the complement was measured on only one occasion, at the time of the renal biopsy, which was performed at varying stages of the disease.

We studied the correlation between the C′3 levels and the different histologic types and found that the level was markedly and permanently lowered only in cases in which the thickening of the capillary walls resulted from dense deposits in the basement membranes or in cases with subendothelial deposits and exclusive presence of complement on immunofluorescence.

Various treatments have been suggested. They are disparate and difficult to analyze. Their effects are described schematically in Table 43 and compared with natural evolution either before treatment or with no treatment.

Steroids have been used in low doses (0.5 to 1 mg./kg./24 hours) in 27 patients. No remission was observed with this treatment. In three patients, a nephrotic syndrome was replaced by a proteinuria coincidental to the administration of steroids. In half the cases there was no alteration in the nephropathy and furthermore there was definite deterioration in 11 other cases. In one patient the deterioration consisted simply of a raised blood urea level; in the other 10, there was hypertension, either isolated or associated with a blood urea level varying between 60 and 100 mg. per 100 ml. These disorders improved when the steroid therapy was stopped.

Table 43. Response of Membranoproliferative Glomerulonephritis
to Different Treatments

Results	Untreated	Steroids	Immunodepressive Agents	Hydroxychloroquine
Remission	9	0	8	1
Amelioration	10	3	12	1
No change	28	13	29	5
Deterioration	18	11	12	3
Total	65	27	61	10

Immunodepressive agents (mainly chlorambucil, sometimes Imuran) were prescribed for 61 patients. In eight cases, remission coincided with administration of these drugs. In 12 patients, there was diminution of the proteinuria. However, in 29 patients there was no change, and in another 12 patients there was definite aggravation of the disease. Antimalarial agents were prescribed for 10 patients, with no apparent benefit.

These therapeutic results are all the more difficult to interpret in the light of the finding of remission in nine cases and amelioration in 10 cases without any treatment whatever.

The prognosis of membranoproliferative glomerulonephritis is poor. With a mean follow-up of 5 years 7 months, 28 patients have died or are on dialysis, and nine patients have already reached the stage of chronic renal failure. Six patients have hypertension, in three cases in addition to proteinuria and in three cases in addition to nephrotic syndrome. Sixteen patients still had a nephrotic syndrome at the last examination, and 34 had proteinuria that was isolated or associated with microscopic hematuria.

A total of 18 patients had complete remission, often of very brief duration and generally at the beginning of the disease. At the last examination, five of these were still in remission. This remission was recent in three patients (1 month, 4 months, and 7 months) but of longer standing in the remaining two (2 years 6 months and 4 years 4 months). One of these two had been treated by immunodepressive agents and the other had never received treatment.

All the deaths resulted from renal failure. Six patients died in the first year and 15 patients within 4 years of onset. In 12 patients, death occurred between 5 and 18 years after the onset. It is worth noting that all but one of the patients who died within three years of onset had a variable percentage of epithelial crescents in their glomeruli in addition to membranoproliferative glomerulonephritis.

In compiling these figures, we have considered as "dead" those patients maintained on hemodialysis or those who have had kidney transplantation. Four patients with a grafted kidney are alive at the present time. Two of these patients, whom we have placed in the group having membranoproliferative glomerulonephritis with dense deposits in the basement membrane, have identical deposits in the grafted kidney on the basement membranes of the glomeruli and tubules, but no mesangial proliferation.

Six patients became pregnant, and four of these developed hypertension, although in two the hypertension regressed. Except for one case of hydatidiform mole, each of these women gave birth to a normal baby.

In most patients, the disease progresses in chronic fashion, with occasional remissions, generally ending in renal failure and death, but the interval from onset to death varies greatly from one patient to another. Figure 60 represents

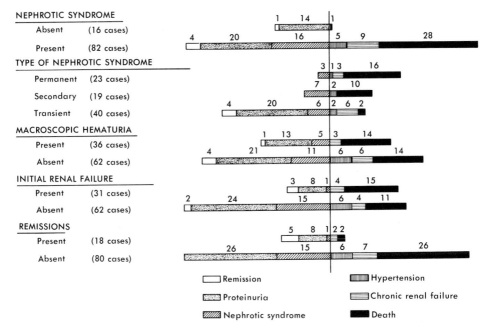

Figure 60. Relationship of prognosis of membranoproliferative glomerulonephritis to clinical signs.

an attempt to analyze the different features of the disease as a function of the evolution in the hope of drawing some conclusions about prognosis. In those patients who present a nephrotic syndrome, the prognosis is poorer if the syndrome is present at onset and if it is permanent (83 per cent with an unfavorable course) than it is in patients in whom the nephrotic syndrome appears later (53 per cent), and the prognosis is very much worse than in patients whose nephrotic syndrome is transient (20 per cent) or who do not develop a nephrotic syndrome at any stage (0 per cent).

Renal insufficiency at the onset is also a poor prognostic sign. Sixty-one per cent of the patients presenting with renal insufficiency have followed an unfavorable course, whereas only 24 per cent of those who did not initially have renal insufficiency have died or currently have chronic renal failure.

In contrast, there is no significant difference between the presence or

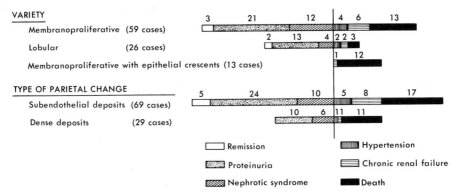

Figure 61. Relationship of prognosis of membranoproliferative glomerulonephritis to histologic type.

absence of complete remission in the course of the disease, or the presence or absence of macroscopic hematuria. So far as histology is concerned, the presence of dense deposits in the basement membranes seems to be a bad sign (Figure 61). The most important point is that the presence of epithelial crescents is a highly significant indication of a poor prognosis, because every one of the children who presented this type of lesion is dead or in chronic renal failure, in contrast to 32 per cent in the group with pure membranoproliferative glomerulonephritis and 20 per cent in the group with lobular glomerulonephritis.

Focal Glomerulonephritis

There are two principal types of focal glomerulonephritis.

Segmental and Focal Glomerulonephritis (99 Cases). In this type of nephropathy, the pathologic glomeruli (rarely constituting more than 30 to 40 per cent) are characterized by segmental involvement of one part of the glomerular tuft. There is both endocapillary and extracapillary proliferation in the involved segment, and there may be a zone of fibrinoid necrosis in the center of the segment. In most cases, the capillary loops are fused to one another and to the adjacent Bowman's capsule by sclerosis. In all cases, the remainder of the tuft is normal (Figure 62).

Half the cases are discovered as part of a systemic disease, notably the Henoch-Schönlein syndrome. In the other half, the nephropathy may be idiopathic or may follow a recent rhinopharyngitis, and the special clinical

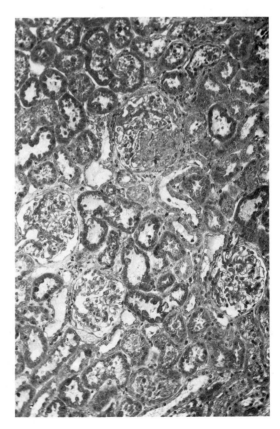

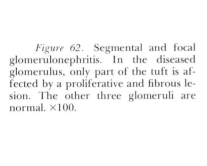

Figure 62. Segmental and focal glomerulonephritis. In the diseased glomerulus, only part of the tuft is affected by a proliferative and fibrous lesion. The other three glomeruli are normal. ×100.

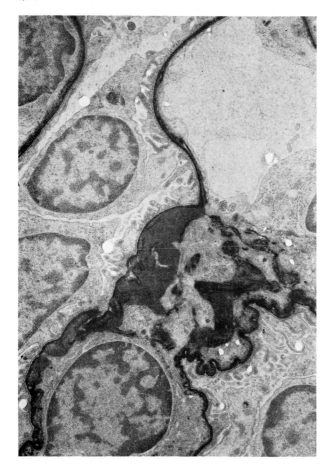

Figure 63. Electron micrograph with silver stain of segmental and focal glomerulonephritis with mesangial deposits of IgA–IgG. These deposits, essentially localized in the intercapillary axes, are easily identified on electron microscopy. ×6000.

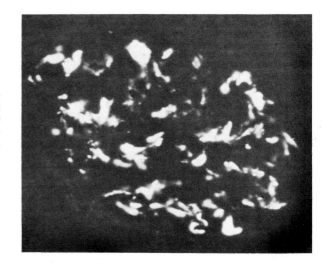

Figure 64. Immunofluorescence of segmental and focal glomerulonephritis. All the glomeruli contain mesangial deposits that fix anti-IgA serum. ×300.

feature is that the patients present with recurrent macroscopic hematuria. It is in this latter group that immunofluorescence techniques have demonstrated mesangial deposits of IgA and IgG (see page 254) (Figure 64). The mesangial localization of the deposits is confirmed by electron microscope studies (Figure 63).[6, 26]

A nephrotic syndrome is very rarely seen with this type of lesion, and when it does occur it is mild, transient, and always accompanied by hematuria. In seven cases, the only clinical manifestation of renal disease was isolated hematuria. Even when it runs a prolonged course, the nephropathy is benign. The only deaths observed in this group were in one patient with rheumatoid purpura who had had many relapses after the renal biopsy, and in one patient with Goodpasture's syndrome, in whom death resulted from pulmonary complications.

Focal Sclerosing Glomerulonephritis (98 Cases).   In these 98 cases, the characteristic feature is the fact that the lesions are focal—that is to say, they affect only a certain percentage of the glomeruli, the remaining glomeruli in most cases being normal.

Two types of lesions have been noted.

1. In 74 patients, the focal disorder is also segmental. In other words, only part of the tuft is affected in any diseased glomerulus, the remainder of the tuft being normal. The other special feature of the lesion is its hyaline character, on the basis of which we have chosen to designate it by the term *focal and segmental hyalinosis* (Figure 65). This type of glomerular lesion has been noted in specimens obtained at various stages from one month to 17 years after the discovery of the disease, but in most cases it was seen during the first two years.

Another special feature of the lesions of segmental hyalinosis is their topography. In 11 patients, only the glomeruli at the corticomedullary junction are involved, and the others are completely normal. A mild diffuse mesangial proliferation may accompany the focal glomerular lesions. The lesion can occasionally extend to include practically the entire glomerulus and may produce a glomerulus that is totally hyalinized.

2. In 24 cases, the focal lesion is characterized by total fibrosis of the affected glomeruli. This is the lesion which we designate by the term *global and focal fibrosis of the glomeruli* (Figure 66). This type of lesion has been noted in biopsy specimens obtained relatively late—after three years in 21 of 24 cases. Some of the glomeruli are normal on light microscopy, whereas others are fibrous, completely hyalinized, small, retractile, containing few cells, and they take up collagen stains. They are scattered in irregular fashion throughout the renal parenchyma. We rate the findings as significant when at least 15 per cent of the glomeruli are fibrous, and especially when there is in addition secondary tubulo-interstitial disease, with bands of fibrous tissue infiltrated in places by round cells or groups of lipophages surrounding atrophic, dedifferentiated tubules (a feature that rules out the diagnosis, in young children, of "congenital glomerulosclerosis").

By careful study of serial sections of renal biopsy material we have found, in nine of these cases, lesions of segmental and focal hyalinosis affecting one or two glomeruli, and these may represent an intermediate stage between the normal glomeruli and the fibrous glomeruli. In one patient there was moderate but diffuse mesangial proliferation in the nonfibrous glomeruli.

We have obtained two or even three biopsies from 25 patients. The results

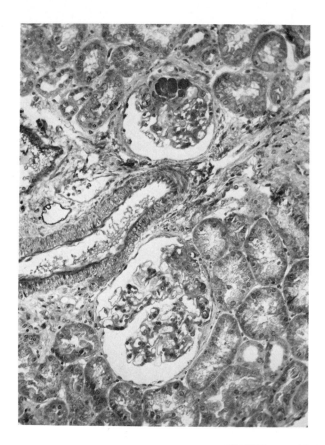

Figure 65. Segmental and focal hyalinization. Note the voluminous deposits of fibrinoid substance in the center of the hyalinized segmental lesions. ×200.

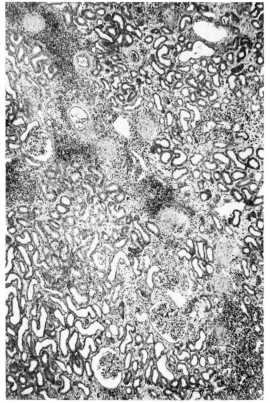

Figure 66. Global and focal fibrosis of the glomeruli. Normal glomeruli coexist with fibrous glomeruli, with focal atrophy of tubules and inflammatory infiltration of interstitial tissue. ×65.

240

of such repeat examinations are variable. In 10 cases, the first biopsy showed optically normal glomeruli, and the focal lesions were not found until the second examination six months to eight years later. In five cases, the first biopsy showed a diffuse mesangial proliferation in all the glomeruli. In the second biopsy, taken six to 18 months later, the hypercellularity had disappeared and the focal lesions were noted for the first time. In the remaining 10 cases, the same type of lesions was noted in both biopsies, with the second biopsy often showing extension of the focal lesions.

In the majority of patients presenting with this type of lesion, the nephropathy is idiopathic, but in a few cases it was discovered following an episode of infectious rhinopharyngitis or after vaccination. This lesion has never been seen in the context of a systemic disease. Most cases present with a nephrotic syndrome (88 cases), with or without hematuria (see page 262), but on occasion the lesions of segmental and focal hyalinosis may be found in patients who present a permanent idiopathic proteinuria with or without hematuria (see page 249).

The prognosis for this type of glomerular nephropathy is poor. With an average follow-up of 6 years, 24 of our patients are dead and seven have chronic renal failure. In the other patients, the nephropathy progressed in chronic fashion, with a persistent nephrotic syndrome or proteinuria and possible periods of remission in 34 patients.

UNCLASSIFIABLE GLOMERULAR LESIONS

In 33 cases, although the glomerular lesions were obvious, they could not be classified in any of the groups just described. Six of these were cases of Alport's syndrome presenting focal hyalinizing and proliferative lesions, with localized reduplication of some of the walls of the capillaries in other glomeruli. Four cases had focal membranoproliferative glomerulonephritis. Some of the glomeruli presented the typical lesions of membranoproliferative glomerulonephritis, but other glomeruli were normal. Because not all of the glomeruli were involved, we did not classify these four cases with the other cases of membranoproliferative glomerulonephritis. There were four cases of extramembranous glomerulonephritis with marked mesangial proliferation. We decided to exclude these four cases because one of the criteria for the definition of extramembranous glomerulonephritis is the absence of endocapillary proliferation. In two cases, spikes were visible on silver staining; in two other cases there were confluent extramembranous deposits. Lastly, there were 19 cases in which the lesions were too advanced for any definite classification.

Conclusion

Apart from the very rare cases of specific glomerulonephritis in which the histologic appearance alone gives a precise diagnosis of the disease, analysis of the facts presented here tends to demonstrate that the only positive conclusion to be drawn from examination of a renal biopsy in a case of glomerular nephropathy concerns the prognosis. It is difficult to be sure of the prognosis when the kidneys are normal on light microscopy or when the glomerular lesions are unclassifiable. On the other hand, a greater degree of certainty is possible for the nonspecific glomerulonephritides.

Table 44. Nonspecific Glomerular Nephropathy: Correlations Between the Glomerular Lesions and the Etiology

Glomerular Lesions		Number of Cases	Sex (Percentage Male)	Nose and Throat Infection		Systemic Disease					Idiopathic
				Hemolytic Streptococci Present	Hemolytic Streptococci Absent	Rheumatoid Purpura	Lupus	Periarteritis Nodosa	Goodpasture's Syndrome	Unidentified Systemic Disease	
Diffuse non-proliferative	Extramembranous glomerulonephritis	50	76	2	5	0	0	0	0	6	37
	"Membranous" glomerulonephritis	10	70	2	1	0	0	0	0	0	7
	Infantile mesangial sclerosis	10	60	0	0	0	0	0	0	0	10
Diffuse proliferative	Pure endocapillary glomerulonephritis	86*	58	25	26	4	1	0	0	1	29
	Endocapillary and extracapillary glomerulonephritis (with focal crescents)	121	52	20	24	48	5	3	0	6	15
	Endocapillary and extracapillary glomerulonephritis (with diffuse crescents)	27†	55	4	5	4	0	3	2	2	7
	Membranoproliferative and lobular glomerulonephritis	106	42	10	32	2	3	2	0	1	56
Focal	Segmental and focal glomerulonephritis	99	70	1	25	36	4	0	2	6	25
	Focal sclerosing glomerulonephritis	98	59	1	24	0	0	0	0	0	73
Total number of cases		607		65	142	94	13	8	4	22	259
Percentage			58	10.9	23.4	15.3	2.1	1.3	0.6	3.6	42.6

*Five of these patients are also included in the category of focal sclerosing glomerulonephritis.
†Eight of these patients are also included in the category of membranoproliferative glomerulonephritis.

Table 45. Nonspecific Glomerular Nephropathies: Correlation Between the Glomerular Lesions and the Symptomatology

Glomerular Lesions	Number of Cases	Isolated Hematuria	Isolated Proteinuria	Proteinuria + Hematuria	Pure Nephrotic Syndrome	Nephrotic Syndrome + Hematuria	Initial Renal Insufficiency	Initial Hypertension
Diffuse non-proliferative								
Extramembranous glomerulonephritis	50	0	0	6	2	42	2	3
"Membranous" glomerulonephritis	10	0	0	3	0	7	1	2
Infantile mesangial sclerosis	10	0	0	0	7	3	6	0
Pure endocapillary glomerulonephritis	86*	0	0	45	4	37	35	36
Diffuse proliferative								
Endocapillary and extracapillary glomerulonephritis (with focal crescents)	121	0	0	57	0	64	48	30
Endocapillary and extracapillary glomerulonephritis (with diffuse crescents)	27†	0	0	7	0	20	18	13
Membranoproliferative and lobular glomerulonephritis	106	0	0	21	3	82	34	24
Focal								
Segmental and focal glomerulonephritis	99	7	0	82	0	10	17	10
Focal sclerosing glomerulonephritis	98	0	6	4	28	60	12	11
Total number of cases	607	7	6	225	44	325	173	129
Percentage		1.1	1	37	7.2	53.5	28.5	21.2

*Five of these patients are also included in the category of focal sclerosing glomerulonephritis.
†Eight of these patients are also included in the category of membranoproliferative glomerulonephritis.

A study of the correlation between the histologic types and the etiology (Table 44) shows:

1. The same histologic appearance may be found in different etiologic circumstances, although it should be emphasized that certain types of lesion are never seen in the course of systemic diseases ("membranous" glomerulonephritis, infantile mesangial sclerosis, focal sclerosing glomerulonephritis).

2. Conversely, a nephropathy appearing in a specific etiologic context may be associated with various types of lesion, rheumatoid purpura being an excellent example.

3. The fundamental point is that it is impossible to find a precise cause in 42.6 per cent of cases of nonspecific glomerular nephropathy.

Study of the correlation between the histology and the clinical features (Table 45) shows that:

1. The same histologic appearance may be found with various patterns of clinical disease. It should be noted, however, that a patient with extramembranous glomerulonephritis, with endocapillary and extracapillary glomerulonephritis with diffuse crescents, with membranoproliferative glomerulonephritis, or with focal sclerosing glomerulonephritis presents clinically with a nephrotic syndrome and hematuria much more often than in any other way.

2. Conversely, a nephropathy with a specific clinical pattern may be associated with various histologic findings, an excellent example of this being the nephrotic syndrome with hematuria. Almost any type of lesion may be found in a patient presenting as a nephrotic syndrome with hematuria.

The fundamental point that emerges from our study is that, whatever the etiology and clinical presentation, there is a close correlation between the histology and the prognosis.

REFERENCES

1. Allen, A. C.: The Kidney. New York, Grune and Stratton, 1951.
2. Bariéty, J., Samarcq, P., Lagrue, G., Fritel, D., and Milliez, P.: Evolution ultrastructurale favorable de deux cas de glomérulopathies primitives à dépôts extramembraneux diffus. Presse Méd. 76:2179, 1968.
3. Bariéty, J., Druet, P., Lagrue, G., Samarcq, P., and Milliez, P.: Les glomérulonéphrites "extramembraneuses." Étude morphologique en microscopie optique, électronique et en immuno-fluorescence. Path. Biol. 18:5, 1970.
4. Bariéty, J., Druet, P., Loirat, P., and Lagrue, G.: Les glomérulonéphrites pariéto-prolifératives. Étude histopathologique en microscopie optique, électronique et en immuno-histochimie de 49 cas. Corrélations anatomo-cliniques. Path. Biol. 19:259, 1971.
5. Berger, J., and Galle, P.: Dépôts denses au sein des membranes basales du rein. Presse Méd. 49:2351, 1963.
6. Berger, J.: IgA glomerular deposits in renal disease. Transplant. Proc. 1:939, 1969.
7. Cameron, J. S., Glasgow, E. F., Ogg, C. S., and White, R. H. R.: Membranoproliferative glomerulonephritis and persistent hypocomplementaemia. Brit. Med. J. 4:7, 1970.
8. Chan, W. C., and Tsao, Y. C.: Diffuse membranous glomerulonephritis in children. J. Clin. Path. 19:464, 1966.
9. Churg, J., Grischman, E., Goldstein, M. H., Yunis, S. L., and Porush, J. G.: Idiopathic nephrotic syndrome in adults. New Eng. J. Med. 272:165, 1965.
10. Churg, J., Habib, R., and White, R. H.: Pathology of the nephrotic syndrome in children. Lancet 1:1299, 1970.
11. Courtecuisse, V., Habib, R., and Monnier, C.: Nonlethal hemolytic and uremic syndromes in children: an electron microscope study of renal biopsies from six cases. Exp. Mol. Path. 7: 327, 1967.
12. Ducrot, H., Tsomi, C., Jungers, P., de Montera, H., Hinglais, N., and Giromini, M.: Étude

anatomo-clinique des glomérulonéphrites extramembraneuses. In Actualités néphrologiques de l'Hôpital Necker. Paris, Flammarion, 1969, p. 115.

13. Ehrenreich, T., and Churg, J.: Pathology of membranous nephropathy. In Sommers, S. C., ed.: Pathology Annual. Vol. 3. New York, Appleton-Century-Crofts, 1968, p. 145.
14. Forland, M., and Spargo, B. H.: Clinicopathological correlations in idiopathic nephrotic syndrome with membranous nephropathy. Nephron 6:498, 1969.
15. Gotoff, S. P., Fellers, F. X., Vawter, G. F., Janeway, C. A., and Rosen, F. S.: The B₁C globulin in childhood nephrotic syndrome. Laboratory diagnosis of progressive glomerulonephritis. New Eng. J. Med. 273:524, 1965.
16. Habib, R., Ducrot, H., Slama, R., and de Montera, H.: Anatomie pathologique de l'amylose rénale, à propos de 14 observations. J. Urol. Nephrol. 64:515, 1958.
17. Habib, R., Michielsen, P., de Montera, H., Hinglais, N., Galle, P., and Hamburger, J.: In G. E. N. Wolstenholme and M. P. Cameron, eds.: Symposium on Renal Biopsy. London, Churchill, 1961, p. 70.
18. Habib, R., Courtecuisse, V., Leclerc, F., Mathieu, H., and Royer, P.: Étude anatomo-pathologique de 35 observations de syndrome hémolytique et urémique de l'enfant. Arch. franç. Pédiat. 26:391, 1969.
19. Habib, R.: Classification anatomique des néphropathies glomérulaires. Pädiat. Fortbildk. Praxis (Karger) 28:3, 1970.
20. Habib, R., and Kleinknecht, C.: The primary nephrotic syndrome of childhood. Classification and clinicopathologic study of 406 cases. In S. C. Sommers, ed.: Pathology Annual. New York, Appleton-Century-Crofts, 1971, p. 414.
21. Habib, R., Kleinknecht, C., and Gubler, M. C.: Extramembranous glomerulonephritis in children. J. Pediat. 82:754, 1973.
22. Hardwicke, J., Blainey, J. D., Brewer, D. B., and Soothill, J. F.: The nephrotic syndrome. Proceedings of the Third International Congress of Nephrology, Washington, D.C. 1966. New York, S. Karger, 1967, p. 69.
23. Hendrickse, R. G., Adeniyi, A., Edington, G. M., Glasgow, E. F., White, R. H. R., and Houba, V.: Quartan malarial nephrotic syndrome. Lancet 1:1143, 1972.
24. Pickering, R. J., Herdman, R. C., Michael, A. F., Vernier, R. L., Fish, A. J., Gewurz, H., and Good, R. A.: Chronic glomerulonephritis associated with low serum complement activity (chronic hypocomplementemic glomerulonephritis). Medicine 49:207, 1970.
25. Kimmelstiel, P., and Wilson, C.: Intercapillary lesions in the glomeruli of kidney. Amer. J. Path. 12:83, 1936.
26. Lèvy, M., and Gubler, M. C.: Hématuries macroscopiques récidivantes idiopathiques et dépôts mésangiaux d' IgA-IgG (maladie de Berger). In Journées parisiennes de Pédiatrie. Paris, Flammarion, 1972, p. 226.
27. Mathieu, H., and Habib, R.: Syndromes néphrotiques congénitaux. In Journées parisiennes de Pédiatrie. Paris, Flammarion, 1968, p. 288.
28. Mery, J. P., and Patte, D.: Le rein de la maladie périodique. In Actualités néphrologiques de l'Hôpital Necker. Paris, Flammarion, 1962, p. 151.
29. Michael, A. F., Drummond, J. N., Vernier, R. L., and Good, R. A.: Immunologic basis of renal disease. Pediat. Clin. N. Amer. 11:695, 1964.
30. Michael, A. F., Herdman, R. C., Fish, A. J., Pickering, R. J., and Vernier, R. L.: Chronic membranoproliferative glomerulonephritis with hypocomplementemia. Transplant. Proc. 1:925, 1969.
31. de Paillerets, F., Habib, R., Loubières, R., Clerc, M., Chapuis, Y., and Assi Adou, J.: Le syndrome néphrotique de l'enfant en Côte-d'Ivoire. Guigoz Scient. Rev. 89:2, 1972.
32. Pirani, C. L., and Manaligod, J. R.: The kidneys in collagen disease. In F. K. Mostofi and D. Smith, eds.: The Kidney. Baltimore, Williams & Wilkins, 1966, p. 147.
33. Pollak, V. E., Rosen, S., Pirani, C. L., Muehrcke, R. C., and Kark, R. M.: Natural history of lipoid nephrosis and of membranous glomerulonephritis. Ann. Intern. Med. 69:1171, 1968.
34. Rosen, J.: Membranous glomerulonephritis: current status. Hum. Path. 2:209, 1971.
35. Royer, P., Habib, R., Vermeil, G., Mathieu, H., and Alizon, M.: Les glomérulonephrites prolongées de l'enfant. Ann. Pédiat. 3:173, 1962.
36. Sohar, E., Gafni, J., Pras, M., and Heller, H.: Familial Mediterranean fever. Amer. J. Med. 43:227, 1967.
37. Vitsky, B. H., Suzuki, Y., Strauss, L., and Churg, J.: The hemolytic-uremic syndrome: a study of renal pathologic alterations. Amer. J. Path. 57:627, 1969.
38. Van Acker, K. J., Van den Drande, J., and Vincke, H.: Membranous proliferative glomerulonephritis. Helv. Paediat. Acta 25:204, 1970.
39. West, C. D., McAdams, A. J., McConville, J. M., Davis, N. C., and Holland, N. H.: Hypocomplementemic and normocomplementemic persistent (chronic) glomerulonephritis; clinical and pathologic characteristics. J. Pediat. 67:1089, 1965.
40. White, R. H. R., Glasgow, E. F., and Mills, R. J.: Clinicopathological study of nephrotic syndrome in childhood. Lancet 1:1353, 1970.

Chapter Three

THE MAJOR SYNDROMES

The clinical expression of glomerular disease is a simple one. It consists in proteinuria, hematuria, hypertension, and signs of renal insufficiency. We have never seen a glomerular nephropathy present solely with an elevated blood pressure or elevated blood urea level, but an isolated proteinuria or isolated hematuria may on occasion be the only manifestation of glomerular disease. In most cases, several or all of these signs are associated with each other. When the proteinuria is considerable, associated hypoproteinemia, hyperlipemia, and edema produce a nephrotic syndrome. This nephrotic syndrome may be "pure" or associated with hematuria, hypertension, or renal insufficiency. The clinical onset may be sudden, in which case we describe it as acute, as in certain acute glomerulonephritides and nephrotic syndromes. Very often the proteinuria is revealed by routine examination of the urine. The onset of the nephropathy may then be regarded as insidious.

The case may go on to complete cure with varying rapidity, as in acute glomerulonephritis with pure endocapillary proliferation or in certain nephrotic syndromes with minimal glomerular lesions. The disease may become chronic or follow various patterns. The process may be continuous, with the same clinical and laboratory features throughout, or the form of the disease may change with time. Its course may be punctuated by complete remissions followed by relapses.

All these "chronic" nephropathies terminate in death from chronic renal failure after a variable period of time. This is seen, for example, in most cases of extramembranous glomerulonephritis, in membranoproliferative and lobular glomerulonephritis, in segmental and focal hyalinosis, and sometimes even in glomerulonephritis with mesangial deposits of IgA and IgG.

Some cases of glomerulonephritis, such as endocapillary and extracapillary glomerulonephritis with diffuse crescents, prove rapidly fatal from terminal renal failure. Paradoxically, this type of nephropathy is often termed "subacute." We prefer to call it malignant glomerulonephritis or glomerulonephritis with rapidly progressive renal failure.

The term "acute" should be applied only to the mode of onset of a nephropathy and not to its curability or noncurability, which can be assessed only on histologic examination. A glomerulonephritis that presents acutely may prove to be chronic or malignant. The term "chronic" should be used only to indicate the type of evolution, never to designate a particular histologic type of glomerular nephropathy. As we saw in Chapter 2 of Part III, the majority of glomerular lesions may be the histologic substratum of a chronic glomerulonephritis. Such a chronic glomerulonephritis may present with any of the signs of glomerular disease (hematuria, proteinuria, isolated or associated with hematuria, nephrotic syndrome) or may be entirely latent.

246

PROTEINURIA*

The discovery of proteinuria has constituted one of the most ancient modes of diagnosing kidney disease. Every nephropathy, whether constitutional or acquired, can produce this symptom. In any proteinuria, six characteristics must be defined: (1) the concentration of proteins per liter; (2) the protein output per 24 hours or per minute; (3) the electrophoretic pattern;[11] (4) the selectivity;[3, 4] (5) the possible association of hematuria, urologic abnormalities, hypertension, pyuria, renal insufficiency, or, conversely, the isolated nature of the proteinuria; (6) when isolated, whether orthostatic or permanent.

Once proteinuria is discovered, a group of examinations with logical organization should be arranged. Most of these do not require admission to hospital.

The clinical history should include the age and circumstances of the discovery, whether at routine examination prior to vaccination or during a test performed for a special reason, such as recent infection, either localized (sore throat, otitis) or generalized (scarlet fever), or the appearance of edema, macroscopic hematuria, dysuria, or purpura. Details of growth and development and the presence of polyuria and polydipsia or any symptoms of hypertension should next be noted. In the family history, particular attention should be paid to any evidence of nephropathy, deafness, or visual disorder in parents and siblings or in other relatives.

The clinical examination should devote particular attention to the presence or absence of edema, the blood pressure, the height (defective growth is an argument in favor of long-standing renal disease), vision, hearing, and the presence of any associated deformities, some of which may point to a particular type of nephropathy—for example, absence of patella and the malformed nails of onycho-osteodysplasia, or the emaciated facies of faciotruncal lipoatrophy.

The initial examination must include measurement of the urinary protein output per 24 hours, a test for orthostatic proteinuria, cytobacteriologic examination of the urine, measurement and electrophoresis of the serum proteins, measurement of the blood urea nitrogen and serum creatinine levels, measurement of endogenous creatinine clearance, a urine concentration test, and intravenous urography with films taken before, during, and after micturition, without compression. In the second stage of investigation, it may be important to determine the exact nature of the proteinuria and its selectivity. Renal biopsy may also be indicated. In the majority of cases, these examinations will reveal the cause of the proteinuria, the prognosis, and the therapeutic indications. Two conditions remain: idiopathic, permanent, isolated proteinuria and isolated, orthostatic proteinuria. In both, the mechanism is obscure, but the prognosis is excellent.

Proteinuria with Hematuria

When glomerulonephritis presents acutely after an infection, it is usual not to perform renal biopsy but to make sure that the serum complement (C'3) returns to normal in less than six to eight weeks and that the urine becomes normal within a year.

---

*This section was written in collaboration with C. Loirat.

Whether there was an acute clinical onset or the proteinuria and hematuria were discovered accidentally, if abnormal urine persists for more than one year a renal biopsy should be performed to determine the particular glomerular nephropathy.

Most nonspecific glomerular lesions can be accompanied by proteinuria and hematuria. We analyzed a series of 607 cases of nonspecific glomerulonephritis.[6] In 225 of these children (37 per cent), the only clinical and laboratory evidence of disease was a *syndrome of "proteinuria with hematuria"* (see Table 45, page 243). In some types, including all cases of pure endocapillary proliferative glomerulonephritis, certain cases of extramembranous glomerulonephritis, and certain cases of segmental and focal glomerulonephritis, the prognosis is good. All the other types of lesion are associated with nephropathies that either evolve in chronic fashion (including extramembranous glomerulonephritis, endocapillary and extracapillary glomerulonephritis with focal crescents, membranoproliferative glomerulonephritis, and segmental and focal hyalinosis) or prove rapidly progressive (such as endocapillary and extracapillary glomerulonephritis with diffuse crescents).

If no glomerular lesions can be detected on light microscopy, the discovery of proteinuria with hematuria in a child should suggest in the main two diagnoses: Berger's disease (mesangial deposits of IgA and IgG) and Alport's syndrome. More refined techniques, including immunofluorescence and electron microscopy, are then essential to determine the exact type of disorder.

Proteinuria Without Hematuria

Isolated proteinuria, predominantly an albuminuria without hematuria, may be seen in renal hypoplasia, in polycystic disease, in urolithiasis, in malformations of the urinary tract, and, above all, in the glomerulopathies that progress in chronic fashion, in which hematuria may be absent. The protein loss in the urine may amount to many grams per day, and the patient will then develop a nephrotic syndrome (see page 258). Two hereditary disorders of metabolism are associated with proteinuria, with an extreme predominance of albuminuria. First is *selective vitamin B_{12} malabsorption* (Imerslund's syndrome), presenting in early childhood with a combination of megaloblastic anemia that responds to cobalamine injection and isolated proteinuria, sometimes with hyperaminoaciduria. For this condition, the renal prognosis is excellent. The second hereditary metabolic disorder is lack of *lecithin-cholesterol acyltransferase*; in this disorder, there is anemia with fatty deposits in the cornea, an elevated total cholesterol content, and absence of esterified cholesterol. The albuminuria is associated with a high level of nonspecific antistreptolysins. Foam cells are found on renal biopsy.

Three conditions require more detailed consideration.

Proteinuria of Tubular Type

This type of proteinuria may be found in tubular acidosis, in idiopathic hypercalciuria, in Bartter's syndrome, in the Fanconi syndrome, and in Lowe's syndrome. Initially, this proteinuria was defined on electrophoresis as a triple globulinuria with traces of albumin. With ultracentrifugation, Sephadex filtration, and immunodiffusion, it has been established that the identifying characteristic of proteinuria of tubular type is the presence of 25 to 60 per cent of proteins of low molecular weight, migrating with the α_2 and β fractions and sometimes with the α_1 and post-gamma fractions. On Sephadex filtration, fractions with peak molecular weight between 10,500 and 44,000 have been isolated, and the majority of these correspond to the proteins present in the plasma. It is generally held that this proteinuria results from failure of tubular reabsorption of plasma proteins.

Permanent Isolated Proteinuria

In the absence of follow-up studies over a sufficiently long period, the long-term prognosis is unpredictable. Permanent isolated proteinuria can be seen at any age, including the first months of life. The proteinuria is generally slight, less than 1 or 1.5 g./24 hours. In an electrophoretic study in 30 of our patients, we found some traces of physiologic type, some traces suggesting a disorder of glomerular permeability, selective or otherwise, traces of tubular type, and in other cases a significant output of light-chain proteins. Any classification was quite impossible. In the absence of renal biopsy the significance of the findings remains entirely hypothetical.

We carried out renal biopsy in 65 children with permanent isolated proteinuria and found the kidney to be normal in 55. It is impossible, however, to draw any conclusions about prognosis because of the absence of follow-up study. In 10 children, segmental and focal hyalinosis (see page 237) (Figure 67) was found in renal biopsy material obtained between nine months and nine years after the discovery of the proteinuria. In one of these patients, an earlier biopsy had revealed minimal glomerular lesions. The lesions of segmental and focal hyalinosis were discovered in a second biopsy, nine years after the first, at a stage in which the patient was developing a nephrotic syndrome and renal failure.

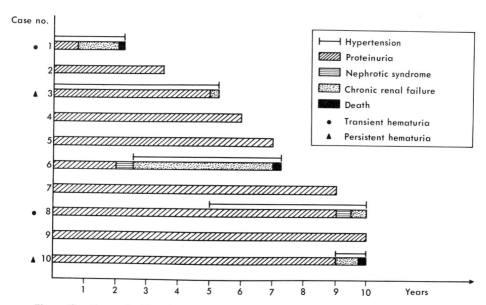

Figure 67. Course in 10 patients with segmental and focal hyalinization presenting with permanent isolated proteinuria.

Five of these patients were boys and five were girls, and the age at which the nephropathy was discovered varied from 2 years to 13½ years (seven patients over the age of 6 years). In six of the patients the proteinuria was strictly isolated. In four patients hematuria developed at some stage.

In all these cases, the proteinuria increased gradually over a period of years. In only two cases there was a mild, transient nephrotic syndrome appearing shortly before the onset of renal failure. In three cases, the proteinuria was accompanied by permanent hypertension. In two other patients, the hypertension did not appear until the terminal stages, at the same time as the renal failure. Three patients died (2 years 3 months, 7 years 3 months, and 10 years) after the discovery of the proteinuria. Two other patients, who have had hypertension for many years, are in moderate renal failure after 5½ years and 10 years, respectively. It would seem that the prognosis is just as poor for this type as for the cases in which the focal lesions are associated with an idiopathic nephrotic syndrome.

Chaptal and associates[5] also emphasize the high incidence of renal lesions which were present in 10 of 19 cases. Antoine and his colleagues[1] found a variety of renal lesions in 23 of 32 cases in adults. There were 10 cases of membrano-proliferative glomerulonephritis, seven of hyalinosis, five of basement membrane disease, and one of endocapillary proliferation, but the findings of this group are not strictly applicable to the problem under discussion, because they included some patients with a hematuria output between 5000 and 10,000 red blood cells per minute. The isolated arteriolar lesions, identical to those of nephroangiosclerosis, which were discovered by Morel-Maroger and his co-workers[14] in 10 of 33 cases, have never been reported in children. Since histologic and follow-up data are still very incomplete, it would seem justifiable to be very guarded about long-term prognosis of permanent isolated proteinuria in children.

The indications for renal biopsy are open to argument. In very young children, in whom the lesions are slight or may be focal, biopsy may provide no useful information. In practice, biopsy is performed when the proteinuria persists for more than one or two years. Definite indications for biopsy include proteinuria greater than 1.5 g./24 hours, microscopic hematuria, a nephrotic syndrome, hypertension, or any deterioration in renal function. We routinely check the degree of proteinuria every month, the urinary cell count every three months, and the other parameters every six or 12 months.

No treatment is envisaged. Activity should not be restricted. *Vaccinations* may be given without taking special precautions. In practice, the BCG and poliomyelitis vaccines are administered in the normal manner. Antitetanus and antidiphtheria vaccines are given with certain precautions. In the prophylaxis of tetanus after receiving a wound, specific gamma globulin is given instead of antitetanus serum. However, children are not vaccinated against smallpox unless it becomes absolutely necessary. Nevertheless, it is by no means certain that our practice in this regard is correct.

Isolated Orthostatic Proteinuria

Proteinuria is regarded as isolated when all the other complementary examinations described above, and the blood pressure, are normal. In orthostatic proteinuria, the urinary protein output is less than 0.1 g./liter during the night but may be as much as 5 or 10 g./liter during the day. The total urinary protein output in 24 hours is rarely more than 1 or 1.5 g. In some cases, orthostatic proteinuria is constant, but in others, probably the majority, it is intermittent.[17]

Orthostatic proteinuria is generally discovered by chance in children over the age of 4 or 5 years, with a particularly high incidence occurring in adolescence.[13] The sexes are affected equally.[17] Electrophoretic analysis of both day and night urine shows that the protein is little if at all selective, and it is of the physiologic type. The protein patterns of the night urine may give a slight indication of disordered glomerular permeability.[12]

Histologic studies in children are few. We have carried out six biopsies, and 14 were reported by Chaptal and associates.[5] In all cases the kidneys appeared normal. In adults, arteriolar lesions have been reported,[14] and varying degrees of glomerular abnormalities were found in 43 per cent of the 56 cases studied by Robinson and his co-workers.[15, 16] The glomerular lesions apparently are more common in cases in which electrophoretic study reveals that the urinary protein is not of the physiologic type.[12]

This condition is usually regarded as benign and is probably a result of a functional disorder rather than a nephropathy. General experience confirms that this opinion is well founded. Mery and associates[13] followed 61 patients for more than five years, 29 of them for more than 10 years, and none of these cases developed either hypertension or renal insufficiency. The same experience has been reported by other groups.[9, 10] In 20 to 30 per cent of cases, the proteinuria disappears, usually within five years of its discovery[10] and in most cases before the age of 25 years.[13] Certain reservations have been expressed by Robinson and associates,[15, 16, 17] because of histologic findings, and also by King.[8] King followed 531 young adults for a mean period of six years and found that the orthostatic proteinuria changed to permanent proteinuria in 18 per cent and hypertension developed in 15 per cent. In fact, some of these patients had hypertension or a malformation of the urinary tract from the beginning and so do not properly belong to the category under discussion.

There would seem to be no need to modify the optimistic attitude generally adopted unless some very prolonged follow-up study should lead to different conclusions. There is no need to restrict activity, and no special precautions are needed for vaccination. Medical supervision should be limited to an annual check on the blood pressure and on the orthostatic character of the proteinuria. Glomerular clearances are reviewed every five years. Renal biopsy is pointless. It has been reported that orthostatic proteinuria disappears on steroid therapy, and this may have some diagnostic significance.[7]

Conclusion

Proteinuria is a symptom, not a disease. It is very often the first indication of urinary disorder and may be the result of any of the diseases of the kidney or urinary tract. The discovery of proteinuria is an absolute indication for a properly organized series of tests. It must be made clear to the family that full investigation at the outset is essential. It still happens all too often that the urine albumin is measured over and over again but this repetition adds nothing to diagnosis, prognosis, or treatment. A series of simple tests will quickly reveal in most cases whether the physician is dealing with a serious nephrologic problem, a permanent solitary proteinuria requiring prolonged and perhaps anxious supervision, or merely a perfectly benign isolated orthostatic proteinuria.

There is still much to be learned about the nature of certain urinary proteins, the mechanism of their renal excretion, and the histologic correlations and prognosis of permanent isolated proteinuria.

HEMATURIA*

Nearly every disease of the kidneys or urinary tract may present with hematuria at some stage. Hence the discovery of hematuria, whether macroscopic or microscopic, is an indication for performing a series of investigations.

The Practical Approach to Hematuria

In taking the history, special attention must be paid to the age at onset, the existence of some precipitating factor such as trauma or infection, the interval between infection and hematuria, any associated pain suggestive of renal colic, symptoms of urinary infection, disorders of micturition, and symptoms suggesting a general disease—especially rheumatoid purpura. It is important to elicit any previous history of hemorrhagic disease and to find out whether any time was spent in a country where schistosomiasis is endemic. An inquiry should be made about any family history of lithiasis or of nephropathy with or without deafness.

Clinical examination should include measurement of height and weight. Recent loss of weight may suggest the presence of a tumor or general disease. Retardation of growth may indicate some long-standing renal condition. The blood pressure is important. Bimanual palpation of the loins may reveal a mass.

In the first instance, a relatively limited investigation is indicated. A plain radiograph of the abdomen and intravenous urography with films taken before, during, and after micturition are essential in all cases unless the diagnosis of acute glomerulonephritis is obvious. In all cases, the urinary sediment is examined and the urine is cultured. Tests for glomerular disorder include measurement of the 24 hour urinary protein output, measurement of the serum proteins and electrophoresis, and measurement of blood urea level and creatinine clearance.

Routine renal biopsy is not justifiable. Regular review is much more logical. This should include a urinary cell count and measurement of 24 hour urinary protein output every three months and measurement of blood urea and creatinine clearance every six to 12 months.

Orientation of the Diagnosis

Glomerular Nephropathy

This rarely presents with isolated hematuria. In only seven cases in our experience was segmental and focal glomerulonephritis revealed by renal biopsy in patients presenting with isolated hematuria.

---

*This section was written in collaboration with C. Loirat, M. Levy, and H. Beaufils.

In most cases, the hematuria, whether macroscopic or microscopic, is but one feature associated with other signs of glomerular disease, especially proteinuria.

There is seldom any problem in the diagnosis of a curable acute glomerulonephritis when there is a history of sudden onset of hematuria one to three weeks after an infection, usually in the upper respiratory tract, and there may be a history of sudden gain in weight or edema, of mild hypertension, of proteinuria, or perhaps of oliguria with a mild nephrotic syndrome. There may be confirmatory evidence in the discovery of hemolytic streptococci in the throat, a raised antistreptolysin titer, or a lowered complement level. The strongest evidence is the regression in a matter of days of the clinical symptoms and signs or of any renal insufficiency or nephrotic syndrome and the return of the complement level to normal in less than 8 weeks. Macroscopic hematuria may persist for several weeks. Microscopic hematuria and the proteinuria that may be associated are the last to disappear, usually in six to 12 months. The long-term prognosis is excellent, and there are very few indications for renal biopsy (see page 271).

The initial picture may be similar in other types of glomerulonephritis, which have a more uncertain prognosis. Hematuria may occur in any glomerular nephropathy, whether idiopathic, following infection, or part of a systemic or congenital disease (such as Alport's syndrome). The particular lesion can be identified only by following the progress of the disease and above all by renal biopsy (including immunofluorescence study) which will distinguish the diffuse glomerulonephritides (extramembranous, membranoproliferative, and endocapillary and extracapillary proliferative), which have doubtful prognoses, from the glomerulonephritides with mesangial deposits of IgA and IgG (with or without segmental and focal glomerulonephritis), which carry a good prognosis.

Hematuria of Nonglomerular Origin

Whenever the diagnosis of glomerular nephropathy is not absolutely definite, the entire urinary tract must be studied. In addition to intravenous urography, it may be necessary to perform cystography by the retrograde or suprapubic puncture technique and also micturating cystography. Arteriography may be indicated in some cases.

Any of the malformations of the urinary tract may present with hematuria. This is sometimes associated with urinary infection, or the hematuria may follow trauma. Intravenous urography is indicated in every case of hematuria with a history of trauma. Notwithstanding its rarity, hematuria associated with frank difficulty in micturition points to tumor of the urogenital sinus (the so-called "botryoid" tumor) (see page 34). Renal tuberculosis is rare in children (see page 144).

Hematuria of vesical origin, associated with cystitis or trigonitis, is fairly rare. It is often, though not always, associated with urinary infection. Cystography may reveal the fine, irregular appearance of granular cystitis. The diagnosis is confirmed by cystoscopy. If there is any question of exposure to schistosomiasis, the urine should be searched for evidence of *Schistosoma*.

If lithiasis and urinary tract malformation are excluded, a metabolic source must be sought. It should be remembered that hematuria accompanied by abdominal pain is very suggestive of lithiasis, even if radiography proves negative, and in such cases metabolic investigations should include measurements of the 24 hour urinary output of calcium and oxalate, the uric acid clearance, and the Brandt test.

All the cystic diseases of the kidney may cause bleeding. A Wilms' tumor may be revealed by hematuria. Hematuria of vascular origin (angioma, telangiectasis) is rare. Hemorrhagic diseases such as hemophilia, thrombocytopenia, and disordered platelet function may be responsible for hematuria.

In an African black child, schistosomiasis must always be considered, and the possibility of sickle cell anemia should be considered in any black child. Hematuria in an infant may be the result of renal vein thrombosis or the large kidney-hematuria syndrome (see page 122).

Recurrent Macroscopic Hematuria

Recurrence of macroscopic hematuria is exceptional in the course of a curable acute glomerulonephritis. It is also very rare during the course of "chronic" glomerulonephritis.

If lithiasis or any urologic cause can be ruled out, the differential diagnosis includes segmental and focal glomerulonephritis with mesangial deposits of IgA and IgG, Alport's syndrome, benign familial recurrent hematuria, and allergic hematuria.

Segmental and Focal Glomerulonephritis with Mesangial Deposits of IgA and IgG (Berger's Disease)

The association of recurrent macroscopic hematuria with segmental and focal glomerulonephritis has been known for a long time.[43] All authors emphasize the benign nature of this nephropathy in children.[20, 21, 26, 27, 31, 32, 34, 38–41]

Immunofluorescence techniques have opened new vistas in this condition. In 1965, Bodian[26] noted the presence of immunoglobulin deposits in all glomeruli examined, and he emphasized the diffusion of the glomerular lesions. It was Berger and his colleagues[6, 7] who showed that the characteristic feature of this nephropathy was the presence of diffuse mesangial deposits that fixed anti-IgA and anti-IgG sera. These deposits are also found in some patients who present a hematuric glomerulonephritis with kidneys that are normal on light microscopy. These mesangial deposits are commonly found in adults,[25, 29, 36, 44] but, unlike our findings in children, there is macroscopic hematuria in only 25 per cent of patients. The nephropathy seems to be more serious in adults, with several cases progressing to terminal renal failure.

Electron microscopy reveals the precise character of the deposits and their mesangial topography. The peripheral capillary loops are normally intact. The discovery of morphologically identical deposits in patients who have not been studied by immunofluorescence[30] raises questions about their significance. It is evidently impossible to predict their immunohistochemical composition, but in practice we have made the diagnosis of glomerulonephritis with mesangial deposits of IgA and IgG in children with recurrent macroscopic hematuria whose kidneys were normal on light microscopy or who presented segmental and focal glomerulonephritis (10 personal cases).

We have seen 33 cases of idiopathic recurrent macroscopic hematuria with mesangial deposits of IgA and IgG. Renal biopsy in these children demonstrated minimal glomerular lesions in 12 cases, segmental and focal glomerulonephritis in 15, and endocapillary and extracapillary glomerulonephritis with focal crescents in six (Table 46). Twenty of the patients were boys and 13 were girls. The youngest was three years old when the hematuria was discovered. Half the cases occurred in children between the ages of 6 and 12 years.

In 23 children, there was no history of any antecedent episode. Seven other children had recurrent nose and throat infections, and one had undergone tonsillectomy. Two children had a definite history of allergy, consisting of eczema in early childhood followed by attacks of asthma. One child had had rheumatoid purpura without renal involvement three years previously.

In the majority (29 cases), macroscopic hematuria was the presenting feature of the nephropathy. In four children, the first episode of hematuria was preceded by proteinuria discovered on routine examination 12 months, six months, two months, and eight days previously.

The hallmark of these hematurias is their recurrent nature, but the interval between recurrences varies from 10 days to two years, often being of many months. It is our impression that recurrence is more frequent in the early stages of the disease. In approximately half the cases, both the first and subsequent attacks of hematuria follow a febrile episode associated with upper urinary tract infection, but only rarely is this proved to be streptococcal (two cases).

It will be recalled that the interval between the development of upper respiratory infection and the appearance of signs of renal disease is eight to 20 days in acute glomerulonephritis, but in Berger's disease it is usually very short, less than 48 hours. In some cases, the sore throat and macroscopic hematuria appear on the same day. Apart from rhinopharyngeal infections, other precipitating factors include effort, intoxications, attacks of asthma, parotitis, and tonsillectomy. In many cases, the hematuria occurs with no discernible cause. Each attack of hematuria is accompanied by a proteinuria that varies from patient to patient and from attack to attack, but the urinary protein loss is rarely more than 1 g./24 hours. Two of our patients did have a proteinuria greater than

Table 46.   The Clinocopathologic Correlations in 33 Cases of Recurrent Hematuria with Mesangial Deposits of IgA–IgG

	Histologic Type		
Symptomatology	M.G.L.*	S.F.G.N.†	E.E.G.N.‡
Recurrent hematuria as an isolated symptom	12	14	3
Recurrent hematuria with initial renal insufficiency	0	1	1
Recurrent hematuria with initial nephrotic syndrome	0	0	2
Total	12	15	6

*Minimal glomerular lesions.
†Segmental and focal glomerulonephritis.
‡Endocapillary and extracapillary glomerulonephritis, type I.

3 g./24 hours, which was associated in one case with a transient nephrotic syndrome and with a more persistent nephrotic syndrome in the other (Table 46).

Renal function is generally normal, but in two of our patients the blood urea level was over 100 mg. per 100 ml. In one this dated from the first attack and in the other it followed a later attack of hematuria. In only one of these children the rise in blood urea level has persisted for several months, and it was accompanied by hypertension.

The attacks of hematuria rarely last for more than two weeks, and in over 60 per cent of cases, the attack lasts no longer than three days.

After the attack, the hematuria becomes microscopic and the proteinuria gradually diminishes, ultimately disappearing completely. In some patients (14 of our cases), the episodes of hematuria can be separated by a period of complete remission. In 16 cases, between the attacks there was either minimal proteinuria (less than 0.5 g./24 hours) or microscopic hematuria, and in three patients the attacks of macroscopic hematuria were superimposed on a continued proteinuria varying from 1 to 6 g./24 hours.

The period of follow-up of these children after the discovery of their nephropathy varies from one to 15 years. None of these children has developed renal failure. In eight children, a proteinuria of more than 0.5 g./24 hours in two cases and more than 1.0 g./24 hours in six cases continued many months after an attack of macroscopic hematuria. At 10 and 15 years after the onset of the disease, two of these eight children had a proteinuria of 3 g./24 hours and 1 g./24 hours, but neither has had an attack of hematuria for many years.

There is a definite relationship between the histologic type and the initial manifestations of the nephropathy, the frequency of attacks of microscopic hematuria, the persistence of proteinuria, and the evolution of the disease. The cases of endocapillary and extracapillary glomerulonephritis have a more severe nephropathy than the patients with segmental and focal glomerulonephritis. None of the 12 patients with minimal glomerular lesions had a urinary protein output greater than 0.2 g./24 hours at the last examination.

Four patients were treated with antibiotics, one with steroids, four by tonsillectomy, and seven by immunodepressive drugs, but treatment did not appear to have any effect on the occurrence of attacks of macroscopic hematuria. One of the seven patients on immunodepressive treatment with chloraminophene had no further hematuria, but relapses occurred in all the other patients during treatment and when treatment was stopped. In three of these cases, immunofluorescence studies on renal biopsy material obtained after stopping treatment revealed characteristic mesangial deposits. At the last analysis of these seven children treated by immunodepressive drugs, four had had no proteinuria or a proteinuria of less than 0.1 g./24 hours, with or without hematuria, two had a greater degree of proteinuria but less than 1 g./24 hours, and one had proteinuria of more than 3 g./24 hours.

Despite certain evidence to the contrary, including the very short interval between the infectious episode and the hematuria, the universally normal complement level, the particular type of immunoglobulin concerned (IgA), and its localization in the mesangium, it seems likely that an immunologic mechanism involving antigen-antibody complexes (see page 207) is responsible because of recent discoveries about complement and the mesangial system. In the classic mechanism of complement activation, the first fraction of complement interacts with the immunoglobulins IgG and IgM. There is recent evidence of the activation of the fraction C′3 by the immunoglobulin IgA.[33]

The mesangial system[42] also plays an important part. Various tracer substances, such as Thorotrast, ferritin, and colloidal iron, injected into the bloodstream have been found in the matrix or in the intracytoplasmic vacuoles of the cells that function in phagocytosis of the residues of glomerular filtration. In certain conditions, the immune complexes follow the same path. Recent experiments[22,28] have shown that immune complexes, formed in equivalence, heavier and less soluble than those formed with excess of antigen, are deposited in the mesangium.

Alport's Syndrome (See Page 37)

Alport's syndrome commonly presents with recurrent macroscopic hematuria. A careful enquiry into the family history, including a urinary cell count and an audiogram in the parents, may point with certainty to a diagnosis of Alport's syndrome. Absence of any family history, the late onset of deafness, and the normality of the glomeruli, especially in the first 10 years of life, may make it very difficult to differentiate this condition from Berger's disease. Negative immunofluorescence results will rule out the disease with mesangial deposits.

Familial Benign Recurrent Hematuria

It is difficult to know how to classify the condition described by McConville and his colleagues[35] as familial benign recurrent hematuria. The cases described by them were not subjected to immunofluorescence study. The condition was defined as recurrent on the basis of microscopic hematuria found at repeated examinations on many days and at different times of the day. It is known that activity provokes a rise in the urinary output of red blood cells, even in a normal person.[18]

Allergic Hematuria

Similar to the case with benign recurrent hematuria, the exact nature of allergic hematuria,[19] ascribed in most cases to the ingestion of some particular food, is not at all clear in the absence of precise histologic information.

Conclusion

The cause of a hematuria may be easy or difficult to determine. It is sometimes obvious, as in lithiasis, in most of the glomerulonephritides, and in hematuria of urologic origin. Conversely, many hematurias remained unexplained until recent years. These were the isolated hematurias, especially recurrent macroscopic hematuria that was difficult to classify exactly, since the urinary tract was normal, there was no trace of stone, there was no familial or auditory evidence of Alport's syndrome, and, most important of all, the renal parenchyma was normal on light microscopy. Immunofluorescence studies have made it clear that a significant number of these cases result from glomerulonephritis characterized by the presence of mesangial deposits of IgA and

IgG. When this examination is negative as well, it may be suspected that the case is one of Alport's syndrome in which the full clinical picture will not be apparent for many years, but it must be recognized that there are still many cases of isolated hematuria that remain totally unexplained.

THE NEPHROTIC SYNDROME*

The nephrotic syndrome is characterized by a collection of symptoms and signs, including edema, significant proteinuria, and disturbances of the serum proteins and lipids, and also a fall in the total serum proteins and a change in the electrophoretic pattern, with lowering of the albumin level and an increase in alpha-2 globulin. There is also a rise in serum lipid levels.

The limits of the nephrotic syndrome are defined differently by different authors. The elements of the nephrotic syndrome may be dissociated, and all stages between frank, complete, nephrotic syndrome and a mild disequilibrium of plasma proteins may exist. We have arbitrarily defined the nephrotic syndrome as the association of a proteinuria greater than 50 mg./kg./day with a serum protein level below 6.0 g. per 100 ml. and a serum albumin below 3.0 g. per 100 ml., whether or not there is edema and hyperlipemia.

The primary phenomenon appears to be the proteinuria. Every major, lasting proteinuria produces a nephrotic syndrome owing to hypoalbuminemia that leads to hypovolemia and hyperaldosteronism on the one hand and, on the other hand, increases the synthesis of protein in the liver, especially the pre-beta lipoproteins, whose hydrolysis is inhibited also.

First described by Bright in 1836, this syndrome was attributed to tubular lesions by Muller, who introduced the term "nephrosis." Munk and subsequently Volhard and Fahr distinguished "lipoid nephrosis" with tubular lesions from "nephritis" accompanied by inflammatory glomerular lesions. Later, Löhlein and then Bell and Dunn emphasized the possibility of glomerular disease. At the same time that clinicians were struck by the great variety in the etiology, clinical presentation, and course of "nephrosis," the practice of renal biopsy revealed that the condition might be associated with very many types of histologic appearance, hence the term "nephrotic syndrome" is preferred to "nephrosis." Electron microscopy and immunofluorescence clarified the situation still further, especially with regard to the lesions of the walls of the glomerular capillaries. It is now possible to make a clinicopathologic classification of nephrotic syndromes.[52] The first step is distinguishing between secondary and primary nephrotic syndromes.

Secondary Nephrotic Syndromes

These are part of an identified general disease or result from some evident cause. Although they represent one third of the cases of nephrotic syndrome seen in adults, in our experience they account for no more than 10 per cent of nephrotic syndromes in children. Half of these are the nephropathies of rheumatoid purpura. Other possible etiologies include amyloidosis, Alport's syn-

---

*This section was written in collaboration with C. Kleinknecht and M. C. Gubler.

drome, systemic lupus erythematosus, and thrombotic microangiopathy. Only thrombotic microangiopathy and amyloidosis can be regarded as specific renal lesions. In the other cases, the etiology is determined by the clinical features or laboratory findings.

Primary Nephrotic Syndromes

Some cases of nephrotic syndrome regarded as primary or idiopathic may follow an episode of infection. However, the length of time elapsing between the primary infection and development of the nephropathy is impossible to define. There may be preceding infection in all the histologic types, and the infection is not associated with any particular clinical pattern; furthermore, the existence of preceding infection may not be recognized in cases seen late in the course of the disease.

There are no specific features to the histologic lesions seen in primary nephrotic syndromes; all of them can be found in patients who have never experienced any changes in the levels of serum lipids or proteins. There is, however, a certain individuality about the lesions, and they generally remain the same type throughout the course of the disease, as we have learned from serial renal biopsies. Each histologic variety is associated with a particular clinical pattern. Analysis of the different clinicopathologic groups shows that there are in fact definite entities. Knowledge of these types is essential both for prognosis and as a guide to therapy. These conclusions are derived from a study of 512 personal cases of primary nephrotic syndrome. The details are given here to illustrate the problems posed by the nephrotic syndrome in childhood (Table 47).

Nephrotic Syndrome with "Minimal Glomerular Lesions"

In 209 cases, histologic study of the renal parenchyma detected no glomerular change visible on light microscopy, with the exception of slight hyper-

Table 47.   Histopathologic Classification of Idiopathic Nephrotic Syndromes in Children (512 Cases)

I. Minimal glomerular lesions (209 cases)	209
II. Focal glomerular sclerosis (88 cases)	
A. *Segmental and focal hyalinization*	64
B. *Global and focal fibrosis of glomeruli*	24
III. Diffuse glomerular lesions (187 cases)	
A. *Extramembranous glomerulonephritis*	44
B. *Proliferative glomerulonephritis*	
Pure endocapillary	41
Endocapillary and extracapillary	20
Membranoproliferative and lobular	82
IV. Unclassifiable glomerular lesions (11 cases)	11
V. Forms peculiar to infants (17 cases)	
A. *Microcystic nephrotic syndromes*	11
B. *Diffuse mesangial sclerosis*	6
Total number of cases	512

trophy of the intercapillary tissue (19 cases) and a minimal increase in the number of mesangial cells (10 cases). In certain cases, there were moderate tubulo-interstitial lesions, which were focal in 28 cases and diffuse in eight cases.

On electron microscopy, the only lesion normally observed is fusion of the pedicels.

The disease may appear at any age, with a definite predominance in young children. More than half the cases appeared before the age of 4 years and two thirds before the age of 5 years. Boys are affected more often (72 per cent) than girls. Seven children had a brother or sister who was also affected. In 80 per cent of cases, edema is the presenting symptom; in the other cases, the proteinuria is discovered by chance at some time before (never more than four months) the appearance of the full nephrotic syndrome.

In most cases, the nephrotic syndrome is gross (Table 48). The proteinuria is selective and the urinary sodium output is very low. Hematuria was found in only 36 per cent of cases, and then it was generally microscopic and transient (47 cases) or intermittent (13 cases). In 13 patients, the hematuria persisted for several months, and it was macroscopic in only three patients. A rise in blood urea (20 cases) or blood pressure (12 cases) is uncommon but does occur. The serum complement (C'3) level is normal. Ten patients had prolonged spontaneous remissions without treatment. Of 181 children treated with steroids, 111 (62 per cent) had a complete remission (full steroid sensitivity); 41 (or 22 per cent) had partial remission, with disappearance of the nephrotic syndrome but persistence of proteinuria (partial steroid sensitivity); and in 29 children (16 per cent) the treatment had no effect (steroid resistance).

Analysis of Figure 68 provides a series of conclusions. In each child, the

Table 48.   The Nephrotic Syndrome with Minimal Glomerular Lesions (209 Cases)*: Maximal Disorders Observed During the Disease

Severity	Edema (Number of Cases)	Proteinuria (Number of Cases)	Serum Proteins (Number of Cases)	Serum Albumin (Number of Cases)	Lipemia (Number of Cases)
+++	89	103	89	52	53
++	80	52	95	72	59
+	24	54	25	12	83
0	16				12
Unknown				73	2

*The severity of the elements of the nephrotic syndrome in this and the following tables is expressed as follows:

Severity	Edema	Proteinuria	Serum Proteins	Serum Albumin	Lipemia
+++	Ascites or anasarca	≥250 mg./kg./day	≤4.0 g. per 100 ml.	≤1.0 g. per 100 ml.	≥2.0 g. per 100 ml.
++	Generalized subcutaneous	100 to 200 mg./kg./day	4.0 to 5.0 g. per 100 ml.	1.0 to 2.0 g. per 100 ml.	1.5 to 2.0 g. per 100 ml.
+	Slight	≤100 mg./kg./day	5.0 to 6.0 g. per 100 ml.	2.0 to 3.0 g. per 100 ml.	0.8 to 1.5 g. per 100 ml.
0	Absent	Nil	≥6.0 g. per 100 ml.	≥3.0 g. per 100 ml.	≤0.8 g. per 100 ml.

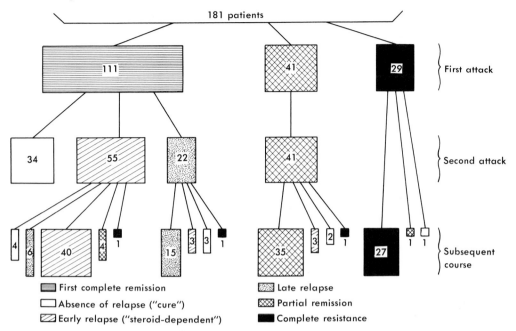

Figure 68. Effect of steroid therapy in 181 patients suffering from nephrotic syndrome with minimal glomerular lesions.

response to treatment follows a specific pattern in most cases. It is extremely rare to find remission in a child who was initially steroid-resistant (a single case in remission for seven years), and it is equally rare to find complete steroid resistance appearing later in a child who is initially steroid-sensitive (two cases). Transient steroid resistance may, however, coincide with episodes of infection. In our series, half of the steroid-sensitive patients are "steroid-dependent"; proteinuria reappears either on stopping treatment or when the dose is diminished below a threshold figure that seldom varies much in any particular patient.

Relapse after two years of complete remission is exceptional. We have seen it on four occasions, after four, five, 10, and 12 years of remission. These relapses always responded rapidly to treatment. The great majority of "cures" (34 of 44) occurred after a single attack.

Immunodepressive drugs were used in 101 patients, starting with the first attack in 18 patients and after steroid treatment in the others. Prednisone in a dose of at least 1 mg./kg./24 hours was used in addition in 51 patients. This treatment has produced remission for more than one year in 68 children. The incidence of remission is related to the previous steroid sensitivity (Table 49), but remission is possible in steroid-resistant patients. This mode of treatment is too recent to allow any assessment of the risk of late relapse. At the present time, 12 children have had relapses, four of them after remissions of two to three years.

The current status of 209 children, followed from one to 10 years, is given in Table 55 (page 271). Of these, 148 are in complete remission, 26 are in partial remission, 21 still have a nephrotic syndrome, and 14 have died. Only three deaths were the result of chronic renal failure, occurring five, six, and eight years after the onset of a steroid-resistant nephrotic syndrome. The other 11 deaths resulted from intercurrent complications. These complications (infection,

Table 49.   Nephrotic Syndrome with Minimal Glomerular Lesions:
Action of Immunodepressive Agents (101 Cases)

Previous Nature of the Nephrotic Syndrome	Total Number of Cases Treated	Complete Remission (Number of Cases)	Partial Remission (Number of Cases)	Failure (Number of Cases)
Total steroid resistance	20	6	3	11
Partial steroid sensitivity	19	13	6	–
Total steroid sensitivity steroid dependence	37	30	2	5
Steroid sensitivity with spaced relapses	7	7	–	–
Not treated by steroids	18	12	2	4
Total	101	68	13	20

thromboembolic accidents, collapse) are in fact common and occur principally in steroid-resistant patients. Certain indices of poor prognosis include total steroid resistance, hematuria (especially if persistent), nonselectivity of the proteinuria (which suggests steroid resistance), and onset at a very early age. Of nine cases of nephrotic syndrome that presented in the first year of life, six were steroid resistant and three proved fatal. Except for the cases appearing very early, a familial history has not indicated a poor prognosis in our series.

Nephrotic Syndrome with "Focal Glomerular Sclerosis"

In 64 cases there were lesions of segmental and focal hyalinosis (see page 237), and 24 cases there were lesions of global and focal fibrosis (see page 239). These focal glomerular lesions were found in 52 boys and 36 girls. In six patients, the nephrotic syndrome was discovered in the first year of life (at birth in two of these), but it can appear at any age, usually before the age of 5 years (55 cases). In six patients the nephrotic syndrome was familial, and in three of these the onset was within the first year of life.

No pathologic antecedent could be found in the majority of cases, although the first symptoms were preceded by an episode of upper respiratory tract infection in 24 children. Four of these followed vaccination. Most patients had edema as well as the altered blood chemistry of the nephrotic syndrome. In seven patients, isolated proteinuria had been noted some time before the onset of the edema. Microscopic hematuria was sought from the onset of the disease in 68 patients and was detected in 33. A moderate and transient rise in blood pressure or blood urea nitrogen level was noted in 11 and 12 cases, respectively.

Once it appears, the nephrotic syndrome is generally gross (Table 50). In the 11 cases in which it was calculated, the index of selectivity[53] revealed moderately selective proteinuria in three cases, slightly selective proteinuria in five cases, and nonselective proteinuria in three cases. In 60 patients, the nephrotic syndrome was accompanied by microscopic hematuria in 52 cases and by macroscopic hematuria in eight cases. The hematuria was permanent in 34 cases and transient in the others. Signs of proximal tubular disorder (glycosuria, hyperaminoaciduria) were found in four patients with normal renal function and

Table 50.   Segmental and Focal Hyalinization: Elements of the
Nephrotic Syndrome (88 Cases)

Elements of the Nephrotic Syndrome	Severity	Presence at Onset (Number of Cases)	Maximal Disorder in the Course of the Disease (Number of Cases)
Edema	Absent	10	0
	Moderate	17	3
	Generalized	47	27
	Anasarca*	14	**58**
Proteinuria (mg./kg./24 hours)	≤100	13	0
	100–250	29	21
	≥250	31	**67**
	Unknown	15	0
Serum proteins (g./100 ml.)	≥6	4	0
	5–6	17	5
	4–5	33	35
	≤4	8	**48**
	Unknown	26	0
Serum lipids (g./100 ml.)	≤0.8	6	0
	0.8–1.5	22	22
	1.5–2.0	20	26
	≥2.0	12	**36**
	Unknown	28	0

*With serous effusions.

in four patients with chronic renal insufficiency. The level of the C′3 fraction of complement was measured in 11 children and found to be normal in all of them.

Apart from purely symptomatic treatment, all our patients were given steroids and some were later treated by immunodepressive drugs. Prednisone was given in an initial dose of 1 to 2 mg./kg./24 hours, then in discontinuous fashion four days a week, in progressively diminishing doses, to be stopped altogether after a period of three to 14 months. In the first attack, 79 patients were treated by steroids alone; 53 of these were totally steroid-resistant (Table 51) and only one patient was improved by subsequent courses of steroids. Three of the steroid-sensitive patients became steroid-resistant after some months or years. All the others remained partially (eight cases) or totally (18 cases) sensitive to steroids.

Fifty-six patients were subsequently treated by immunodepressive drugs.

Table 51.   Segmental and Focal Hyalinization: Effects of First
Steroid Treatment in 79 Patients

Response to Steroids	Number of Cases	Percentage of Total Number of Cases
Complete sensitivity to steroids	6	8
Steroid sensitivity with steroid dependence	12	15
Partial sensitivity to steroids	8	10
Resistance to steroids	53	67

The drugs used were basically chlorambucil alone or associated with mechlorethamine, much more rarely azathioprine and cyclophosphamide (the latter generally for periods longer than six months). Thirty of these patients did not respond at all to treatment; in 13 patients, the nephrotic syndrome disappeared but proteinuria persisted; and in 13 patients, complete remission was observed. These results appear to be independent of the drug used. They are, however, interesting to analyze as a function of the initial steroid sensitivity (Table 52). Of 35 patients who were totally steroid-resistant, 28 derived no benefit from immunodepressive treatment and three obtained complete remission. In contrast, all the patients partially or totally sensitive to steroids in the first attack of the disease were improved by immunodepressive drugs; nine had prolonged, complete remission, and eight others had a stable, incomplete remission.

Intercurrent complications are particularly common, being seen in 24 patients. Nine of these patients suffered infections that were sometimes recurrent and often severe, including streptococcal septicemia (one case), typhoid fever (two cases), bronchopneumonia (one case), purulent peritonitis (one case), extensive skin infection (five cases), urinary infection (one case), and lymphangitis in a lower limb (one case). None of these infections proved fatal. In four children, attacks of edema were accompanied by intense abdominal pain, leading to laparotomy and the removal of a normal appendix. Five patients developed venous thrombosis of a lower limb that was extensive and proved fatal in one patient, with another developing arterial thrombosis. Five other children died of a complication (acute adrenal failure, uncontrollable diarrhea, acute hemorrhagic pancreatitis, malignant influenza, and sudden death).

Our patients have been followed for periods varying from three months (early accidental death) to 17 years, with a mean of 9 years 5 months. We have found that the disease follows one of two fundamental patterns (Table 53). In 54 patients, the nephrotic syndrome progressed without interruption. Sixteen patients died of renal failure after the nephrotic syndrome had been present for many years. Six patients died from some intercurrent complication, five of these a few months after the onset of the disease. Four survivors at present are in renal failure and two others have hypertension. In 19 patients, the nephrotic syndrome persists unchanged. Lastly, in seven patients in this group, the nephrotic syndrome continued, unresponsive to treatment, for many months

Table 52. Segmental and Focal Hyalinization: Response to Immunodepressive Agents in 56 Patients, Most of Whom were Previously Treated with Steroids

Response to Immunodepressive Agents	Number of Cases	Response to Steroids			
		Sensitivity	Partial Sensitivity	Resistance	Untreated
Complete remission	13	8	1	3	1
Partial remission	13	4	4	4	1
Failure	30	0	0	28	2
Total	56	12	5	35	4

Table 53.   Segmental and Focal Hyalinization: Clinical Course in 88 Cases

Clinical Course	Permanent Nephrotic Syndrome	Relapsing Nephrotic Syndrome
Number of cases	54	34
Death from nonrenal causes	6	0
Death from renal disease	16	0
Renal failure and/or hypertension	6	1
Persistence of nephrotic syndrome	19	7
Persistence of isolated proteinuria	2	11
Complete remission	5	15
Follow-up of survivors	5 years 3 months	8 years 2 months

or even years and then became progressively less serious, until there was only isolated proteinuria, and five of the patients went on to complete remission. In the second group, of 34 patients, the nephrotic syndrome occurred in attacks separated by complete or incomplete remissions. When last examined, all patients had normal renal function. One has hypertension, seven still have a nephrotic syndrome, 11 have isolated proteinuria, and 15 have obtained complete remission.

Overall, the prognosis for a nephrotic syndrome with focal glomerular lesions appears poor. Of 88 patients, 22 are dead, three have hypertension, and four are in renal failure, after a follow-up period averaging six years. Twenty patients, followed for a similar length of time, are in complete remission, with normal renal function.

Certain features have a definite prognostic significance. Permanent hematuria, complete steroid resistance, and the absence of complete remissions in the course of the disease are all signs of an unfavorable prognosis. In our series, all the deaths occurred in the group with a permanent nephrotic syndrome. A histologic feature of prognostic significance is global and focal fibrosis. Sixty-two per cent of the patients with this type of lesion belong to the group with relapsing nephrotic syndromes. The disease progresses more slowly in the patients with global and focal fibrosis than in the patients with segmental and focal hyalinization. In the latter group, five years after the onset of the disease, 11 of 35 patients have died, while 17 patients with global and focal fibrosis are still alive. We have chosen, nevertheless, to analyze the two groups together because of their very similar clinical patterns.

Nephrotic Syndrome with Diffuse Glomerular Lesions

Extramembranous Glomerulonephritis.   The clinical description of patients with extramembranous glomerulonephritis (with or without a nephrotic syndrome) is given elsewhere (see page 220). The nephrotic syndrome, mild in most cases, was present from the onset in 31 children and appeared later in the disease in 13 other patients. In every case except two, there was an accompanying hematuria, but this persisted throughout the period of observation in only 11 cases. Only in the last group did we find an unfavorable evolution (two dead, three in chronic renal failure).

Endocapillary Proliferative Glomerulonephritis (See Page 225). Apart from the cases (15 in our series) of obvious "acute" glomerulonephritis in which the nephrotic syndrome was always transient and the prognosis excellent, the course is difficult to predict in this group. In some cases, the clinical evolution is very similar to that of the nephrotic syndromes with minimal glomerular lesions. However, in most cases, in our experience, the disease pursues a prolonged course, with a severe and lasting nephrotic syndrome that is steroid-resistant and accompanied by hematuria. In five cases of this type, a second renal biopsy revealed focal glomerular lesions.

Endocapillary and Extracapillary Proliferative Glomerulonephritis. The high incidence of nephrotic syndrome with this type of lesion has already been emphasized (see page 228). An infectious etiology was noted in half of the 20 patients concerned. Hematuria was macroscopic in 11 cases, and greater than 100,000 red cells per minute in the remainder. In the seven cases in which the extracapillary proliferation was slight, the nephrotic syndrome was mild and transient; rarely it was associated with a brief initial renal insufficiency. All the patients in this group pursued a favorable course. Five patients were cured after periods varying from 18 to 30 months, and the remaining two still have proteinuria three years after the onset.

In contrast, when the extracapillary proliferation involves more than 80 per cent of the glomeruli (13 cases), the nephrotic syndrome is often severe and lasting, having appeared at the onset of the disease in 10 of our patients and at a later stage in the other three. The particular feature of this group is the presence of renal insufficiency. This appeared early in 10 patients and at a later stage in the other three, but, once it appeared, it persisted throughout the course of the disease, ending in death, usually within one year. Treatment with prednisone or immunodepressive agents proved ineffective.

Membranoproliferative and Lobular Glomerulonephritis. The clinical features of membranoproliferative and lobular glomerulonephritis (with or without nephrotic syndrome) have been described elsewhere (see page 229). The nephrotic syndrome was usually permanent and accompanied by hematuria, and it was present throughout the period of observation in 23 patients; it was a late feature but a permanent one in 19 cases. In the last group (40 cases), the nephrotic syndrome was intermittent or transient. The outcome was unfavorable in 83 per cent of the patients who had a permanent, complete nephrotic syndrome. Fifty-three per cent of the patients who developed a nephrotic syndrome as a secondary feature and 20 per cent of those with a transient nephrotic syndrome went on to chronic failure or death.

Forms Peculiar to Infancy (17 Cases)

All the types so far described are common to adults and children, but in 17 cases we have found lesions that seem peculiar to the young infant.

"Microcystic" Nephrotic Syndrome (11 Cases) (See Page 47). In this type, the only abnormality is cystic dilatation of the proximal convoluted tubules, diffuse and irregular in one patient but localized to the deep cortex in the others. All the other elements of the renal parenchyma, most notably the glomeruli, are normal. In one patient, nephron microdissection confirmed the moniliform character of the dilatations of the proximal convoluted tubule, which are characteristic of this curious condition.[4, 12] The clinical pattern was the same in all

11 cases. The placenta was large and the nephrotic syndrome appeared in the first four months of life, often in the first days. The patient did not respond to treatment with steroids or immunodepressive drugs. The complications are extremely severe, including infections (peritonitis, purulent pericarditis, pneumonia), profuse diarrhea, extreme malnutrition, and thrombosis of the renal veins. The condition is always rapidly fatal. Death occurred in less than one year in every case, always from intercurrent complications, never from progressive renal failure.

Diffuse Mesangial Sclerosis (Six Cases) (See Page 51). In six patients, the mesangium was invaded by fibrillary sclerosis with no hypercellularity, and all the glomeruli were involved. In advanced cases, the glomerular tuft takes on the appearance of a fibrous ball surrounded by a corona of epithelial cells. In all six cases the nephrotic syndrome appeared during the first year of life, in one case presenting at birth. In four cases, the syndrome was familial. All the patients died of renal failure before the age of three years.

Comparison of the Principal Varieties of Nephrotic Syndrome

Virtually all the primary nephrotic syndromes are represented by four major histologic groups: minimal glomerular lesions, focal glomerular lesions, extramembranous glomerulonephritis, and membranoproliferative and lobular glomerulonephritis. The clinical features and course of the disease vary with the histologic type.

Clinical Features

Membranoproliferative and lobular glomerulonephritides are distinguished from the three other groups by having a later age of onset. We have never seen this variety before the age of 2 years and rarely before the age of 5 years. Another distinguishing feature of this group is the higher proportion of girls affected (Table 54). A familial history is found only in nephrotic syndrome with minimal or focal glomerular lesions. A patient with permanent proteinuria may develop a nephrotic syndrome only after having had, for a considerable length of time, a diffuse glomerulonephritis (extramembranous glomerulonephritis, or

Table 54. Age at Onset and Distribution According to Sex in the Principal Varieties of Nephrotic Syndrome in Children (346 Cases)

Histologic Type	Onset Before 5 Years	Onset Between 5 and 10 Years	Onset After 10 Years	Percentage of Males
Minimal glomerular lesions (209 cases)	63 per cent	26 per cent	11 per cent	72 per cent
Focal glomerular lesions (88 cases)	62 per cent	21 per cent	17 per cent	59 per cent
Extramembranous glomerulonephritis (44 cases)	46 per cent	27 per cent	27 per cent	76 per cent
Membranoproliferative and lobular glomerulonephritis (82 cases)	8 per cent	26 per cent	66 per cent	42 per cent

membranoproliferative and lobular glomerulonephritis). With minimal or focal glomerular lesions, the interval from discovery of the disease to the development of a nephrotic syndrome is rarely more than four months.

The nephrotic syndrome is severe only for minimal and focal glomerular lesions. A patient with serous effusions, a serum albumin level below 1.0 g. per 100 ml., serum lipids above 2.0 g. per 100 ml., and a very low urinary sodium output is virtually certain to belong to one of these two groups. The proteinuria is not very selective except in the group with minimal glomerular lesions.

Macroscopic hematuria is generally seen only in diffuse glomerulonephritis. Conversely, the absence of hematuria at the onset and confirmed at repeated examinations is evidence in favor of minimal glomerular lesions but is not enough to rule out focal lesions. Furthermore, when hematuria does develop in a nephrotic syndrome with minimal glomerular lesions, it is transient in most cases.

Early renal failure is common in membranoproliferative and lobular glomerulonephritis but rare with minimal and with focal glomerular lesions (10 and 12 per cent). Renal failure occurred in only two of all the patients who had glomerulonephritis with extramembranous deposits. Initial hypertension is common in membranoproliferative and lobular glomerulonephritis but very rare in the other varieties. Lowering of the C′3 fraction of serum complement was found only in membranoproliferative and lobular glomerulonephritis.

Response to Treatment

If steroid therapy is instituted in the first attack, it will produce complete remission in the majority of cases with minimal glomerular lesions, in a small number of cases with focal glomerular lesions, and in some cases of glomerulonephritis with extramembranous deposits. Sensitivity to steroids is definite and reproducible only in the minimal and the focal glomerular lesions. Steroid sensitivity is doubtful in extramembranous glomerulonephritis, and the membranoproliferative and lobular glomerulonephritides are steroid-resistant.

The efficacy of immunosuppressive drugs seems to be well established in minimal glomerular lesions and in certain cases of focal glomerular lesions. A particular value of these drugs is that they allow interruption of steroid therapy in steroid-dependent patients. Any good effect is less evident in extramembranous glomerulonephritis. Immunodepressive drugs have produced no remissions in membranoproliferative and lobular glomerulonephritis.

Course of the Disease

Complete remission is possible in any case, but the incidence of complete remission differs greatly in the various groups. In the diffuse glomerulonephritides, remission sets in progressively, is rarely repeated, and seems to be independent of treatment. Only patients with minimal or focal glomerular lesions have numerous relapses, punctuated by remissions that are generally induced by treatment. "Cures," or at least very prolonged remissions, occur essentially with minimal glomerular lesions and with extramembranous glomerulonephritis. The "cures" seen in the other groups are fewer in number and the follow-up period is too short to be certain that the cure is genuine.

An unfavorable course is much more common in the focal glomerular

lesions (38 per cent) and in membranoproliferative and lobular glomerulonephritis (41 per cent) than in minimal glomerular lesions (seven per cent) or
extramembranous glomerulonephritis (eight per cent). With diffuse glomerular
lesions, death always results from progressive renal failure. In cases with minimal or focal glomerular lesions, death may stem from intercurrent complications.

Conclusion

The primary nephrotic syndrome in children is represented by two main
groups, "nephrosis" and nephrotic syndromes associated with diffuse glomerulonephritis.[52]

"Nephrosis"

In our experience, "nephrosis" represents fewer than 50 per cent of the
primary nephrotic syndromes seen in childhood. This is certainly a falsely low
figure; the actual value should be of the order of 90 per cent in an unselected
series.[60] These "nephroses" have a predilection for boys, in whom the nephrotic
syndrome is often extremely severe. Two types of clinical course can be distinguished.

In the first type, by far the most common, the proteinuria is selective,[47]
the hematuria may be obvious or slight and transient, and the condition is
generally sensitive to steroids and to immunosuppressive drugs. These patients
never go on to renal failure. The gravity of the disease is linked to the appearance of complications, especially infection and thromboembolism.[50, 54] The
disorders of hemostasis that accompany the nephrotic syndrome predispose
to clotting disorders. The patient may be cured after a single attack or after
several attacks with varying intervals. As a rule, renal biopsy reveals minimal
glomerular lesions, but 11 patients in our series, in whom the disease progressed
over many years, had focal glomerular lesions. However, the prognosis is still
good in the latter group, with renal function remaining normal after periods
of from 14 to 18 years.

In the second type, there is nonselective proteinuria, frequent hematuria,
and total resistance to steroids. The prognosis is poor. The kidney may appear normal, but in most cases it presents focal glomerular lesions. Renal failure is common, sometimes preceded by tubular disorders. Of the immunosuppressive drugs, azathioprine is ineffective,[45] but there is some evidence that
chlorambucil and cyclophosphamide may produce complete remission. However, the follow-up periods are too short to be sure that such remission is
definitive.

The relationship between minimal and focal glomerular lesions is not clear.[51]
Most authors[46, 55] regard focal lesions as a development of nephrotic syndromes
with minimal glomerular lesions. In fact, in both of these types, the etiologic
circumstances (age, sex) and the clinical presentation are very similar. In one
third of cases, the clinical course is absolutely the same in both groups, and
characteristically there are repeated attacks that are sensitive to steroids.
Focal lesions may be found at a later biopsy in patients whose first biopsy had
shown only minimal glomerular lesions.[46, 51, 55] In two thirds of the cases, however, the presence of hematuria, the total steroid resistance, the nonselectivity

of the proteinuria, the relentless progression to renal failure, and the early discovery of focal lesions on renal biopsy all constitute considerable evidence that this is a different histologic and clinical entity.[51, 53]

It is true that all the features just mentioned can be found in patients with minimal glomerular lesions, but in view of the fact that focal lesions are often confined to the juxtamedullary zone, it is possible that they may be present but unrecognized, and they may be discovered on a second biopsy. There is no doubt that a close relationship exists between these two groups of patients.

Diffuse Glomerulonephritis

In this group, which includes extramembranous glomerulonephritis and the proliferative glomerulonephritides (endocapillary, membranoproliferative, lobular, and endo- and extracapillary forms) the nephrotic syndrome may dominate the clinical picture, but it is never very severe. In addition, it is often transient. The proteinuria is only slightly if at all selective. There is nearly always an associated hematuria.

In the early years of the disease, there is often improvement, generally spontaneous, in the nephrotic syndrome, in the hematuria, and in renal function, if this was affected initially. Complete and sometimes lasting remissions may occur, especially in extramembranous glomerulonephritis. The long-term prognosis, however, is often poor. Steroid therapy is ineffective and may be poorly tolerated.[57] The effect of immunosuppressive drugs is still a subject of debate.[45, 59] Lowering of the C′3 fraction of complement is characteristic of membranoproliferative glomerulonephritis.[49, 58]

Prognosis

The overall prognosis of the nephrotic syndrome in our series is poor. Twenty-five per cent of the children are dead or have renal failure. Death from renal failure occurs in 100 per cent of cases of extracapillary glomerulonephritis with diffuse crescents, but in only seven per cent of cases of "nephrosis," the largest group. No more than 1.5 per cent of children with nephrotic syndromes owing to minimal glomerular lesions die of renal failure, the remaining deaths resulting from intercurrent complications. It is obvious that the prognosis varies considerably with the histologic type (Table 55).

Knowledge of the histology is essential for proper choice of treatment. All cases of "nephrosis" must be treated initially by steroids in appropriate dosages. If steroids prove ineffective or if the patient is steroid-dependent, there are serious risks to prolonging the steroid therapy. The use of immunosuppressive drugs is then justified because of their effectiveness in certain cases, but the dangers of using these drugs are not yet clearly established. It has been shown that in all varieties of diffuse glomerulonephritis, steroid therapy is useless and even dangerous; in addition, the beneficial effect of immunosuppressive drugs has not yet been established.

Granted these facts, should *renal biopsy* be performed in every child with a nephrotic syndrome? In a large number of cases, the overall clinical picture and laboratory findings point with some certainty to the histologic type. A pure nephrotic syndrome, without hematuria, with very selective proteinuria, appearing in a child between the ages of 1 and 8 years, is almost certainly the

Table 55.   Overall Prognosis of Primary Nephrotic Syndromes in Children
(507 Cases)

Histologic Type	Total Number of Cases	Unfavorable Course	Persistent Abnormalities	Cure
Minimal glomerular lesions	209	14	47	148
Focal glomerular lesions	88	29	39	20
Glomerulonephritis with extramembranous deposits	44	5	21	18
Glomerulonephritis with pure endocapillary proliferation	41	7	12	22
Glomerulonephritis with endocapillary and extra-capillary proliferation	20	13	2	5
Membranoproliferative and lobular glomerulonephritis	82	37	41	4
Microcystic kidney	6	6	–	–
Diffuse mesangial sclerosis	6	6	–	–
Unclassifiable	11	9	2	–
Total	507	126	164	217

result of minimal glomerular lesions and is very likely to be steroid-sensitive and to have a good prognosis. In such a case, it is perfectly reasonable to institute steroid therapy without direct histologic evidence and to refrain from renal biopsy unless, for example, steroid-resistance is encountered. On the other hand, persistent hematuria, initial renal insufficiency and hypertension, poorly selective proteinuria, and total resistance to steroids add up to a picture suggesting either focal glomerular lesions, if the nephrotic syndrome is very severe, or proliferative glomerular lesions, if the serum complement level is lowered. None of these features, however, has an absolute value, and renal biopsy remains the best criterion of prognosis and the best guide to treatment.

ACUTE GLOMERULONEPHRITIS OR THE SYNDROME OF "POSTINFECTIOUS GLOMERULONEPHRITIS OF ACUTE ONSET"*

The condition generally appears one to three weeks after infection of the upper respiratory tract or of the skin by beta-hemolytic streptococci. The onset is sudden, with hematuria, often macroscopic, proteinuria, and sometimes edema. There may also be oliguria, hypertension, or a nephrotic syndrome.

Incidence

This is almost impossible to determine, because there are probably a large number of mild and fleeting cases that are not seen in hospital. Indeed, asymptomatic cases, diagnosed by the discovery of microscopic hematuria on routine

---

*This section was written in collaboration with C. Loirat.

examination of the urine, represent 50 per cent of cases in general studies of the population carried out during certain epidemics.[68]

Etiology

The first symptoms of glomerulonephritis occur as a rule one to three weeks after an infectious episode. A sore throat is the most common cause. Other respiratory tract infections, including sinusitis, pneumonia, otitis, and also scarlet fever, may be concerned. In underdeveloped countries, septic dermatitis is still a common cause of glomerulonephritis.[68]

The responsible infection is nearly always a beta-hemolytic streptococcus of group A. Only the so-called nephritogenic types are concerned—usually type 12, more rarely types 2, 4, 6, 19, 25, 31, and 49. In practice, it is often impossible to prove that the infection was streptococcal; the discovery of hemolytic streptococci in the throat is rare nowadays because the majority of patients with a sore throat have been given antibiotics. McCrory[69] found hemolytic streptococci in 20 per cent of patients who had been given antibiotics and in 47 per cent of patients who had not been given antibiotics. Another inconstant finding is an elevation in the antistreptolysin titer beginning one to three weeks after the infection, reaching a maximum between the third and fifth weeks, and returning to normal in two or three months. We found an elevated antistreptolysin titer in 60 per cent of our patients; Chaptal and associates[63] give a figure of 50 per cent, whereas McCrory[69] gives a figure of 87 per cent. Evidence of streptococcal infection would probably be found in a larger number of cases by simultaneously investigating other streptococcal antibodies, such as antihyaluronidase, antistreptokinase, and antidiphosphopyridine-nucleotidase. Certain strains of streptococcus may be weak stimulators of antibody production, and the use of antibiotics may diminish the antigenic stimulation. It is very likely that other etiologic agents also occur. Endocapillary proliferative glomerulonephritis has been observed as a complication of chickenpox[70] and of certain viral infections, especially with the ECHO 9 virus.[61] These different etiologic factors explain why the disease may be seasonal (in winter or early spring), sporadic, or epidemic (in families or schools).

Age at Onset

The disease appears in older children. In our own experience, the average age was 8 years 11 months, and the youngest patient was aged 2 years 3 months. Although some cases have been reported in very young children (youngest was 8 months old[69]), acute glomerulonephritis is unlikely to occur before the age of 2 years. Some authors report a preponderance of boys,[62, 69] but this is not a constant finding.[68]

Variations in Presentation

The diagnosis is obvious in cases presenting the full classical picture, occurring one to three weeks after a sore throat, with proteinuria, macroscopic hematuria, possibly oliguria (urinary output less than 300 ml./m.^{2}/day), with a gain in weight, sometimes mild edema, and moderate hypertension. The child often has gastrointestinal disorders, such as nausea, vomiting, and abdominal pain, but he is rarely feverish and his general condition usually remains good.

However, these various symptoms may appear in an isolated fashion. Most often there is proteinuria or macroscopic hematuria, and sometimes there may be edema and abdominal pain. It is in the initial stage that acute glomerulonephritis may pose a difficult diagnostic problem and require urgent treatment to save the patient's life. The condition may present with oliguria or anuria and, if not correctly treated, may prove fatal from acidosis, hyperkalemia, and above all the cerebral and cardiovascular complications of water and salt overloading. Acute glomerulonephritis may present with convulsions[64] or with other manifestations of cerebral edema, such as blindness. We have had one case that presented with acute asystole and pulmonary edema, and there are several reports in the literature of similar cases.

These neurologic and cardiovascular manifestations are usually linked to water and salt overloading in an oliguric or anuric child. In such cases there is an increase in weight, edema, and hypertension, but the severity of the manifestations contrasts with the relatively mild hypertension. The systolic blood pressure is no more than 150 mm. Hg, and the diastolic blood pressure is generally between 80 and 120 mm. Hg. In the majority of cases, the diagnosis is indicated by a history of recent sore throat, oliguria, and the discovery of proteinuria and hematuria. It is not always possible to obtain a history of preceding infection, and there are varieties with minimal urinary abnormalities,[67, 71] in which there is oliguria but no proteinuria (or only slight and transient proteinuria), or microscopic hematuria, although the neurologic and cardiovascular complications are extremely serious. In such cases, it is vital to consider the possibility of acute glomerulonephritis, because in practice this may be an indication for peritoneal dialysis. Lowering of the $C'3$ fraction of serum complement is important evidence in favor of a diagnosis of acute glomerulonephritis.

The use of the term "acute glomerulonephritis" to describe all these cases is not entirely a happy choice. In practice, the word "acute" is used in a twofold sense: to designate the mode of onset of the disease, and to indicate favorable prognosis, with disappearance of the various abnormalities in several months at most. In fact, the evolution of the disease is known only in retrospect, and the observed condition might better be described by such terms as "postinfectious glomerulonephritis of acute onset" or "postinfectious acute nephritic syndrome." Some such term would have the advantage of not prejudging the evolution of the disease in patients whose initial symptoms may indeed be similar, but in whom the long-term or short-term prognosis may be guarded. A study of 139 patients belonging to this group, who presented signs of glomerulonephritis with an acute onset following infection, reveals that the prognosis in such cases is not always favorable, even in children. In this study, we have included only those patients with diffuse proliferative glomerulonephritis.

Histopathology

The most common variety is *diffuse endocapillary proliferative glomerulonephritis.* We have studied 49 cases. This figure represents fewer than half of the cases seen and does not reflect the true picture because this histologic variety is always associated with curable acute glomerulonephritis and in our department such cases are submitted to biopsy only relatively infrequently. The essential lesion is the mesangial proliferation. The exudative character (the presence of large numbers of polymorphonuclear cells) and the presence of "humps" (small, spaced extramembranous deposits on the epithelial aspect of the basement membrane) are evident only in early biopsy material, obtained before the end of the first month of the disease. During the second month, the polymorphonuclear cells and the humps disappear, and only the mesangial proliferation remains. In turn, the proliferation disappears and the histologic appearances return to normal after an interval varying from two months to two years. Some authors have reported the persistence of histologic abnormalities and of deposits of IgG and of B₁C for more than two years,[74] but this is unusual.

In addition to this mesangial proliferation and segmental sclerosis of the glomerular tuft, with deposits limited to certain capillary walls, there may be extracapillary proliferation, nearly always in the most affected segments of the tuft. This is the condition that we designate by the term *endocapillary and extracapillary glomerulonephritis with focal crescents.* We have divided this into two types, depending on the number of glomeruli involved. In type 1 fewer than 30 per cent of the glomeruli are affected, whereas in type 2 between 30 and 80 per cent of the glomeruli are affected. We have studied 36 cases. In 14 cases, there were large and circumferential epithelial crescents in all the glomeruli. The term *endocapillary and extracapillary glomerulonephritis with diffuse crescents* is applied to this type of lesion. In 40 cases, in addition to the mesangial proliferation, there were deposits thickening the walls of the glomerular capillaries (subendothelial or dense deposits) with *(lobular glomerulonephritis)* or without *(membranoproliferative glomerulonephritis)* nodular sclerosis of the mesangium.

Clinical Features

Diffuse Endocapillary Proliferative Glomerulonephritis (49 Cases)

Our series includes 30 boys and 19 girls. There was evidence of streptococcal infection in 26 cases. In the other cases, the nephropathy appeared eight to 20 days after some upper respiratory infection or febrile sore throat, in which the streptococcus could not be incriminated with certainty. In every patient, the onset was sudden, with proteinuria and hematuria which was accompanied, in certain cases, by a nephrotic syndrome or hypertension, and/or signs of renal failure.

Initial Period. A variable degree of renal insufficiency is common (31 cases). Total anuria was observed in only three cases and for only a short period (two, three, and five days). Oliguria persisting for several days was noted on 13 occasions. In 15 cases, there was a rise in the blood urea nitrogen, even though the urinary output did not fall. Only in two of the 15 cases did the blood urea level rise above 200 mg. per 100 ml. The renal insufficiency lasted for one month in one case, for three months in two cases, and for six months in one case; in the remaining 27 cases, renal function returned to normal in a few days. Hypertension was present in 29 of the 49 cases; it was moderate in 24 and more severe in five patients, in whom initial treatment had perhaps been inadequate. Hypertension was transient in most cases, the blood pressure returning to normal in a few days as the salt and water overload was corrected. An elevated blood pressure did, however, persist for three months in one patient and for four months in another.

Hematuria was a constant feature. There was macroscopic hematuria, often the presenting symptom, in 36 cases, and microscopic hematuria in 13 cases. Hematuria that was macroscopic in the beginning usually became microscopic in a period of one or two months. Proteinuria was present in all cases. In 14 patients, the proteinuria was never more than 1 g./24 hours, but it was greater than this in the 35 other cases. The proteinuria was sufficiently great in 15 of these patients to produce a nephrotic syndrome, but the nephrotic syndrome was never gross. In no case did the serum proteins drop below 5.0 g. per 100 ml. In 10 patients, the nephrotic syndrome was transient and the blood protein levels returned to normal in less than 15 days. The nephrotic syndrome persisted for two months in one patient, for three months in two patients, and for four months in two patients. Edema, usually mild and transient, was found in 26 patients.

Long-term Prognosis. The various symptoms and signs disappeared spontaneously in every patient. Of 34 patients who were followed for more than six months, 25 had no urinary abnormality at the end of the six months. In most of these patients, the proteinuria was very slight after two months, and the last sign to disappear was the hematuria. In seven patients, the urinary signs (proteinuria, proteinuria with hematuria, isolated hematuria) disappeared before the end of the first year. Isolated hematuria persisted for 13 months in one patient, and there was periodically recurrent macroscopic hematuria over a period of four years in one other patient, who had had a particularly severe

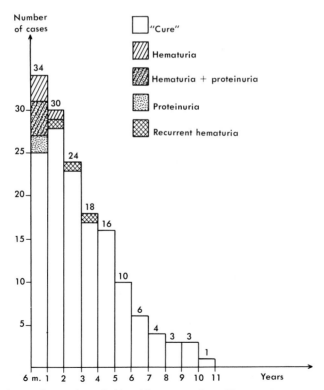

Figure 69. Acute glomerulonephritis with pure endocapillary proliferation. Course of 34 cases followed for periods ranging from six months to 11 years.

acute glomerulonephritis, with the initial rise in blood urea nitrogen persisting for three months.

These 34 patients were followed for a period varying from one to 11 years (Figure 69), and, within the limits of this follow-up, all patients recovered completely, as has been reported in other studies.[72] Recurrent glomerulonephritis is rare,[73] but we had the opportunity to perform renal biopsy in two patients who relapsed 20 and 25 months after the initial attack. In both, there had been complete recovery from the first attack in less than six months.

Endocapillary and Extracapillary Glomerulonephritis with Focal Crescents (36 Cases)

Our series includes 20 boys and 16 girls. Upper respiratory tract infection preceded the onset of the kidney disease in all patients, but this infection was proved to be streptococcal in only 16.

Initial Stage. Signs of renal insufficiency were present in 25 patients. Initial anuria was noted on six occasions, lasting only one day in two patients, and in the other four persisting for seven days, 11 days, 13 days, and 23 days. Eight patients had oliguria, which never lasted longer than eight days. In the remaining 11 patients, there was a rise in the blood urea nitrogen, with no diminution of urinary output. In 20 of the 25 patients, the signs of renal insufficiency disappeared rapidly, but return to normal renal function took one month in one case, three months in one case, four months in one case, nine months in one case, and one year in one case.

The blood pressure was elevated in 14 patients. It returned rapidly to normal in eight cases, but the hypertension persisted for more than a month in six patients. All the patients had hematuria, which was macroscopic in 22. In 32 of the 36 patients, the urinary protein output was more than 1 g./24 hours, and the serum protein levels fell below 5.5 g. per 100 ml. in eight patients. The nephrotic syndrome disappeared in less than one month in four of the eight but persisted for three months in two and for five months in the remaining two. Six patients developed a nephrotic syndrome secondarily after intervals varying from 20 days to four months. This was transient in four patients and prolonged in two (six months and eight months). Edema was noted in 18 patients and was severe in some of them.

Long-term Prognosis. We were able to follow 27 patients for more than six months (see Figure 70), and six of these were clinically cured before the end of the first year. In two other patients, the urine became completely normal after 14 and 18 months, respectively. In a follow-up period as long as 11 years in some cases, seven patients seem definitively cured. There was, however, one patient whom we regarded as cured when his urine became completely normal nine months after the onset of the disease, but after 11 years of complete remission (during which time his urine was repeatedly found to be protein-free), he developed chronic renal insufficiency with a proteinuria of 3 g./24 hours and severe hypertension. One to seven years after the onset of the nephropathy, the remaining 19 patients still have signs of renal disease, most often proteinuria, but sometimes proteinuria with microscopic hematuria though with normal renal function.

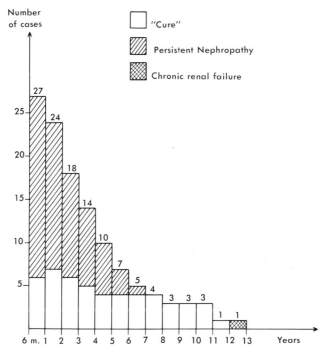

Figure 70. Acute glomerulonephritis with endocapillary and extracapillary proliferation and focal crescents. Course of 27 patients followed for periods ranging from six months to 13 years.

Endocapillary and Extracapillary Glomerulonephritis with Diffuse Crescents (14 Cases)

Our series includes seven boys and seven girls. In all 14 there was a previous episode of upper respiratory tract infection, which proved to be streptococcal in eight.

Initial Stage. There were signs of severe renal failure in most of these patients (11 cases). Five patients were anuric from the outset. The anuria lasted only two days in one of these patients, but in the other four it lasted 14 days, 20 days, and one month (two cases). Two patients had oliguria for less than two weeks. In the four remaining patients, there was an elevated blood urea nitrogen without a drop in urinary output. Secondary renal failure developed in three patients after intervals of two to three months. In all but one of these patients, once renal failure appeared, it persisted until the child died.

A secondary nephrotic syndrome, sometimes severe, appeared in six patients after intervals of one to four months. In four cases, this nephrotic syndrome persisted until death occurred, between five and 15 months after onset of the disease. In the other two patients, the nephrotic syndrome lasted six and eight months. These two patients subsequently died after intervals of 2 years 10 months and 3 years 7 months. Edema was noted in 10 patients but was severe in only one.

Long-term Prognosis. With one exception, all the patients died with terminal renal failure and severe hypertension after a variable interval, usually less than 15 months (11 cases). The single exception was a patient who was treated early by anticoagulants and cyclophosphamide, in whom the blood urea nitrogen level returned to normal after two months, and whose only abnormality at seven months is isolated proteinuria of 1.5 g./24 hours. Two patients survived longer, for 2 years 10 months and for 3 years 7 months, although there were signs of renal insufficiency throughout the illness.

Membranoproliferative Glomerulonephritis (40 Cases)

There were 24 girls and 16 boys with this condition. A history of upper respiratory tract infection, often febrile, was found in all cases but proved to be streptococcal in only 10.

Initial Stage.   Sixteen patients presented signs of initial renal insufficiency, and two of these had oliguria. Initial anuria was never seen in this group. The blood urea level never rose above 200 mg. per 100 ml. and usually returned to normal in less than one month, although signs of renal insufficiency persisted for two to six months in five patients.

Initial hypertension, usually moderate, was noted in 16 cases. In most cases, the blood pressure returned to normal in the first month of the illness. In four patients, the hypertension was prolonged for five or six months before the pressure returned to normal, and one patient had persistent hypertension until death occurred from terminal renal failure two and a half years after the onset of the disease. All but three of the patients had hematuria.

Except for five patients, the urinary protein was always greater than 1 g./ 24 hours, and this was accompanied by an initial nephrotic syndrome in 15 cases. In 11 of the cases, the nephrotic syndrome was severe, with serum protein levels below 5.0 g. per 100 ml. A secondary nephrotic syndrome appeared in 12 patients. In half of these, the nephrotic syndrome appeared at the end of one month, in five cases it appeared between two months and six months, and in the last case it appeared at 10 months.

Long-term Prognosis.   Except for three patients who underwent complete remission at 11 months, two and a half years, and four years, respectively, and who remain in remission with a follow-up of 10 months, 2 years, and 2 years 8 months, all the patients have persistent evidence of nephropathy, leading to terminal renal failure in 10 and to chronic renal insufficiency in two.

Modalities of Evolution of the Disease

It can be seen from Table 56 that the symptoms in the initial stage of the disease are very similar in all four types of acute glomerulonephritis, and only their frequency varies. The evolution, on the other hand, differs greatly, and it is possible to distinguish three clinical types according to the modalities of evolution of the disease.

Form with Acute Onset that is Curable

Essentially these are cases of diffuse endocapillary glomerulonephritis. However, we have observed eight "cures" in 34 cases of endocapillary and extra-capillary glomerulonephritis with focal crescents. The cure is apparently definitive in seven of these children, but the eighth patient is now in terminal renal failure after a period of complete remission of 11 years (Figure 68).

Table 56. Glomerulonephritis of Acute Onset After Infection: Clinicopathologic Correlation in the Initial Stage

Histologic Type	Number of Cases	Hematuria		Proteinuria (g./24 hours)		Nephrotic Syndrome	Renal Failure		Hypertension
		Macro-scopic	Micro-scopic	<1	>1		With Oliguria	Without Oliguria	
Pure endocapillary glomerulonephritis	49	36	13	14	35	15	16	15	29
Endocapillary and extracapillary glomerulonephritis with focal crescents	36	22	14	4	32	8	14	11	14
Endocapillary and extracapillary glomerulonephritis with diffuse crescents	14	8	6	0	14	5	7	4	3
Membranoproliferative and lobular glomerulonephritis	40	18	19	5	35	15	2	14	16
Total	139	84	52	23	116	43	39	44	62

In this group, the lowering of the C'3 fraction of complement is transient, with the level returning to normal in a period of weeks.

Form with Acute Onset Progressing to Chronic Disease

This includes most of the cases of endocapillary and extracapillary proliferative glomerulonephritis with focal crescents and the membranoproliferative and lobular glomerulonephritides. In the group of 27 patients followed for more than six months in whom renal biopsy had revealed endocapillary and extracapillary glomerulonephritis with focal crescents, 19 continued to have proteinuria, some for many years (Figure 69 and Table 57). In the group of 38 patients with membranoproliferative and lobular glomerulonephritis, 35 patients have signs of persistent nephropathy, with the condition deteriorating in 12 patients after a variable length of time (Table 57).

Persistent lowering of the C'3 fraction of serum complement is evidence in favor of this type of glomerulonephritis.

Form with Acute Onset Leading to Rapidly Progressive Renal Failure

This group consists exclusively of cases of endocapillary and extracapillary glomerulonephritis with diffuse crescents. The natural history of this type of nephropathy is discussed elsewhere (see page 282). The course of the disease is in no way modified by the fact of preceding infection.

It is obvious from this analysis that there is a correlation between the histologic appearance and the course of the disease in cases of glomerulonephritis that begin acutely after an infectious episode. Renal biopsy should, however, probably be reserved for cases presenting one of the following alarm signals: prolonged anuria (more than five days); renal insufficiency (creatinine clearance below 60 ml./min./1.73 m.^{2} and serum creatinine level above 1.5 mg. per 100 ml., repeatedly confirmed) beyond the first month; persistence of a nephrotic syndrome beyond the first month, or, especially, the secondary onset of a neph-

Table 57. Glomerulonephritis with Acute Onset After Infection: Correlation Between Histologic Type and Course of the Disease

Histologic Type	Number of Cases Followed for More Than 6 Months	Cure	Persistent Nephropathy	Unfavorable Course
Pure endocapillary glomerulonephritis	34	33	1	0
Endocapillary and extracapillary glomerulonephritis with focal crescents	27	7	19	1
Endocapillary and extracapillary glomerulonephritis with diffuse crescents	14	0	1	13
Membranoproliferative and lobular glomerulonephritis	38	3	23	12
Total	113	43	44	26

rotic syndrome; persistence of hypertension beyond two weeks; persistence of a very low level of complement (C'3) beyond the second month;[65, 66, 75] persistence of a urinary protein output greater than 1 g./24 hours beyond the sixth month and of microscopic hematuria for more than 12 to 18 months; recurrence of macroscopic hematuria a considerable time after the initial attack (which is suggestive of Berger's disease — see page 254).

Conclusion

The term "acute glomerulonephritis" is useful but ambiguous. The ambiguity derives from the fact that there is often an implicit assumption of a good prognosis, with disappearance of all the different abnormalities in a matter of months. This notion would be justified if "acute glomerulonephritis" could be reserved for curable acute glomerulonephritis characterized by pure diffuse endocapillary proliferation. However, there are other types of glomerulonephritis (membranoproliferative, endocapillary and extracapillary proliferative) that may present in a very similar fashion, with an equally acute onset, perhaps following a streptococcal infection, for which the prognosis must be more guarded. It does, of course, remain to be proved that all the forms of acute glomerulonephritis which we have observed are in fact different expressions of the same disease and not different diseases. Many authors hold the view that membranoproliferative and lobular glomerulonephritis has nothing in common with acute glomerulonephritis, a term which they reserve exclusively for curable glomerulonephritis of acute onset.

PROLONGED OR CHRONIC GLOMERULONEPHRITIS

We can present here only a brief summary of the relevant facts and ideas that are scattered through many chapters of this section of the work.

Cases of prolonged glomerulonephritis are manifested clinically by proteinuria-hematuria, and/or a nephrotic syndrome, and/or chronic renal insufficiency with or without hypertension. The disease may be discovered by chance at a routine urine examination or during one of the episodes that mark the course of the condition, such as a nephrotic syndrome, hematuria, hypertension, or uremia. The condition evolves over many years, sometimes more than a decade, with the possibilities of obtaining amelioration or even apparent clinical cure, or, conversely, of undergoing aggravation. Sometimes there is an obvious etiologic factor, such as systemic disease or streptococcal infection, but in most cases the etiology is obscure.

Increased comprehension of prolonged glomerulonephritis has been achieved from advances in immunology and in histopatholgy, especially the use of renal biopsy, electron microscopy, and immunofluorescence. In consequence, the general notion of prolonged or chronic glomerulonephritis has given way to better defined clinicopathologic and immunologic entities, so that the prognosis and sometimes the indications for treatment can be more clearly assessed. This is why it has seemed preferable to describe the various entities in detail: diffuse membranoproliferative glomerulonephritis (see page 229), diffuse extramembranous glomerulonephritis (see page 220), focal chronic glomerulonephritis (see page 237), the chronic form of the hemolytic-uremic syndrome, and the nephropathies of systemic diseases (see page 302).

GLOMERULONEPHRITIS WITH RAPIDLY PROGRESSIVE RENAL FAILURE (MALIGNANT GLOMERULONEPHRITIS)

Various names have been given to this type of glomerular nephropathy, including subacute glomerulonephritis,[89] acute oliguric glomerulonephritis,[78, 83] rapidly progressive glomerulonephritis,[77, 84] and malignant glomerulonephritis.[82] The definition of the condition rests exclusively on the course of the disease. The onset is usually acute, with signs of renal insufficiency of varying severity, with or without oliguria, but the onset may also be insidious, with renal failure appearing as a secondary feature. The characteristic of this form of glomerulonephritis is the irreversible nature of the renal failure, progressing relentlessly to terminal uremia in a matter of months, rarely more than 18 months. In every case, histologic examination of the kidney reveals the lesions of endocapillary and extracapillary glomerulonephritis, and so the condition is a clinicopathologic entity.

Rapidly progressive or malignant glomerulonephritis has been described mainly in adults, and we have been able to find only 14 cases in children described in the literature,[76, 78–80, 83, 87, 88] but in fact the condition is not uncommon in children. Habib[81] found 22 cases in a series of 344 children with nonspecific glomerulonephritis. These 22 cases form the basis for our description of this type of glomerulopathy.

Pathologic Anatomy

In the 22 cases reported here, the characteristic glomerular lesion was a variable degree of mesangial proliferation associated with huge epithelial crescents (endocapillary and extracapillary glomerulonephritis with diffuse crescents) (see page 228).

In 80 to 100 per cent of glomeruli, Bowman's space is filled by a proliferation of epithelial cells derived to a large extent from the parietal leaf of Bowman's capsule. Among these cells, in recent lesions, were found large fibrinoid deposits, and in the older lesions there were collagen fibrils. Variable changes were seen in the walls of the glomerular capillaries. In seven cases, the picture was that of a membranoproliferative glomerulonephritis with the addition of epithelial crescents, and in five of the seven there was a "dense deposit in the basement membranes." In 13 cases, the lesions of the capillary walls were more irregular and haphazard and seemed to result from mesangial invasion, with progressive sclerosis rather than true deposition.

Any similarity in these lesions is only apparent; their diversity is even more evident on immunofluorescence study. Most of the cases in this series were observed before immunofluorescence techniques were available, but studies in recent cases have revealed that the only constant characteristic of these lesions is fixation of antifibrin serum in the epithelial crescents. Fixations within the tuft are very variable.

Sometimes there is no fixation at all. At other times the appearance is that of a membranoproliferative glomerulonephritis, with subendothelial deposits or with dense deposits in the basement membranes (see page 229). In some cases there is fixation of anti-IgG and anti-B_1C sera in separate granules, as in acute glomerulonephritis. In one case we found a linear fixation, as occurs in Goodpasture's syndrome. In this case, there were circulating anti-basement membrane antibodies. It may be that any type of glomerular nephropathy may be "accompanied" by crescents and that the crescents are responsible for the grave character of the condition.

Clinical Features (Table 58)

In our 22 cases, there were 12 girls and 10 boys, ranging in age from 5 to 15 years, with the exception of one child aged two and a half years. Etiology

Table 58. Comparison of Clinical Features in the Three Types of Endocapillary and Extracapillary Proliferative Glomerulonephritis

Types	I	II	III
Number of cases	21	20	22
Male/female ratio	10/11	8/12	10/12
Etiologic circumstances			
Systemic disease	7	9	7
Unidentified	3	2	2
Postinfectious	6	6	7
Idiopathic	5	3	6
Presenting symptoms			
Oliguria	1	1	1
Hematuria, edema	3	4	0
Macroscopic hematuria	10	8	3
Edema	3	2	10
Maximal proteinuria			
<5 g./liter	12	8	5
>5 g./liter	9	10	14
Total proteins			
<6.0 mg. per 100 ml.	10	12	17
>7.0 mg. per 100 ml.	5	1	2
Edema			
Absent	13	11	1
Moderate	8	7	14
Severe	0	2	7
Nephrotic syndrome			
Frank	5	7	16
Biochemical	5	5	4
Hypertension			
Absent	14	12	2
Initial	3	2	3
Progressive	1	2	15
Renal failure			
Absent	8	5	0
Initial	9	9	17
Secondary	4	6	5
Transient	12	10	0

was very variable. In seven cases, the nephropathy followed a streptococcal infection. In seven other cases, the nephropathy was a renal manifestation of systemic disease (see page 302) – rheumatoid purpura in four and periarteritis nodosa in three. In the remaining eight cases no etiological factor could be discovered; in six of these, the nephropathy was isolated, but in the other two there were associated extrarenal signs (arthralgia, elevated sedimentation rate, hypergammaglobulinemia) suggesting a systemic disease of indeterminate nature.

The dominant feature is a permanent proteinuria accompanied by a nephrotic syndrome in the majority of cases, associated with hematuria and, above all, with signs of renal insufficiency that may appear early or late. The serum protein levels were always low, except for two cases in which they were elevated (8.2 and 8.5 g. per 100 ml.). A nephrotic syndrome was present at some stage in 20 patients; in four of these it was purely biochemical, but in the remaining 16 it was frank, and in four of the children the edema was gross.

This nephrotic syndrome tends to diminish or even disappear as the renal insufficiency develops. Hematuria is constant and permanent, sometimes macroscopic (nine cases), sometimes microscopic (eight cases). In five patients, macroscopic and microscopic hematuria alternated. Hypertension was present from the outset in three patients and developed gradually in 15. In these 18 cases, the hypertension persisted until death. Hypertension became manifest in the terminal stages in only two cases. Hematologic abnormalities included severe anemia in eight cases and leukocytosis in nine.

Every patient showed signs of renal insufficiency, and this presented early in 17 cases, with urinary output diminishing to anuria in five. The oliguria persisted for a variable length of time; it gave way to a frank nephrotic syndrome in four of the patients, and in the other case it persisted until death after six weeks. In the remaining 12 children, urinary output was maintained, and the renal insufficiency was accompanied by a nephrotic syndrome appearing at an early stage in 11 patients.

The signs of renal insufficiency appeared secondarily after several weeks in five patients in whom the only clinical features up to that time had been a glomerulonephritis with a nephrotic syndrome.

There are two remarkable features about the course of the disease. The mode of onset is not uniform. In 17 cases the picture was that of sudden acute renal insufficiency, sometimes severe, but usually with the urinary output maintained. In five patients, the clinical onset was much more insidious, resembling a glomerulonephritis with a complete nephrotic syndrome, and chronic renal insufficiency set in secondarily, generally before the end of the third month. Either way, once the renal insufficiency appears, it persists until death.

Sixteen of the patients died before the end of the seventh month (Figure 71) and the six remaining children died after 10 months, 15 months, 16 months, 17 months, and 20 months. It should be noted in this regard that the 22 patients were seen over a period of 15 years and the differences in length of survival may be explained in many cases by developments in therapeutic methods.

It is very difficult to analyze the results of treatment in our series in view of the great diversity of type and duration of treatments used and the fact that therapy was introduced at very different stages in different patients.

All the children were treated with a special diet, and seven were put on

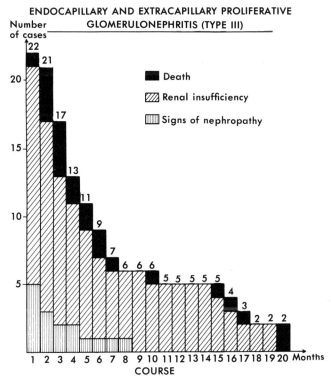

Figure 71. Rapidly progressive glomerulonephritis. Course in 22 cases.

peritoneal dialysis. Nine patients received prednisone or immunosuppressive drugs or both; one patient received indomethacin in addition. There was transient improvement in one patient treated with mechlorethamine hydrochloride (Caryolysine), in one patient with prednisone, and in one patient with indomethacin, but there was no other evidence of benefit from any treatment.

There is little difference between the cases reported here and those in the literature.[76, 78-80, 83, 87, 88] The 14 cases recorded in children include eight in boys and six in girls and the age at the onset of the disease varied from 2 to 14 years. In five cases, the nephropathy appeared in the context of a systemic disease. The remaining nine cases were either idiopathic or followed an infection. In eight patients the onset was sudden, with oliguria, and in the other six cases the onset was insidious. All the children died after an interval varying from 23 days to two years. The glomerular lesions reported were of the endocapillary and extracapillary proliferative type. The same evolutional modalities are noted in adults,[90] but a sudden onset with oliguria seems more common in adults, and their survival time is generally shorter. Hamburger gives the survival as six months. Certain cases have been reported as following a favorable course with or without treatment. One should be very circumspect in the analysis of such observations. In view of the constant association of the histologic lesion of endocapillary and extracapillary glomerulonephritis and the clinical condition of glomerulonephritis with rapidly progressive renal failure, certain authors tend to make the *clinical* diagnosis on the renal biopsy findings. But, as we have shown,[81] only type 3 endocapillary and extracapillary glomerulo-

nephritis—in which at least 80 per cent of the glomeruli present a circumferential extracapillary proliferation—is rapidly fatal. When the extracapillary proliferation is focal (types 1 and 2) the nephropathy, whose onset may be very
similar to that of malignant glomerulonephritis (Table 58), generally pursues
a less severe course; we have even seen several cases go on to spontaneous cure.
In any interpretation of a favorable evolution, it is important to define accurately
the histologic type.

Although there is considerable evidence that a malignant glomerulonephritis may develop in a very short period of time, many authors suggest the
possibility of exacerbation of a preexisting renal disease or of "superimposition"
of acute glomerulonephritis on some long-standing and unrecognized nephropathy.[80]

All the published series refer to a variety of etiologic circumstances, but in
many cases the etiology remains obscure.[77] In addition to the etiologic factors
already cited, we should mention Goodpasture's syndrome, rare in children,
which usually presents as a glomerulonephritis with very rapidly progressive
renal failure (see page 318).

Has the etiology any significance in the clinical picture of the disease, the
evolutional modalities or the histopathologic characteristics of the lesions observed? In an attempt to answer this question, we have analyzed the different
clinical and laboratory findings as a function of the etiologic circumstances in
our series of 22 patients but we have not found any differences among the
clinical pictures in the various circumstances. It does seem, however, that early
renal insufficiency with or without anuria occurs more frequently in the systemic
diseases, whereas the nephrotic syndromes with a secondary renal failure occur
more often in postinfectious or idiopathic glomerulonephritis. The histologic
appearance that we regard as membranoproliferative glomerulonephritis with
epithelial crescents is found exclusively in the primary renal diseases, mainly
those following infection, sometimes in idiopathic cases.

Eight of the nine patients who presented a nephropathy associated with
systemic disease died within six months, whereas only seven of 12 patients with
postinfectious or idiopathic glomerulonephritis died within this period. It is
apparent that the etiologic circumstances do play a definite part in the evolutional modalities and in the duration of the disease.

Both in our own series and in cases reported by other authors, steroids
and immunosuppressive agents seem to be of no value in the treatment of
malignant glomerulonephritis, but, on the other hand, heparin therapy is
now thought to have distinct possibilities of success.[85, 86] Very recently, we have
used the same treatment as Horvath and his associates (see page 339, Horvath
et al.[12]) in two children with severe glomerulonephritis, in whom renal biopsy
revealed endocapillary and extracapillary glomerulonephritis with diffuse
crescents. The immediate improvement in renal function was spectacular, but
we do not yet know how long it will continue.

Conclusion

Malignant glomerulonephritis is defined by two characteristics, one clinical
and the other histologic. The clinical feature is the rapid progression and the
irreversibility of the renal failure once it appears. The histologic feature is the

presence of circumferential epithelial crescents in more than 80 per cent of the glomeruli. Two evolutional modalities are possible: (1) an acute onset with initial renal insufficiency (with or without oliguria), which becomes rapidly progressive, or (2) an insidious onset as a glomerulonephritis with a nephrotic syndrome and the secondary development of renal failure that progresses remorselessly to terminal uremia in a short period.

The value of heparin therapy has yet to be established, but no other commonly used treatment (steroids or immunosuppressive agents or a combination of the two) is of any value.

REFERENCES

PROTEINURIA

1. Antoine, B., Symvoulidis, A., Dardenne, M., de Montera, H., and Bach, J. F.: L'état de protéinurie permanente isolée. I. Diversité histologique. Presse Méd. 77:9, 1969.
2. Antoine, B., Symvoulidis, A., Dardenne, M., de Montera, H., and Bach, J. F.: L'état de protéinurie permanente isolée. II. Stabilité évolutive. III. Signification nosologique. Presse Méd. 77:51, 1969.
3. Cameron, J. S., and Blandford, G.: The simple assessment of selectivity in heavy proteinuria. Lancet 2:242, 1966.
4. Cameron, J. S.: Histology, protein clearances, and response to treatment in the nephrotic syndrome. Brit. Med. J. 4:352, 1968.
5. Chaptal, J., Jean, R., Bonnet, H., and Pages, A.: Étude histologique du rein dans 33 cas de protéinurie isolée de l'enfant. Arch. franç. Pédiat. 23:385, 1966.
6. Habib, R.: Classification of glomerulonephritis based on morphology. In P. Kincaid-Smith, T. A. Mathew, and E. L. Becker: Glomerulonephritis. New York, John Wiley & Sons, 1973.
7. Herdman, R. C., Michael, A. S., and Good, R. A.: Postural proteinuria, response to corticoid therapy. Ann. Intern. Med. 65:286, 1966.
8. King, S. E.: Diastolic hypertension and chronic proteinuria. Amer. J. Cardiol. 9:669, 1962.
9. Lagrue, G., Bariéty, J., Druet, P. H., and Milliez, P.: Les protéinuries, Paris, Sandoz, 1969.
10. Lecocq, F. R., McPhaul, J. J., and Robinson, R. R.: Fixed and reproducible orthostatic proteinuria. V. Results of a five year follow-up evaluation. Ann. Intern. Med. 64:557, 1966.
11. Manuel, Y., and Revillard, J. P.: Study of urinary proteins by zone electrophoresis. Methods and principles of interpretation. In Proteins in Normal and Pathological Urine. New York, Karger, 1970, p. 153.
12. Manuel, Y., Revillard, J. P., François, R., Traeger, J., Gaillard, L., Salle, B., Freycon, M. T., and Borentain, I.: Trace proteinuria. In Proteins in Normal and Pathological Urine. New York, Karger, 1970, p. 198.
13. Mery, J. P., Berger, J., Milhaud, A., and Crosnier, J.: La protéinurie orthostatique. A propos de 300 observations. Rev. Prat. (Paris), 11:3115, 1961.
14. Morel-Maroger, L. Leroux-Robert, C., Amiel, C., and Richet, G.: Étude histologique de 33 cas de protéinurie isolée. Fréquence des dépôts hyalins et fibrinoïdes dans les artérioles rénales. Nephron 4:13, 1967.
15. Robinson, R. R., Glouer, S. N., Philippi, P. J., Lecocq, F. R., and Langelier, P. R.: Fixed and reproducible orthostatic proteinuria. I. Light microscopy studies of the kidney. Amer. J. Path. 39:291, 1961.
16. Robinson, R. R., Ashworth, C. T., Glouer, S. N., Philippi, P. J., Lecocq, F. R., and Langelier, P. R.: Fixed and reproducible orthostatic proteinuria. II. Electron microscopy of renal biopsy specimens from 5 cases. Amer. J. Path. 39:405, 1961.
17. Robinson, R. R.: Postural proteinuria. In Proteins in Normal and Pathological Urine. New York, Karger, 1970, p. 224.

HEMATURIA

18. Alyea, E. P., Parish, H. M., and Durhan, N. C.: Renal response to exercise: urinary findings. J.A.M.A. 167:807, 1958.
19. Amman, P., and Rossi, E.: Allergic hematuria. Arch. Dis. Child. 41:539, 1966.
20. Arneil, G., Lam, C., and McDonald, M.: Recurrent haematuria in 17 children. Brit. Med. J. 2:233, 1969.

21. Ayoub, E., and Vernier, R.: Benign recurrent hematuria. Amer. J. Dis. Child. *109*:217, 1965.
22. Bari, W., Taylor, J., and Germuth, F.: The pathogenesis of focal immune complex glomerulo-nephritis (abstract). Fed. Proc. *29*:236, 1970.
23. Berger, J., Neuveu, T., Morel-Maroger, L., and Antoine, B.: Localisation des immunoglobulines et du fibrinogène dans les lésions glomérulaires. *In* Actualités néphrologiques de l'Hôpital Necker. Paris, Flammarion, 1967, p. 161.
24. Berger, J.: IgA glomerular deposits in renal disease. Transplant. Proc. *1*:939, 1969.
25. Berger, J., Yaneva, H., and Hinglais, N.: Les glomérulonéphrites focales. *In* Actualités néphro-logiques de l'Hôpital Necker. Paris, Flammarion, 1968, p. 141.
26. Bodian, M., Black, J., Kobayashi, N., Lake, B., and Schuler, S.: Recurrent hematuria in child-hood. Quart. J. Med. *34*:359, 1965.
27. Cameron, A.: Renal biopsy in recurrent hematuria. Arch. Dis. Child. *39*:299, 1964.
28. Dreesman, L., Senterfit, L., and Germuth, F.: Experimental immune complex disease: antibody level, immune complex size and pattern of glomerular alteration (abstract). Fed. Proc. *29*: 3285, 1970.
29. Druet, P., Bariéty, J., Bernard, D., and Lagrue, G.: Les glomérulopathies primitives à dépôts mésangiaux d'IgA et d'IgG. Etude clinique et morphologique de 52 cas. Presse Méd. *78*: 583, 1970.
30. Galle, P., and Berger, J.: Dépôts fibrinoïdes intercapillaires. J. Urol. Néphrol. *68*:123, 1962.
31. Gervais, M., and Drummond, K.: L'hématurie récidivante chez l'enfant. Un. Méd. Canada *99*: 1234, 1970.
32. Glasgow, E., Moncrieff, M., and White, R.: Symptomless hematuria in childhood. Brit. Med. J. *2*:687, 1970.
33. Gotze, O., and Muller-Eberhard, H.: The C′3 activation system: an alternative pathway of complement activation. J. Exp. Med. *134*:90, 1971.
34. Hendler, E., Kashgarian, M., and Hayslett, J.: Clinicopathological correlation of primary hematuria. Lancet *1*:458, 1972.
35. McConville, J. M., West, C. D., and McAdams, A. J.: Familial and non-familial benign hema-turia. J. Pediat. *69*:207, 1966.
36. Morel- Maroger, L., Leathem, A., and Richet, G.: Glomerular abnormalities in non-systemic dis-ease: relationship between light microscopy and immunofluorescence in 433 renal biopsies. Amer. J. Med. *53*:70, 1972.
37. Northway, J.: Hematuria in children. J. Pediat. *78*:381, 1971.
38. Ross, J.: Recurrent focal nephritis. Quart. J. Med. *29*:391, 1960.
39. Roy, L., Fish, A., and Michael, A.: "Benign hematuria." A review of 22 patients with light and immunopathologic studies (abstract). Amer. Soc. Nephrol., 1971, p. 66.
40. Singer, D., Hill, L., Rosenberg, H., Marshall, J., and Swenson, R.: Recurrent hematuria in childhood. New Eng. J. Med. *279*:7, 1966.
41. Van Acker, K., and Mestdagh, J.: Benigne recurrende hematuria. Maandsch Kindergeneesk. *36*:157, 1968.
42. Vernier, R., Mauer, S., Fish, A., and Michael, A.: Les cellules mésangiales dans les glomérulo-néphrites. *In* Actualités néphrologiques de l'Hôpital Necker. Paris, Flammarion, 1971, p. 37.
43. Volhard, F., and Fahr, T.: Die Brightsche Nieren Krankheit. Berlin, Springer, 1914.
44. Zollinger, H. U., and Gaboardi, F.: Verzögerte Heilung einter diffusen intra- und extracapil-laren Glomerulonephritis mit IgA-Depots. Virchow. Arch. (Path. Anat.) *354*:349, 1971.

NEPHROTIC SYNDROME

45. Abramowicz, M., Barnett, H. L., Edelmann, C. M., Greifer, I., Kobayashi, C., Arneil, G. C., Barron, B. A., Gordillo, G., Hallman, N., and Tiddens, H. A.: Controlled trial of azathioprine in children with nephrotic syndrome. Lancet *1*:959, 1970.
46. Berger, J., de Montera, H., and Hinglais, N.: Comment évoluent les lésions rénales des malades atteints de syndrome néphrotique. *In* Actualités néphrologiques de l'Hôpital Necker. Paris, Flammarion, 1966, p. 265.
47. Cameron, J. S.: Histology, protein clearance and response to treatment in the nephrotic syn-drome. Brit. Med. J. *4*:352, 1968.
48. Giles, H., Pugh, R. C. B., Darmady, E. M., Stranack, F., and Wolff, L. I.: The nephrotic syn-drome in early infancy: a report of three cases. Arch. Dis. Child. *32*:167, 1957.
49. Gotoff, S. P., Fellers, F. X., Vawter, G. F., Janeway, C. A., and Rosen, F. S.: The beta-1C globulin in childhood nephrotic syndrome. Laboratory diagnosis of progressive glomerulonephritis. New Eng. J. Med. *273*:524, 1965.
50. Habib, R., Courtecuisse, V., and Bodaghi, E.: Thrombose des artères pulmonaires dans les syn-dromes néphrotiques de l'enfant. J. Urol. Néphrol. *74*:349, 1968.
51. Habib, R., and Gubler, M. C.: Les lésions glomérulaires focales des syndromes néphrotiques idiopathiques de l'enfant. A propos de 49 observations. Nephron *8*:382, 1971.

52. Habib, R., Kleinknecht, C., and Royer, P.: Le syndrome néphrotique primitif de l'enfant. Classification et étude anatomique de 406 observations. Arch. franç. Pediat. 28:277, 1971.

53. Hayslett, J. P., Krassner, L. S., Bensch, K. G., Kashgarian, M., and Epstein, F. H.: Progression of "lipoid nephrosis" to renal insufficiency. New Eng. J. Med. 281:181, 1969.

54. Lieberman, E., Heuser, E., Gilchrist, G. S., Donnell, G. N., and Landing, B. H.: Thrombosis, nephrosis and corticosteroid therapy. J. Pediat. 73:320, 1968.

55. McGovern, V. J.: Persistent nephrotic syndrome: a renal biopsy study. Austr. Ann. Med. 13: 306, 1964.

56. Oliver, J.: Microcystic renal disease and its relation to "infantile nephrosis." Amer. J. Dis. Child. 100:312, 1960.

57. Sharpstone, P., Ogg, C. S., and Cameron, J. S.: Nephrotic syndrome due to primary renal disease. II. A controlled trial of prednisone and azathioprine. Brit. Med. J. 2:535, 1969.

58. West, C. D., McAdams, A. J., Conville, J. M., Davis, N. C., and Holland, N. H.: Hypocomplementic and normocomplementic persistent (chronic) glomerulonephritis, clinical and pathologic characteristics. J. Pediat. 67:1089, 1965.

59. White, R. H., Cameron, J. S., and Trounce, J. R.: Immunosuppressive therapy in steroid-resistant proliferative glomerulonephritis accompanied by the nephrotic syndrome. Brit. Med. J. 2:853, 1966.

60. White, R. H. R., Glasgow, E. F., and Mills, R. J.: Clinicopathological study of nephrotic syndrome in childhood. Lancet 1:1353, 1970.

ACUTE GLOMERULONEPHRITIS

61. Burch, G. E., Chu, K. C., and Sohal, R. S.: Glomerulonephritis induced in mice by ECHO 9 virus. New Eng. J. Med. 279:1420, 1968.

62. Callis, L., Castello, F., and Garcia, L.: Histopathological aspects of acute diffuse glomerulonephritis in children. Helv. Paediat. Acta 22 (Suppl. 16):3, 1967.

63. Chaptal, J., Jean, R., Habib, R., Bonnet, H., Pagès, A., and Dumas, R.: Glomérulonéphrite post-infectieuse de l'enfant. Confrontations anatomo-cliniques au cours de l'évolution. Arch. franç. Pédiat. 24:907, 1967.

64. Fleischer, D. S., Voci, G., Garfunkel, J., Purugganan, H., Kirkpatrick, J., Wells, C. R., and De Elfresch, A. E.: Hemodynamic findings in acute glomerulonephritis. J. Pediat. 69:1054, 1966.

65. Herdman, R. C., Pickering, R. J., Michael, A. F., Vernier, R. L., Fisch, A. J., Gewurz, H., and Good, R. A.: Chronic glomerulonephritis associated with low serum complement activity (chronic hypocomplementic glomerulonephritis). Medicine 49:207, 1970.

66. Humair, L. M.: B_1C globulin and complement in nephritis. Serological and immunological studies in acute, chronic, membranous and lupus glomerulonephritis. Helv. Med. Acta 34: 279, 1968.

67. Kandall, S., Edelmann, C. M., Jr., and Bernstein, J.: Acute poststreptococcal glomerulonephritis. A case with minimal urinary abnormalities. Amer. J. Dis. Child. 118:426, 1969.

68. Kaplan, E. L., Anthony, B. F., Chapman, S. S., and Wannamaker, L. W.: Epidemic acute nephritis associated with type 49 streptococcal pyoderma. I. Clinical and laboratory findings. Amer. J. Med. 48:9, 1970.

69. McCory, W. W.: Natural history of acute glomerulonephritis in children. In J. Metcoff: Acute glomerulonephritis. Boston, Little, Brown & Co., 1967, p. 15.

70. Minkowitz, S., Wenk, R., Friedman, E., Yuceoglu, A. M., and Berkovich, S.: Acute glomerulonephritis associated with varicella infection. Amer. J. Med. 44:489, 1968.

71. Mozziconacci, P., Attal, C., Pham-Huu-Trung, M. T., Boisse, J., Guy-Grand, D., and Féron, J. F.: Glomérulonéphrite aiguë avec encéphalopathie hypertensive et manifestations urinaries mineures. Ann. Pédiat. 15:352, 1968.

72. Perlman, L. V., Herdman, R. C., Kleinman, H., and Vernier, R. L.: Poststreptococcal glomerulonephritis. A ten year follow-up of an epidemic. J.A.M.A. 194:63, 1965.

73. Roy, S., Wall, H. P., and Etteldorf, J. N.: Second attacks of acute glomerulonephritis. J. Pediat. 75:758, 1969.

74. Treser, G., Ehrenreich, T., Ores, R., Sagel, I., Wasserman, E., and Lange, K.: Natural history of "apparently healed" acute poststreptococcal glomerulonephritis in children. Pediatrics 43:1005, 1969.

75. West, C. D., Northway, J. D., and Davis, N. C.: Serum levels of B_1C globulin, a complement component, in nephritic, lipoid nephrosis, and other conditions. J. Clin. Invest. 43:1507, 1964.

MALIGNANT GLOMERULONEPHRITIS

76. Allen, D. M., Diamond, L. K., and Howell, D. A.: Anaphylactoid purpura in children. Amer. J. Dis. Child. 99:833, 1960.

77. Bacani, R. A., Velasquez, F., Kanter, A., Pirani, C. L., and Pollak, V. E.: Rapidly progressive glomerulonephritis. Ann. Intern. Med. *69*:463, 1968.
78. Berlyne, G. M., and Baker, S. B.: Acute anuric glomerulonephritis. Quart. J. Med. *33*:105, 1964.
79. Brun, C., Gormsen, H., Hilden, T., Iversen, P., and Raaschou, F.: Kidney biopsy in acute glomerulonephritis. Acta Med. Scand. *160*:155, 1958.
80. Edelmann, C. M., Grifer, I., and Barnett, H. L.: The nature of kidney disease in children who fail to recover from apparent acute glomerulonephritis. J. Pediat. *64*:879, 1964.
81. Habib, R.: Classification anatomique des néphropathies glomérulaires. Pädiat. Fortbildungskurse *28*:3, 1970.
82. Hamburger, J.: Les glomérulonéphrites malignes. *In* Entretiens de Bichat. Paris, Expansion Scientifique Française, 1956, p. 231.
83. Harrison, V. V., Loughridge, L. W., and Milne, M. D.: Acute oliguric renal failure in acute glomerulonephritis and polyarteritis nodosa. Quart. J. Med. *33*:39, 1964.
84. Heptinstall, R. H.: Pathology of the Kidney. London, Churchill, 1966.
85. Herdman, R. C., Edson, J. R., Pickering, R. J., Fish, A. J., Marker, S., and Good, R. A.: Anticoagulants in renal disease in children. Amer. J. Dis. Child. *119*:27, 1970.
86. Kincaid-Smith, P.: Anticoagulants in "irreversible" acute renal failure. Lancet *2*:1360, 1968.
87. Manassero, J., Vaillaud, J. C., Paglia, R., and Geneste, F.: A propos d'un cas de glomérulonéphrite aiguë dite maligne. Pédiatrie *25*:221, 1970.
88. McCluskey, R. T., and Baldwin, D. S.: Natural history of acute glomerulonephritis. Amer. J. Med. *35*:213, 1963.
89. Sarre, H.: Nierenkrankheiten. Stuttgart, Thieme, 1967.
90. Sonsino, E., Nabarra, B., Kazatchkine, M., Hinglais, N., and Kreis, H.: Les glomérulonéphrites prolifératives extracapillaries dites "glomérulonéphrites malignes." *In* Actualités néphrologiques de l'Hôpital Necker. Paris, Flammarion, 1972, p. 119.

For additional recent information, see:

a. Lewy, J. E., Salinas-Madrigal, L., Herdson, P. B., Pirani, C. L., and Metcoff, J.: Clinico-pathologic correlations in acute poststreptococcal glomerulonephritis. Medicine *50*:453, 1971.

Chapter Four

HEMOLYTIC UREMIC SYNDROME

The hemolytic uremic syndrome is the most common cause of acute renal failure in infants. The characteristic clinical picture makes the diagnosis easy. There is hemolytic anemia of the microangiopathic type, a hematuric or anuric nephropathy, and thrombocytopenia, which are always present. Less constant findings include convulsions and hypertension.

Various names have been applied to the condition, such as acute glomerulonephritis with anemia, nephro-anemic syndrome, and nephro-hemolytic syndrome, but the term most widely used is hemolytic uremic syndrome. The clinical picture may be found with many types of histologic lesion, including (1) the cortical necrosis described in 1955 by Gasser and associates,[9] who were the first to use the term "hemolytic uremic syndrome"; (2) an exclusively renal thrombotic microangiopathy described by us in 1958;[14, 28] and (3) thrombotic microangiopathy with vascular lesions disseminated throughout many organs, characteristic of Moschowitz's disease or thrombotic thrombocytopenic purpura. Obviously the condition is common, because we have seen more than 60 cases, and many hundreds are reported in the literature. Although the clinical and histologic features of the hemolytic uremic syndrome are well known, many questions remain to be answered, in particular about the etiology, the pathophysiology, and the treatment.

Etiology

The sexes are affected equally. The syndrome may occur in small epidemics, and this has been particularly striking in Argentina, France, and Wales. There is also a seasonal incidence, the maximal incidence in our experience being in August and September. The involvement of more than one member of the family has been reported on several occasions. Cases included identical twins, two brothers and sisters in two families, and two first cousins who were in frequent contact, in whom the disease appeared simultaneously.

Despite this evidence in favor of some infection, etiologic studies have largely proved negative, although various viruses have been isolated, including the type A_4 virus by Glasgow, arbovirus by Gianantonio in Argentina, and myxovirus in one of our cases. Recently Mettler[24] found, in two children with the hemolytic uremic syndrome and one adult with thrombotic thrombocytopenic purpura, a microorganism classed as a microtatobiote, of the order Rickettsia and family Bartonellacea. This organism can be transmitted to mice and reproduces the clinical syndrome in the rhesus monkey. The vector apparently is a mite.

Other possible etiologic factors should be recalled. The hemolytic uremic syndrome has appeared after a vaccination in some cases. There may be some abnormal immune factor. A case has occurred in a child with a nephrotic syndrome treated with prednisone and chlorambucil; another case occurred in a child of 16 months suffering from agammaglobulinemia with alymphocytosis. These facts have encouraged some authors to attempt to relate the hemolytic uremic syndrome to the Shwartzman phenomenon.

Clinical Features

We have described the clinical features in detail in recent articles in which we reported on 37 children with the hemolytic uremic syndrome.[15–17, 22] The disease attacks infants who previously were well; more rarely it occurs in older children. After a brief prodromal period there is a sudden onset, with simultaneous hemolytic anemia and renal disorder.

Prodromal Features

The prodromal stage may last from a few hours to several days. The most common symptoms in this stage are gastrointestinal disorders. Diarrhea is quite characteristic of the syndrome in infants. There is also abdominal pain, vomiting, and sometimes hematemesis, but only rarely is melena seen. Fever occurs in half of the cases. The rise in temperature is generally moderate, to 38° or 39° C. There may be enlargement of the lymph nodes or a rash. The syndrome may also set in without any prodromal symptoms.

Principal Signs

The characteristic feature of the acute phase is the simultaneous appearance of the principal symptoms, thus excluding the idea that the uremia might be caused by the hemolytic anemia, or vice versa.

Hemolytic Anemia.   The anemia is rapid in onset and very severe; it may worsen in subsequent exacerbations. The red blood count may fall to 2 million per cubic millimeter in a period of 24 hours. The hemolytic nature of the anemia is revealed by the high level of reticulocytes in the circulating blood and the erythroblastosis in the bone marrow, the passage of normoblasts into the peripheral blood, the fall in haptoglobin level, and the finding of large amounts of iron in liver, spleen, and kidney at autopsy. Generally, the serum bilirubin level is only slightly elevated.

The red blood cells are very deformed, and there are numerous schizocytes. Although the erythrocyte deformities are not specific, they are very important in the clinical context because of their intensity and frequency. These deformities are a constant feature of the syndrome.[3]

There are no Heinz bodies, no antibodies, no abnormal hemoglobin, and no abnormal erythrocyte enzymes. The hemolysis is extracorpuscular, as shown by the fact that red cells transfused from a healthy person into a patient have a diminished half-life, whereas red blood cells from a patient transfused into a healthy subject have a normal half-life. Brain and his colleagues believe that the erythrocyte distortions and the hemolysis are linked with lesions of the red blood cells produced during their passage through arterioles affected by thrombosis.[3]

In addition to the anemia, there is often a considerable leukocytosis, with the passage of immature white cells (meta-myelocytes, myelocytes and even lymphoblasts) into the peripheral blood. The hemolytic anemia can last for a variable length of time. In infants, in most cases, it does not last more than 20 days. In older children it may last for more than a month, with successive exacerbations that are not necessarily associated with aggravation of the renal disorders. The initial hyperleukocytosis often gives way to leukopenia with eosinophilia.[22]

Disorders of Hemostasis.   These disorders are an almost constant feature, often appearing at the onset of the disease. More rarely, they are first seen in later exacerbations. Disorders of hemostasis are manifested by purpura, cutaneous ecchymoses, and gastrointestinal bleeding. Cerebral hemorrhage is rare, but we have seen one case of meningeal hemorrhage. The bleeding time is frequently prolonged. In nearly every case, there is a considerable thrombocytopenia, with a platelet count below 100,000 per cubic millimeter. The half-life of the platelets is diminished. This thrombocytopenia rarely persists for more than eight days.

Investigation of the coagulation factors gives results that vary from patient to patient and in the same patient from day to day. The results depend to a large extent on the stage at which the investigation is performed. Some authors[2, 3] have found abnormalities of the coagulation factors suggesting intravascular coagulation—decreases in factor V, factor VIII, and fibrinogen levels. In reality, there are never major abnormalities comparable to those found in disseminated intravascular coagulation—for example, those that are secondary to septicemia. There is, however, nearly always an increase in fibrin degradation products.

These abnormalities, along with the diminished half-life of labeled fibrinogen observed in some cases[20] and the histopathologic findings, all suggest that localized intravascular coagulation plays a part in the pathophysiology of the syndrome.

Renal Disorder.   The renal syndrome appears *at the same time* as the anemia and is manifested either by signs of acute glomerulonephritis with or without oliguria or by total anuria.

When the urinary output is maintained, there is nearly always hematuria, often macroscopic, and the proteinuria that is always present may be sufficient to produce a nephrotic syndrome with edema. The blood urea level is nearly always very high at the first examination. These symptoms may regress in a matter of days, but equally may continue for many months, with successive exacerbations.

The C'3 fraction of serum complement is normal in most cases, although at times it has been found to be lowered.[20]

Anuria at the very outset is particularly common in infants. The few milliliters of urine that are passed contain a very large number of red blood cells. The biochemical abnormalities are those of any anuria, and there is a special risk of hyperkalemia because of the hemolysis. This oliguria rarely lasts for more than 10 days. We have, however, observed a return of diuresis after two or even three weeks. In these cases there is naturally a fear of cortical necrosis and all that this diagnosis implies.

Cardiovascular Signs.   The blood pressure is elevated in more than half of the cases. This hypertension may appear in the initial stages. It is generally moderate, with a systolic blood pressure around 140 mm. Hg, but it may be more severe and can sometimes lead to cardiac failure, which then dominates the clinical picture and may even be a mode of presentation of the disease. The hypertension may be related to overhydration, especially in the anuric infant, but can persist after correction of the overhydration, especially in older children, and it then constitutes evidence of hyperreninemia and in some cases may be an indication for bilateral nephrectomy. The hypertension may occur at a later stage, when the signs of renal involvement appear stable or may even be in regression.

Neurologic Signs. These are particularly common in infants. Convulsions may occur at the onset of the disease. The cerebrospinal fluid is generally normal. These complications are not necessarily the result of spread of the vascular disorder to the brain but in most cases are linked to the metabolic disorders secondary to the acute renal failure. Such sequelae as simple abnormalities of the electroencephalogram and convulsions are possible but rare.

Associated Signs. The gastrointestinal disorders of the prodromal period often persist, as does a moderate fever. Melena adds a note of gravity to the clinical picture. Hepatosplenomegaly, enlargement of the lymph nodes, and various eruptions may be seen. Subicterus may be noted in older children.

Evolution

Modern progress in the symptomatic treatment of acute renal failure has considerably transformed the prognosis of this condition. It is interesting in this regard to compare our figures for the last three years (Table 59) with those reported in 1969.[16, 17, 22] The evolution should be considered separately for infants and for older children.

The majority of children under the age of 2 years recover without ill effects. A variable degree of renal failure persists in cases complicated by cortical necrosis (10 to 15 per cent of cases). Only one of our recent cases proved fatal, and this was in a boy with diffuse cortical necrosis.

After the age of 2 years, the prognosis is not so good; two thirds of the cases go on to progressive renal failure with malignant hypertension. It is important to emphasize that in a follow-up over many years we have never seen a relapse of the hemolytic uremic syndrome, nor any deterioration in renal function in

Table 59. Hemolytic Uremic Syndrome: General Course of 25 Patients Seen from 1969 Through 1973

	Age	
	Before 2 Years (20 Patients)	After 2 Years (5 Patients)
Complete cure at May 1, 1973	15	2
Kidney disorders		
Chronic renal failure	2	1
Maintenance dialysis	1	1
Neurologic disorders	1	—
Dead	1	1

patients clinically cured after the acute episode. Hypertension and later neurologic complications have, however, been reported.[12]

Diagnosis

The association of hemolytic anemia and renal symptoms may be observed in other circumstances. It is easy to exclude hemolytic anemia traceable to autoantibodies or to a congenital abnormality of hemoglobin or of erythrocyte enzymes. These anemias are rarely accompanied by acute renal insufficiency, and the prognosis is generally good. The diagnosis may be more difficult in older children with other types of glomerular nephropathy accompanying a hemolytic anemia, as can happen with lupus nephritis. Finally, some cases of malignant hypertension can be accompanied by microangiopathic anemia and rapidly progressive renal failure, underlining the difficulties of diagnosis if the history is not known.[27]

Pathologic Anatomy[5, 6, 11, 16, 28, 29]

The basic lesion of the hemolytic uremic syndrome is in all cases a thrombotic microangiopathy. This lesion has already been defined (see page 217) with

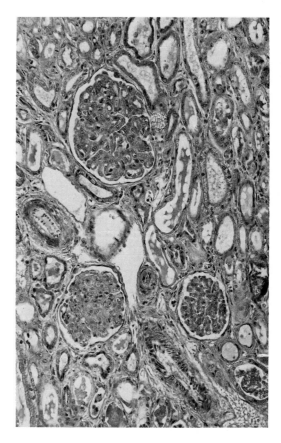

Figure 72. Hemolytic uremic syndrome. The glomeruli are affected in an irregular manner by the lesions of thrombotic microangiopathy. The lumen of the arteriole near the center of the picture is obstructed by endothelial swelling.

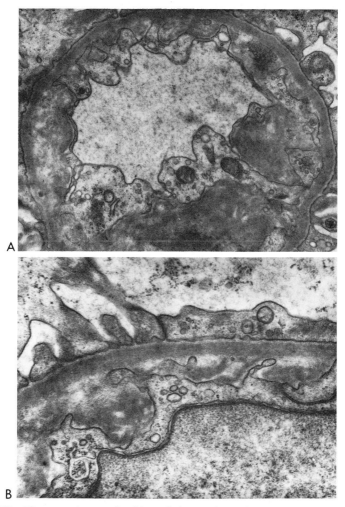

Figure 73. Electron micrograph of hemolytic uremic syndrome with thrombotic microangiopathy. The lesions appear principally on the endothelial aspect of the glomerular capillary. *A,* Swelling of the subendothelial zone is clearly visible. ×10,500. *B,* A clear space can be seen between the basement membrane and the endothelium. ×13,500.

the specific glomerular lesions. The association with arteriolar lesions is constant, although these may vary in intensity and extent. Various anatomic pictures may be noted. Sometimes the thrombotic microangiopathy is *localized exclusively to the kidney,* but this is by no means the type most frequently seen in infants. Sometimes the microangiopathy is accompanied by *cortical necrosis* that does not differ macroscopically from renal cortical necrosis without the hemolytic uremic syndrome. This cortical necrosis may be diffuse, bilateral, and asymmetric, or it may occur in a variable number of small nodular foci. It is sometimes associated with hemorrhagic infarction of the pyramids. Cortical necrosis seems to be more common in infants than in older children. Sometimes the thrombotic microangiopathy is associated with *diffuse arteriolar lesions in other organs,* including the brain, intestines, lungs, adrenals, and spleen. We have found this latter variety only in older children, and it appears to be particularly common in adults.[23, 29]

The nosologic relationship between the various types of lesions is not yet certain. It is probable that these lesions are identical in nature but variable in degree and extent. Study of the renal parenchyma of patients suffering from the hemolytic uremic syndrome may be helpful in assessing the ultimate prognosis. There is in fact a strict correlation between the severity of the histologic lesions and the severity of the renal disorder. In our experience, although not all the patients who presented with initial anuria had cortical necrosis, all of those with cortical necrosis presented with anuria, and in most the anuria was prolonged. It is only in this latter group that renal sequelae have been noted.

The discrete nature and focal character of the lesions of thrombotic microangiopathy are remarkable in the benign forms in which recovery is rapid. The

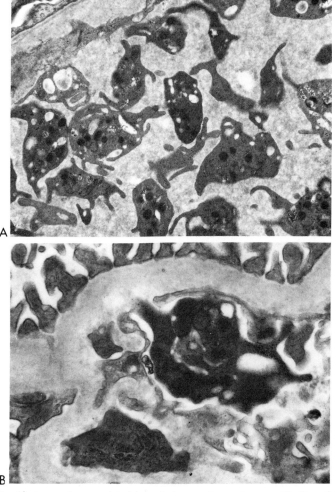

Figure 74. Electron micrograph of hemolytic uremic syndrome with thrombotic microangiopathy. *A,* Masses of platelets can be seen within the lumen of the glomerular capillaries. ×6000. *B,* The platelets even seem to be infiltrating across the pores of the endothelium. ×15,000.

lesions are more diffuse in the severe types. Nonetheless, and despite the mortality rate observed before 1969 in this group, it seems to us that in the cases in which the thrombotic microangiopathy is exclusively renal, even when the glomerular lesions are extensive and there is initial anuria, the prognosis is favorable, especially in infants.

This raises the question of the fate of the glomerular lesions. We lack the evidence to be certain, but in the three cases in which we performed serial biopsies we have observed disappearance of the lesions of the glomerular capillaries, whereas the more severely damaged glomeruli were completely fibrosed. It thus seems likely that the endothelial lesions so characteristic of the disease are reversible.

Pathophysiology

In the hemolytic uremic syndrome, there is very probably a process of intravascular coagulation. But this is only an intermediary mechanism, and the factor that triggers it off must be determined.[21] Many sequences have been suggested to explain the pathogenesis. The view currently held is that the initial lesion in the endothelium of the arterioles, most often in the kidneys, is caused by a virus or some other etiologic agent. The endothelial lesion would then trigger in situ a process of intravascular coagulation with thrombus formation. The general consequence would be a moderate and short-lived consumption of platelets and coagulation factors on the one hand, and on the other hand destruction of the red blood cells and possibly also of platelets as they pass through the regions of the lesions, by a mechanism that has been well studied by Brain and his colleagues.[3] The local consequence in the damaged organs would be an ischemia, whose degree would depend on the severity of the lesions. The hemolytic uremic syndrome would thus be analogous to the Shwartzman phenomenon, in which the vascular lesions seem to play an important part in pathogenesis.[10] Recently, another hypothesis has been suggested,[20] according to which the hemolytic uremic syndrome is the expression of an antigen-antibody conflict within the kidney, comparable to rejection in renal homotransplantation, with, as a consequence, aggregation of platelets, secondary deposition of fibrin, thrombocytopenia, and microangiopathic anemia.

Treatment

Specific Treatment

In the absence of a precise etiology, specific treatment rests on the hypothesis that there is a process of intravascular coagulation in the hemolytic uremic syndrome. The logical treatment then is to use heparin to prevent the formation of new fibrin deposits or to accelerate the process of fibrinolysis by plasminogen activators.

It is difficult, however, to analyze the results of treatment because of the very great variability in the severity of renal involvement and the impossibility of assessing the degree of this involvement in most cases. Early renal biopsy might permit such distinction, but it is difficult to envisage this procedure because of the risks involved.

Heparin therapy has been used for some years.[3, 7, 19, 25] It is impossible to be certain that the treatment is effective in view of the unpredictable course of the untreated disease and the absence of any controlled trials. Despite this uncertainty, heparin therapy is widely used.

In practice the daily dose of heparin in infants is 8 to 10 mg./kg./24 hours injected continuously into a vein by means of a pump. The therapy is controlled by measuring the clotting time twice a day, using micromethods.

Treatment is generally continued for 10 to 15 days. Monitoring the level of fibrin degradation products might be helpful in deciding when to stop treatment. If there is a risk of hemorrhage from some therapeutic maneuver, such as peritoneal dialysis, for example, the action of the heparin should be neutralized by protamine immediately before the particular procedure. Heparin therapy is resumed immediately afterwards. There is a considerable risk of cerebral hemorrhage if the blood pressure is very high and cannot be reduced.

Treatment by fibrinolysis activators has been used by some workers, but here again there is no real proof of the effectiveness of the therapy.[26] Either streptokinase or urokinase may be used. These products activate plasminogen, converting it into plasmin, and thus they dissolve the fibrin in the thrombi. They may be injected intravenously. They have a rapid and short-lived action. Unlike streptokinase, urokinase has the advantage that it does not give rise to the formation of antibodies; it acts directly on the plasminogen, whereas the action of streptokinase is indirect. It forms with plasminogen an activator that in turn acts on the transformation of plasminogen into plasmin. This mode of action requires high doses to eradicate all the circulating plasminogen. There is a risk of producing hemorrhage, and so close monitoring is essential. We have only limited experience with this type of treatment, a treatment that requires the help of a competent hematology laboratory.[13]

Various other treatments have been suggested, such as aspirin and dipyridamole (Persantine), which impede platelet aggregation. All authors agree that steroid therapy is ineffective.

Symptomatic Treatment

Early and intensive treatment of the acute renal failure has considerably improved the prognosis of the hemolytic uremic syndrome in infants. This treatment, which consists essentially in peritoneal dialysis, is described elsewhere (see page 352).

Hypotensive drugs may be necessary to control the blood pressure (see page 412).

The anemia should be treated by transfusions, often repeated, of packed red cells when the red cell count falls below 3 million per cubic millimeter. There is some risk to transfusion in the presence of hypertension or hyperkalemia. Transfusion may be carried out under the protection of peritoneal dialysis.

The neurologic complications may be secondary to water intoxication, in which case they are improved by peritoneal dialysis. They may require the use of anticonvulsant drugs, such as diazepam (Valium).

When the patient goes on to terminal renal failure, it may be possible to place the child on a hemodialysis-transplantation program. In such cases, the presence of malignant hypertension is an indication for bilateral nephrectomy. We have never seen recurrence of the hemolytic uremic syndrome after transplantation.

Conclusion

The hemolytic uremic syndrome of children is a well-defined clinicopathologic entity with a remarkably constant clinical pattern. The lesions are often localized exclusively to the kidney and may lead to cortical necrosis. However, the lesions may extend to other organs, and the picture is then one of thrombotic thrombocytopenic purpura.

Despite the evidence for an infectious and in particular a viral etiology and the extensive studies in this field, the problem of the etiology of the hemolytic uremic syndrome is not resolved. It is probable that the syndrome can be provoked by many infectious agents.

Further studies are needed to discover the precise role of intravascular coagulation in determining the lesions. The discovery of circulating endothelial cells at the onset would be further evidence in favor of the primary character of the damage to the endothelium of the arterioles and capillaries.

Remarkable progress has been made with symptomatic treatment. However, there is still uncertainty about the efficacy of treatment with heparin and with fibrinolysis activators.

REFERENCES

1. Anthony, P. P., and Kaplan, A. B.: Fatal haemolytic uremic syndrome in two sibs. Arch. Dis. Child. *43*:316, 1968.
2. Avalos, J., Vitacco, M., Penalver, J., and Gianantonio, C.: Coagulation studies in the hemolytic-uremic syndrome. J. Pediat. *76*:538, 1970.
3. Brain, M. C., Baker, L. R. I., McBride, J. A., Rubenberg, M. L., and Dacie, J. V.: Treatment of patients with micro-angiopathic hemolytic anemia with heparin. Brit. J. Haemat. *15*:603, 1968.
4. Campbell, S., and Carre, I. J.: Fatal hemolytic uremic syndrome and idiopathic hyperlipemia in monozygotic twins. Arch. Dis. Child. *40*:654, 1965.
5. Churg, J., Loffler, D., Paronetto, F., Rorat, E., and Barnett, R. N.: Hemolytic uremic syndrome as a cause of postpartum renal failure. Amer. J. Obstet. Gynec. *108*:253, 1970.
6. Courtecuisse, V., Habib, R., and Monnier, C.: Nonlethal hemolytic and uremic syndromes in children; an electron microscope study of renal biopsies from six cases. Exp. Mol. Path 7: 327, 1967.
7. Egli, F., Stalder, G., Gloor, F., Duckert, F., Koller, F., and Hottinger, A.: Heparintherapie des hämolytisch-urämischen Syndroms. Helv. Paediat. Acta *24*:13, 1969.
8. Fison, T. N.: Acute glomerulonephritis in infancy. Arch. Dis. Child. *31*:101, 1956.
9. Gasser, C., Gautier, E., Steck, A., Siebenmann, E. E., and Oeschlin, R.: Hämolytisch urämische Syndrom: bilaterale Nierenindennekrosen bei acuten erworbenen hämolytischen Anämien. Schweiz. Med. Wschr. *85*:905, 1955.
10. Gaynor, E., Bouvier, C., and Spaet, T. H.: Vascular lesions: possible pathogenic basis of the generalized Shwartzman. Science *170*:896, 1970.
11. Gervais, M., Richardson, J. B., Chiu, J., and Drummond, K. N.: Immunofluorescent and histologic findings in the hemolytic uremic syndrome. Pediatrics *47*:352, 1971.
12. Gianantonio, C. A., Vitacco, M., Mendilaharzu, F., and Gallo, G.: The hemolytic-uremic syndrome. J. Pediat. *72*:757, 1968.
13. Guillin, M. C., Boyer, C., Beaufils, F., and Lejeune, C.: Traitement par la streptokinase dans deux cas de syndrome hémolytique et urémique. Arch. franç. Pédiat. *30*:401, 1973.
14. Habib, R., Mathieu, H., and Royer, P.: Maladie thrombotique artériolocapillaire du rein chez l'enfant. Rev. Franç. Et. Clin. Biol. *3*:891, 1958.
15. Habib, R., Mathieu, H., and Royer, P.: Le syndrome hémolytique et urémique chez l'enfant. Nephron *4*:139, 1967.

16. Habib, R., Courtecuisse, V., Leclerc, F., Mathieu, H., and Royer, P.: Etude anatomopathologique de 35 observations de syndrome hémolytique et urémique de l'enfant. Arch. franç. Pédiat. 26:391, 1969.
17. Habib, R., Leclerc, F., Mathieu, H., and Royer, P.: Comparison clinique et anatomo-pathologique entre les formes mortelles et curables du syndrome hémolytique et urémique. Arch. franç. Pédiat. 26:417, 1969.
18. Hagge, W. W., Holley, K. E., Burke, E. C., and Stickler, G. B.: Hemolytic uremic syndrome in two siblings. New Eng. J. Med. 227:138, 1967.
19. Kaplan, B., Katz, J., Kravitz, M. B., and Laurie, A.: An analysis of the therapy in 67 cases of the hemolytic-uremic syndrome. J. Pediat. 78:420, 1971.
20. Katz, J., Lurie, A., Kaplan, B. S., Kravitz, J., and Metz, J.: Coagulation findings in the hemolytic-uremic syndrome of infancy: similarity to hyperacute renal allograft rejection. J. Pediat. 78:426, 1971.
21. McKay, D. G.: Disseminated intravascular coagulation: an intermediary mechanism of disease. New York, Harper & Row, 1965.
22. Mathieu, H., Leclerc, F., Habib, R., and Royer, P.: Etude clinique et biologique de 37 observations de syndrome hémolytique et urémique. Arch. franç. Pédiat. 26:369, 1969.
23. Mery, J. P., Grünfeld, J. P., Watchi, J. M., and de Montera, H.: Insuffisance rénale aiguë avec microangiopathie thrombotique chez l'adulte. In Actualités néphrologiques de l'Hôpital Necker. Paris, Flammarion, 1967.
24. Mettler, N. E.: Isolation of a microtatobiote from patients with hemolytic-uremic syndrome and thrombotic thrombocytopenic purpura and from mites in the United States. New Eng. J. Med. 281:1023, 1969.
25. Moncrieff, M. W., and Glasgow, E. F.: Hemolytic-uremic syndrome treated with heparin. Brit. Med. J. 3:188, 1970.
26. Monnens, L., Kleynen, F., Van Munster, P., Schretlen, E., and Bonnerman, A.: Coagulation studies and streptokinase therapy in the hemolytic-uremic syndrome. Helv. Paediat. Acta 27:45, 1972.
27. Sraer, J. D., Morel-Maroger, L., Beaufils, P., Ardaillou, N., Helenon, C., and Richet, G.: Les insuffisances rénales d'origine vasculaire. Etude de 25 cas. J. Urol. Néphrol. 78:317, 1972.
28. Royer, P., Habib, R., and Mathieu, H.: La microangiopathie thrombotique du rein chez l'enfant. Ann. Pédiat. (Paris) 36:572, 1960.
29. Vitsky, B. H., Suzuki, Y., Strauss, L., and Churg, J.: The hemolytic-uremic syndrome: a study of renal pathologic alterations. Amer. J. Path. 57:627, 1969.

A list of references published prior to 1969 can be found in: Arch. franç. Pédiat. 26:369–391, 417, 1969.

Chapter Five

GLOMERULAR
NEPHROPATHIES IN
SYSTEMIC DISEASE*

The glomerular nephropathies of systemic disease do not differ in any way in their clinical, pathological, or biochemical features from the idiopathic glomerular nephropathies described in the preceding chapters. The only special feature is the etiology. The nephropathy is accompanied by a collection of associated signs suggesting what is conveniently called a "systemic disease." These signs include rashes, arthralgia, abdominal pain, hemoptysis, leukocytosis, an elevated sedimentation rate, and hypergammaglobulinemia. The systemic disease may be easily identified on clinical grounds (rheumatoid purpura, Goodpasture's syndrome), or special investigations, such as a search for LE cells, immunoelectrophoresis, and the detection of antinuclear, antierythrocyte, antileukocyte, or antiplatelet antibodies may be required to diagnose systemic lupus erythematosus. Histologic studies may be necessary for the diagnosis of periarteritis nodosa. In many cases, the diagnosis may be revealed only at *autopsy.* In some cases, however, despite presumptive evidence in favor of a systemic disease, this disease cannot be demonstrated by any of the current diagnostic criteria. This is the situation that we have designated in Table 44 (page 242) by the term "unidentified systemic diseases."

In this chapter, we shall study the principal glomerular nephropathies of the systemic diseases, as well as shunt nephritis and Goodpasture's syndrome. The only ones found frequently in children are the renal manifestations of rheumatoid purpura. In our experience, these account for 15 per cent of glomerular nephropathies.

THE NEPHROPATHIES OF RHEUMATOID PURPURA

The incidence of nephropathy in Henoch-Schönlein purpura is difficult to establish. Estimates vary from 22 to 66 per cent, depending on the authors and the method of selecting patients. We have studied the characteristics of the nephropathy in 60 personal cases of rheumatoid purpura.[20] The 60 patients selected had all presented a renal disorder in the course of a typical Henoch-

---

*This chapter was written in collaboration with M. Levy and M. F. Gagnadoux.

Schönlein purpura, characterized by petechial purpura with or without edema, arthralgia with or without swelling, and abdominal pain with or without melena.

Clinical Features (Table 60)

Renal complications are seen more often in boys than in girls (38 boys and 21 girls in our series), with the highest incidence occurring in children about the age of 6 or 7 years.

An upper respiratory tract infection, sometimes streptococcal, precedes the appearance of the Henoch-Schönlein purpura in one third of cases; a similar figure has been reported by other authors.[1, 12, 16] Other predisposing causes have been recorded, including drugs,[10, 12] vaccination,[16, 17, 33] primary tuberculous infection,[16, 33] and insect bites.[14]

In our series, the nephropathy was discovered in 86 per cent of cases in a matter of weeks or even days after the onset of the disease, but it may be detected very much later.[14] It is generally held that renal disease does not precede the appearance of the general Henoch-Schönlein syndrome, but three of our cases and one reported by Herdman and associates[23] suggest that in fact the renal lesion may occur first. A constant feature of the nephropathy is hematuria; this was macroscopic in 90 per cent of our cases, but apparently it is more often microscopic in adults.[14] Proteinuria is sometimes absent,[8, 12, 14] and when present it can vary considerably in degree. In some cases, we have found urinary protein output greater than 2 g./24 hours at the very first examination or after some weeks. When a nephrotic syndrome is seen,[2, 8, 12, 14, 19, 28, 31, 42] as in more than half of our patients, it is nearly always purely biochemical. The nephrotic syndrome appeared early in 23 cases; in eight children, it appeared three to nine months after the onset of the nephropathy and in two other patients it appeared at 18 and 19 months after the onset. In most cases, the nephrotic syndrome was short-lived, but in 10 patients it persisted to the stage of chronic or terminal renal failure. Many authors have reported an episode of renal insufficiency at the onset,[10, 12, 14, 15, 18, 28] and peritoneal dialysis has sometimes been necessary.[15] In most cases, this renal insufficiency is transient, but it can prove irreversible.[12, 14] Three of our patients presented this type of rapidly progressive course and died six weeks, four and a half months, and 15 months after the onset of the disease. Renal insufficiency may appear secondarily after some months, and in our experience this carries a poor prognosis.[34]

There may be hypertension in the initial stage.

The serum complement (C'3) level is generally normal,[1, 14, 15, 32] but rarely it may be lowered.[11, 23] In all 15 cases in which we estimated the serum complement, it proved normal.

The successive attacks of rheumatoid purpura, which vary in number and interval from case to case, may or may not be accompanied by further renal complications. Gary and associates,[15] for example, found the creatinine clearance to be reduced by 30 per cent and hematuria to be increased in two patients two days after each recurrence of skin purpura. It is also possible that the reappearance of macroscopic hematuria is traceable to a new, purely renal localization of the disease.

The course of the nephropathy of rheumatoid purpura is far from being identical in all cases, and results reported in different series vary considerably.

This variation depends to a great extent on the selection of patients. The percentage of patients cured is given as 90 per cent by Comellini and Berni,[10] as 46 per cent by Meadow and colleagues,[28] as 40 per cent by Fillastre and colleagues,[14] as 34 per cent by Cream and co-workers,[12] and as 27 per cent by Bernhardt and associates.[8] Death from renal failure is rare, usually occurring either in the first months of the nephropathy[2, 12, 14, 24, 26, 28, 33] or after many years.[8, 12, 14, 24] In our series, 22 children recovered completely, whereas in 29 others a varying degree of chronic nephropathy persisted. The remaining nine patients are dead. All the children who did poorly had a permanent nephrotic syndrome.[20]

Histopathology

Histologic study of renal biopsy material reveals the great variety of glomerular lesions that can occur in the Henoch-Schönlein syndrome[20, 28, 35] (Table 60). In our 60 cases, we found minimal glomerular lesions in one case, diffuse endocapillary proliferative glomerulonephritis in three cases, focal segmental glomerulonephritis in 24 cases (Figure 75), diffuse proliferative glomerulonephritis with focal crescents involving less than 30 per cent of the glomeruli in 14 cases (type I endocapillary and extracapillary glomerulonephritis), diffuse proliferative glomerulonephritis with focal crescents involving between 30 and 80 per cent of the glomeruli in 12 cases (type II endocapillary and extracapillary glomerulonephritis), diffuse proliferative glomerulonephritis with diffuse crescents in four cases (type III endocapillary and extracapillary glomerulonephritis) (Figure 76), and membranoproliferative glomerulonephritis in two cases.

Clinicopathologic correlation demonstrates the value of renal biopsy in establishing the prognosis of the renal complications of rheumatoid purpura. There does not appear to be any correlation between the severity of the nephropathy and such clinical features as age, sex, etiology, extrarenal (especially abdominal) manifestations, however severe they may be, or the time at which the nephropathy appears. There is a definite correlation between the histologic type and the severity of the proteinuria in the first months. A urinary protein output greater than 2 g./24 hours rarely occurs in the first months of segmental and focal glomerulonephritis (two cases in 12), whereas the protein output is always more than 2 g./24 hours in cases of endocapillary and extracapillary proliferative glomerulonephritis and membranoproliferative glomerulonephritis. Similarly, the incidence, the severity, and the persistence of a nephrotic syndrome increases with the severity of the histologic lesion. On the other hand, initial renal insufficiency, macroscopic hematuria, and the appearance of a nephrotic syndrome, even at a late stage, are not always indicative of a poor prognosis.

There is a close correlation between the course of the disease and the histologic type (Table 61). Seventeen patients with milder glomerular lesions recovered. However, none of the children with type II or type III endocapillary and extracapillary glomerulonephritis or membranoproliferative glomerulonephritis recovered completely, and in these groups the mortality was 50 per cent. One of the children with segmental and focal glomerulonephritis went on to terminal renal failure after five years; after biopsy, he had

(Text continued on page 308)

Table 60. Clinicopathologic Correlation in 60 Cases of Nephropathy of Rheumatoid Purpura

Histologic Type	Number of Cases	Hematuria	Hematuria with Proteinuria	Hematuria with Nephrotic Syndrome	Appearance of Renal Failure		Early Hypertension
					Early	Late	
Minimal lesions	1	1	—	—	—	—	—
Diffuse endocapillary proliferative glomerulonephritis	3	—	3	—	1	—	—
Segmental and focal glomerulonephritis	24	—	18	6	—	1	2
Endocapillary and extracapillary glomerulonephritis							
Type I	14	—	4	10	2	—	1
Type II	12	—	1	11	2	3	2
Type III	4	—	—	4	4	—	—
Membranoproliferative glomerulonephritis	2	—	—	2	1	—	1
Number of cases	60	1	26	33	10	4	6

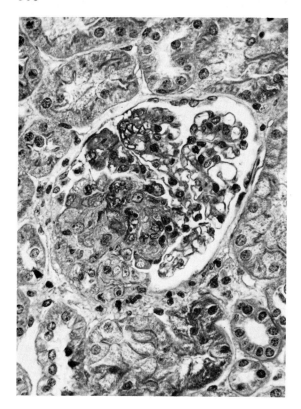

Figure 75. Nephritis of rheumatoid purpura. Appearance of segmental and focal glomerulonephritis. Note the presence of a mass of fibrin in the center of the segmental lesion. ×500.

Figure 76. Nephritis of rheumatoid purpura. Appearance of endocapillary and extracapillary proliferative glomerulonephritis. ×80.

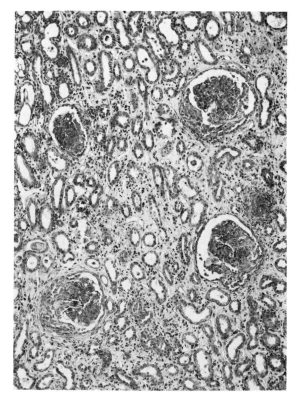

Table 61. Nephropathy of Rheumatoid Purpura: Course and Effect of Treatment

Histologic Type	Number of Cases	Cure	Persisting Signs				
			Minimal Proteinuria	Proteinuria (≥1 g/24 h)	Renal Insufficiency		Death from Renal Failure
					Mild	Severe	
Minimal lesions	1	1	—	—	—	—	—
Diffuse endocapillary proliferative glomerulonephritis	2	2	—	—	—	—	—
Segmental and focal glomerulonephritis	12	7 (1)*	3	1	—	—	1
Endocapillary and extracapillary glomerulonephritis							
Type I	11	7 (6)	2 (2)	2 (2)	1	—	3
Type II	11	—	4 (3)	2 (2)	—	1 (1)	4 (1)
Type III	4	—	—	—	—	—	1
Membranoproliferative glomerulonephritis	1	—	—	—	—	—	—
Number of cases	42†	17	9	5	1	1	9

*Figures in parentheses indicate the number of patients given immunodepressive treatment.
†This table includes only those cases in which renal biopsy was performed in the first six months of the disease.

many subsequent attacks of rheumatoid purpura, which were probably responsible for the aggravation of the renal lesions.

It is apparent that renal biopsy is essential for the evaluation of prognosis, a fact that has been confirmed by many authors.[2, 9, 14, 21, 25, 31] A word of caution is necessary: the histology is a reliable guide to prognosis only if there are no recurrent attacks of the disease after renal biopsy, because such attacks can cause aggravation of the renal lesions.

In the past 10 years, many authors have studied the nephritis of rheumatoid purpura by *immunofluorescence*,[3–7, 13, 14, 22, 23, 26, 29, 30, 38] and their results are similar to our own.[20] Apart from the exceptional cases in which there is no fixation of serum,[1, 18] deposits of immunoglobulin, complement, or fibrinogen can be seen in all the glomeruli, whatever the histologic picture on light microscopy. The subsequent fate of these deposits is variable; some persist for years, signifying progression of the nephropathy, others diminish[23] or disappear.

The deposits occur mainly in the mesangium but may extend throughout the basement membrane of the glomerular capillary. These facts have been confirmed by electron microscopy by Urizar and his colleagues;[38] in the hyperplastic intercapillary tissue, there is augmentation of the mesangial material, infiltration by neutrophil polymorphonuclear cells, and presence of osmiophilic masses corresponding to deposits of immunoglobulin. These same deposits can be seen in the enlarged subendothelial space.

Of the immunoglobulins, the presence of IgA, reported by many authors,[3, 4, 14, 26, 40] should be emphasized; according to Berger,[6] IgA is rarely found except in the nephropathies of systemic lupus erythematosus and in a particular type of nephropathy characterized by mesangial deposits of IgA and IgG.[5] The presence of intercapillary deposits of IgA, IgG, B_1C, and fibrinogen seems to be specific to the nephropathy of rheumatoid purpura, and, if this is confirmed, it might be important for diagnosis in cases in which a renal disorder appears in an atypical clinical situation or as the first localization of the disease.

The presence of these deposits suggests an immunologic mechanism[27, 38, 41] in which the immune complexes formed in the circulating blood may — because of their structure or their size or both — be taken up by the mesangial cells, where they would then induce an inflammatory reaction. Urizar and Herdman[39] believe that abnormalities of coagulation may play an important part; this hypothesis is suggested by certain experimental studies[36, 40] and also by the discovery of fibrin deposits in the mesangial axes in five patients with Henoch-Schönlein syndrome who had no nephropathy.[39]

Treatment

Steroids appear to be ineffective in treating the nephropathy. Many authors have reported good results from treatment with immunosuppressive agents.[14, 18, 30, 37, 42] In our series, 22 patients were treated by chlorambucil; nine of these recovered, one died of renal failure, and the remaining 12 still have evidence of chronic renal disease, although in some cases this is slight. These results are hardly decisive, and in the absence of proper comparative studies, it is difficult to come to any conclusion about the effectiveness of these drugs. In practice, we use these drugs only in patients with relatively severe glomerular lesions (types II and III endocapillary and extracapillary glomerulonephritis).

Some authors advise the use of anticoagulants.[11, 23] We have recently had some success with these drugs in treating the severe forms, but it would be premature to come to any conclusion.

THE NEPHROPATHIES OF PERIARTERITIS NODOSA

Although rare, periarteritis nodosa does occur in children and has even been found in infants under the age of one year. Forty cases in infants have been described in the literature.[43, 47, 48, 50, 52] As in adults, the clinical picture is very variable, and renal complications are not constant, but, when they occur, they are serious. This is an essential feature of the disease.

Clinical Features

When periarteritis nodosa affects the kidneys there is an often considerable proteinuria and sometimes edema. A nephrotic syndrome is very rare. There are also microscopic or macroscopic hematuria, renal insufficiency of variable severity that may go on to terminal renal failure, and nearly always severe hypertension that is often "malignant." Hypokalemia is seen in many of these patients. The nephropathy most often follows a clinical picture typical of periarteritis nodosa, including fever, cachexia, polynuclear leukocytosis, diffuse and intense arthralgia and myalgia, purpura, erythema, sometimes subcutaneous nodules, neuropsychic disorders, and abdominal, respiratory, and cardiac symptoms. In other cases, the signs of renal disease are predominant or even virtually isolated. The diagnosis may then be difficult without histologic confirmation.

Histopathology[45, 46, 49]

Since the classic work of Dawson and associates,[44] two forms of periarteritis — macroscopic and microscopic — are usually distinguished.

Macroscopic Form (Figure 77)

The macroscopic type corresponds to the classic form of the disease as described by Kussmaul and Maier. There are three principal characteristics.

1. Arteries of a particular caliber are involved. These are essentially the large caliber arteries with considerable muscle in their walls: the interlobar and arcuate arteries, which are often affected at bifurcations. Interlobular arteries can be affected, but the renal artery and its main branches are rarely involved.

2. Arterial lesions coexist at different stages. Typical acute lesions, including fibrinoid necrosis of the wall and a perivascular granuloma, can be found side by side with "intermediate" lesions, in which are noted mingled areas of necrosis, fibrosis, rupture of elastic membranes, and some perivascular infiltration, and also cicatricial lesions in which the damaged musculoelastic wall has been replaced by fibrous tissue containing few cells, whereas the lumen is obstructed by lesions of endarteritis and by thromboses that are recanalized to varying degrees. A constant finding is that these lesions are segmental and nodular.

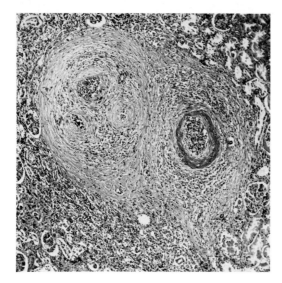

Figure 77. Periarteritis nodosa, macroscopic form. The glomeruli are normal. Different stages of the characteristic vascular lesions of periarteritis nodosa exist side by side. ×50.

3. There usually are no glomerular lesions, but there may sometimes be lesions of glomerular ischemia secondary to arterial obstruction,[45] and, in some cases, glomerular changes secondary to the severe hypertension that is so common in these patients. In addition to these three fundamental features, there may be foci of ischemic atrophy or infarction.

Microscopic Form (Figure 78)

The microscopic form has much in common with the condition described by Rich and Gregory as a hypersensitivity angiitis.[51] The three characteristics

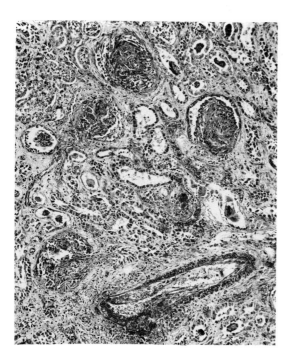

Figure 78. Periarteritis nodosa, microscopic form. Endocapillary and extracapillary proliferative glomerulonephritis. Note the segmental character of the disease of the arcuate artery. ×80.

that distinguish it from the macroscopic form are well defined. The arteries mainly involved are the small caliber (interlobular and preglomerular) arteries.

All the lesions are in the same acute necrotic stage. This is true in the severe and rapidly fatal forms. In the more chronic or artificially prolonged forms, however, we have found that, as in the macroscopic form, arterial lesions may coexist at different stages.

The glomeruli are always affected. As in other systemic diseases, all types of glomerular lesions may be found. Most often there is diffuse proliferative glomerulonephritis. In our experience, the lesions most commonly found are the endocapillary and extracapillary proliferative glomerulonephritides with focal or diffuse crescents, but we have recently seen two cases of membrano-proliferative glomerulonephritis in which the only special feature was the degree of proliferation of the endothelial cells, which was much more marked than the proliferation of the mesangial cells.

Personal Experience

Our experience is based on a study of 11 cases with a confirmed diagnosis seen over a period of 20 years, in children whose ages varied from 2½ to 15

Table 62. Personal Series of Nephropathy of Periarteritis Nodosa (Macroscopic Form, Cases 1 to 4; Microscopic Form, Cases 5 to 11)

Case	Sex	Age (Years)	Predominant Signs	Proteinuria	Hematuria	Nephrotic Syndrome	Renal Insufficiency	Hypertension	Glomerular Histology	Duration of Disease	Cause of Death
1	F	2	Coma	+	+	0	±	?	Normal	6 days	Convulsions
2	F	6	Purpura, Neur. s.	+	?	0	+	+	Normal	1 month	Hypertension
3	F	7	Nodules, Neur. s.	?	+	0	?	+	Hypertensive disease	8 months	Cachexia
4	F	7	Pains	+	0	0	+	+	Hypertensive disease	2 months	(Sudden death)
5	F	12	Purpura, Neur. s.	+	+	0	+	+	E.E. type III	2 months	Renal failure
6	F	5	Neur. s.	+	+	0	+	+	E.E. type III	2 months	Renal failure
7	M	11	Pains, Purpura	+	+	0	+	+	E.E. type III	1½ months	Renal failure
8	M	6	Pains, Purpura	+	+	0	+	+	E.E. type II	2 months	Hypertension
9	M	9	Pains, Purpura	+	+	0	0	+	Membranoproliferative	2 months	Hypertension
10	F	14	Purpura, nodules	+	+	0	+	+	Membranoproliferative	2 months	Hypertension
11	F	9	Purpura, arthralgia	+	+	0	0	0	E.E. type I	12 years	Cardiac failure

Neur. s.: Neurologic signs; E.E.: endocapillary and extracapillary proliferation.

years (Table 62). We have found that the two histologic types just described correspond to two somewhat different clinical pictures. This seems logical in view of the fact that the basic distinction between the two forms is the presence or absence of glomerulonephritis.

Macroscopic Form

Four of our cases were of the macroscopic type. In the first case, the child was not seen until she was virtually moribund, and the diagnosis was made only at autopsy. The three other cases presented with very severe hypertension; signs of renal disease, especially an elevated blood urea level, were present but less permanent. Associated signs were few, but included some cutaneous signs, muscular pain, and neurologic disorders, largely owing to the hypertension. Every case proved more or less rapidly fatal. It should, however, be noted that all these cases were seen before 1955, when modern therapeutic measures, especially those for controlling hypertension, were not available.

Microscopic Form

The seven remaining cases in our series belong to this group.

In six of the seven cases, the clinical presentation was very suggestive of rheumatoid purpura, including severe abdominal pain with melena, arthralgia, purpura, and hematuric nephropathy, and indeed nearly all these patients were admitted to the hospital with a diagnosis of rheumatoid purpura. It was the patient's very poor general condition, the severity of the renal failure, and the hypertension that led to the clinical diagnosis of periarteritis nodosa. Only one case presented as a purely renal disease, developing like a malignant glomerulonephritis, and in this case the diagnosis was made only at autopsy.

The condition proved rapidly fatal (two months or more) in six of the seven cases, including the most recent ones. Death resulted from terminal uremia or malignant hypertension or both. The seventh case took a different course; there were recurrent attacks of fever accompanied by purpura and arthralgia over a period of 11 years; during one of these attacks there were mild signs of renal disorder, proteinuria, and microscopic hematuria, without a rise in either blood pressure or blood urea level. The renal signs disappeared after treatment with steroids and synthetic antimalarial drugs and did not recur up to the time of the patient's death from pulmonary and cardiac complications.

This clinical course is well correlated with the glomerular lesions discovered on histologic examination. The three patients who died of renal failure had endocapillary and extracapillary glomerulonephritis with diffuse crescents; the three patients who died of malignant hypertension had somewhat less severe glomerular lesions, either type II endocapillary and extracapillary proliferation or membranoproliferative glomerulonephritis. In the seventh case, which pursued a more benign course, there was relatively slight extracapillary proliferation.

To propose two totally different clinicopathologic varieties would not, however, be justified. In fact, in a "microscopic" form in which the glomerular lesions are not marked, the nephropathy may go on to a second stage in which the clinical picture and course follow the pattern of the classic disease of

Kussmaul-Maier; on the other hand, in a "macroscopic" form, in which there is serious glomerular damage owing to hypertension or to ischemia, major renal failure may develop and dominate the prognosis.

Treatment

The treatment is the same as that for periarteritis nodosa in adults. Steroid therapy is thought to give the best results, but its principal effect is probably on the extrarenal manifestations. Care must be taken not to aggravate or produce hypertension. Steroid therapy may prove easier to manage with the more effective hypotensive agents currently available.

The synthetic antimalarial drugs have been used with success in certain cases, in association with steroid therapy. This combination proved beneficial in one of our cases (case 11), but the nephropathy was not severe. It would seem logical to try the immunosuppressive drugs, such as chlorambucil and azathioprine, in view of the gravity of the disease, but these drugs have not been proved to be effective. We used them in two patients in our series, but they were of no avail in preventing the fatal outcome. Treatment has proved very disappointing and all our patients have died.

The majority of authors share this pessimism in cases with renal involvement. There is only one recently published report[52] of a child with serious renal involvement who responded to treatment, but the follow-up period is short.

THE NEPHROPATHIES OF SYSTEMIC LUPUS ERYTHEMATOSUS (SLE)

Systemic lupus erythematosus is relatively rare in children. The condition presented before the age of 15 years in 18 per cent of 242 cases reported by Meislin and Rothfield.[64] In adults, renal involvement is clinically manifest in 50 per cent of cases, but in series of SLE routinely submitted to biopsy, histologic lesions are found in the kidney in at least 70 per cent of cases. In children, the incidence of renal complications has been reported as 100 per cent by Royer,[68] as 89 per cent of 35 cases by Cook and associates,[56] as 65 per cent of 42 cases by Meislin and Rothfield,[64] and as 26 per cent of 35 cases by Jacobs.[60] Different criteria for selection of material may explain the variations in these figures. In most cases, the nephropathy appears early in the first year of the disease, but it may occur later. The nephropathy may be the presenting feature, as in 6 per cent of Meislin and Rothfield's cases.[64] There is considerable evidence that lupus is a disease of immune origin[62–64] (see page 157). There is also some evidence of a viral origin.[55, 58]

Clinical Features

There is no special clinical pattern to the renal manifestations of SLE. There is always proteinuria, and often a nephrotic syndrome is present. Hematuria, hypertension, and renal insufficiency are less common. Leukocyturia is thought to be a suggestive finding.

The particular feature of this nephropathy is that it occurs in a very specific clinical context, including skin eruptions (typically in a butterfly pattern), arthralgia, and sometimes nervous, pulmonary, cardiac, and hematologic disorders. The skin eruptions and arthralgia occur in more than 80 per cent of cases. There does not seem to be any correlation between the gravity of the renal complications and the severity of other systemic lesions; rapidly progressive forms of the disease involving many viscera may be associated with very benign nephropathies. In some cases, in contrast, the nephropathy may be isolated or predominant, and it is then important to take a careful history of any previous skin, joint, or other systemic disorders. Immunologic evidence, such as the discovery of LE cells or nuclear antibody, may be very important in the diagnosis.

Histopathology

Except for the hematoxylin bodies of Gross, there is nothing specific about the histologic appearance of lupus, and it is only the association of certain fundamental lesions (karyorrhexis, wire loops, foci of fibrinoid necrosis in the zones of hypercellularity) that is suggestive. The histologic appearances of lupus nephropathy are very diverse; there is not one but many lupus glomerulopathies, with very different clinical patterns. This notion is fundamental to the understanding of the different possible courses of the disease. Based on the work of Baldwin and colleagues,[54] Pollak and Pirani,[67] and Méry and colleagues,[65] four principal types of glomerular disease in lupus may be distinguished (see page 157).

Minor Disorders of the Renal Parenchyma

These are seen in about 30 per cent of cases. The kidney may appear absolutely normal on light microscopy, or it may present small zones of endothelial or mesangial hypercellularity and localized thickenings of the basement membrane. Even if the kidney looks normal, light microscopy may reveal small osmiophilic deposits on one or another aspect of the basement membrane or in the mesangium. In such cases, even if the kidney is normal on light microscopy, immunofluorescence techniques reveal fixation of immunoglobulin (principally IgG), either in the mesangium or along the capillary walls.[53, 61, 66]

Segmental and Focal Glomerulonephritis

This occurs in about 25 per cent of cases. These segmental lesions include endocapillary and extracapillary cell proliferation and foci of fibrinoid necrosis in the zones of hypercellularity. Immunofluorescence reveals fixation of IgG and sometimes IgA, IgM, and B_1C;[53, 54, 61, 66] this fixation is not focal but diffuse, occurring in all the glomeruli. It is of a granular nature and occurs in an irregular pattern along the capillary walls.

Diffuse Proliferative Glomerulonephritis

The diffuse proliferative glomerulonephritides (endocapillary and extracapillary or membranoproliferative) (Figure 79) are found in 30 to 45 per cent of cases. Immunofluorescence gives the same appearance as in focal glomerulonephritis, but the deposits may be larger.

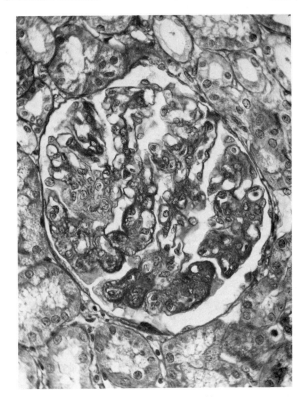

Figure 79. Systemic lupus erythematosus. Membranoproliferative glomerulonephritis with voluminous intermembranoendothelial deposits (wire-loop lesions). ×330.

Extramembranous Glomerulonephritis

This form, which does not differ in any way from the idiopathic varieties of extramembranous glomerulitis, occurs in eight to 25 per cent of cases.

Clinicopathologic Correlations

There is evidence from recent studies[54, 65] that each of these histologic types corresponds to a different clinical picture and, even more important, to a different pattern of evolution.

When kidney lesions are slight or absent, the renal complications amount to little more than a mild proteinuria or slight microscopic hematuria. In this form, the prognosis appears to be very good, and aggravation of the renal lesions is quite exceptional.

In focal glomerulonephritis, symptoms are generally mild, consisting of perhaps a moderate proteinuria and microscopic hematuria. Nephrotic syndrome, hypertension, and renal insufficiency are rare. The prognosis in this variety seems to be good; there were no deaths from renal causes in the series of 14 cases of Baldwin and colleagues,[54] Estes and Christian[57] recorded a five year survival rate of 70 per cent. It is possible, however, for the lesions to deteriorate and become diffuse.

The *diffuse proliferative glomerulonephritides* are associated with much more serious clinical disorders; proteinuria and hematuria are more severe, and a nephrotic syndrome and hypertension are common, as is renal insufficiency progressing to terminal renal failure in a few years. The prognosis for these forms is poor (25 per cent five year survival in Estes and Christian's series[57]). There is evidence that prolonged administration of steroids in high doses may be beneficial.

In extramembranous glomerulonephritis, there is usually considerable protein-uria, often accompanied by hematuria, frequently by a nephrotic syndrome. The course and prognosis are intermediate between the focal and the diffuse proliferative forms; renal insufficiency is less common, and there may be spontaneous remissions.

Personal Experience (Table 63)

Our experience is relatively slight, being confined to 11 cases of SLE with renal complications. Ten of these were submitted to renal biopsy. All the patients were girls, and in 10 of the 11 cases the onset was after the age of 9 years. All but one had cutaneous lupus at some stage, and eight suffered from joint pains.

Only one of our patients suffered from an isolated nephropathy for a period of five years, after which a butterfly rash appeared on the skin and LE cells were found in the blood.

The renal biopsy material from our patients confirmed most of the reports in the literature. We had three patients with segmental and focal glomerulo-nephritis, four with endocapillary and extracapillary glomerulonephritis, and three with membranoproliferative glomerulonephritis, one of whom had voluminous extramembranous deposits. In most of our patients, there was a very clear-cut correlation between the histologic type, the clinical pattern, and course of the nephropathy.

In the three cases of *segmental glomerulonephritis* (cases 1, 2, and 3 in Table 63) the disease presented initially as a very mild disorder with minimal pro-teinuria and microscopic hematuria. All three patients improved rapidly under treatment with steroids and synthetic antimalarial drugs, and this favorable evolution continued for three to eight years.

Follow-up was possible in only one of the cases (case 4) with *endocapillary and extracapillary glomerulonephritis*. At a time of complete clinical remission, renal biopsy revealed regression of the lesions. The patient had presented with a nephrotic syndrome and had been treated with steroids in high doses.

The course was more variable in the three cases of *membranoproliferative glomerulonephritis*. Two (cases 8 and 9) had considerable proteinuria and hema-turia to begin with, and, in addition, case 8 had the laboratory features of a nephrotic syndrome and renal insufficiency. After a follow-up period of five to seven years, these patients are both in complete remission, without any treatment having been given to patient number 9. In contrast, one of our pa-tients (case 10) had a period of remission of several years, then developed progressively a nephrotic syndrome with renal insufficiency and hypertension. She died after 12 years. The last patient pursued a very similar course to that of case 10, but we have no histologic data for this patient.

Our limited experience confirms the good prognosis of the focal forms, but it would seem that the prognosis is more difficult to assess in cases of SLE with membranoproliferative glomerulonephritis.

Table 63. Personal Series of 11 Cases of Lupus Nephropathy in Children

Case	Sex	Age (Years)	Hematuria	Proteinuria	Nephrotic Syndrome	Renal Failure	Hypertension	Treatment	Course	Histologic type
1	F	13	+	±	0	0	0	Steroids + Hydroxychloroquine	Regressive	S.F.
2	F	14	+	+	0	0	0	Steroids + Hydroxychloroquine	Regressive	S.F.
3	F	17	+	±	0	0	0	Steroids + Hydroxychloroquine	Regressive	S.F.
4	F	9	+	+	+	0	0	Steroids	Regressive	(1) E.E. type I (2) S.F.
5	F	10	+	+	0	0	0	?	?	E.E. type I
6	F	15	0	+	0	0	0	0	?	E.E. type II
7	F	11	+	+	0	0	0	Steroids	?	E.E. type II
8	F	13	+	+	±	0	0	Steroids + Hydroxychloroquine	Regressive	Membranoproliferative
9	F	13	+	+	±	0	0	Steroids + immunodepressive drugs	Regressive	Membranoproliferative
10	F	3	+	+	+	+	+	Steroids + Hydroxychloroquine	Death at 15 years	Membranoproliferative
11	F	10	+	+	+	+	+	Steroids + Hydroxychloroquine	Death at 18 years	?

S.F.: segmental and focal glomerulitis; E.E.: endocapillary and extracapillary proliferative glomerulonephritis.

Treatment

Opinions are still very divided about the efficacy of the various treatments proposed.

Many authors have extolled the value of steroids given in high doses over long periods. In fact, their effectiveness should be judged as a function of the histologic type of renal disorder. Many authors[54, 65, 68] consider that steroids are of little value in minimal lesions or extramembranous forms, whereas in the proliferative varieties, especially the diffuse types, the prolonged use of steroids in high dosage does seem to be beneficial.[54, 59, 65, 68] We cannot draw any definite conclusions from our own very limited experience, but it would seem logical in treating a relatively severe nephropathy to try steroid therapy in fairly high doses (2 mg./kg. of prednisone), possibly given every second day for some months, after which a lower maintenance dosage is given.[65]

The synthetic antimalarial drugs have often been used (especially in our own patients), usually associated with or alternating with steroid therapy. It is hard to come to any conclusion about the effectiveness of the antimalarial agents because of the concomitant use of steroids. The possibility of retinal complications must constantly be kept in mind.

It is tempting to try the immunodepressive drugs because of the probable immunologic origin of the disease. There is encouraging experimental evidence provided by the effectiveness of "preventative" treatment by cyclophosphamide in the glomerulonephritis of NZB/W mice.[63] Some successes have been reported in man, but in most cases the drugs have been used in association with large doses of steroids. In the absence of any statistical study of their activity as a function of the histologic lesions, it is impossible to come to any definite conclusion about the value of this treatment. In one of our cases (case 9), chlorambucil seemed to be beneficial, but in the three other cases (cases 8, 10, and 11) in which we tried immunodepressive agents, we had to discontinue treatment at a very early stage because of severe leukopenia.

GOODPASTURE'S SYNDROME

The association of glomerulonephritis and hemorrhagic pulmonary disease described for the first time in 1919 by Goodpasture[71] is exceptional in children[74, 75, 77] (Table 64). Over 100 cases have been reported in young adults.[70, 76]

The pulmonary disorder is characterized by hemoptysis associated with the x-ray finding of cloudy opacities, predominantly perihilar, caused by repeated intra-alveolar hemorrhage. The renal manifestations often appear later and include hematuria, proteinuria, and rapidly progressive renal failure. Histologic examination of the kidney reveals a glomerulonephritis that is initially focal and necrotic (Figure 80). A very large number of the glomeruli are involved, and there is endocapillary and extracapillary proliferation. The prognosis is usually poor, but some cases of stabilization or cure have been reported. Other cases have been managed successfully by bilateral nephrectomy, hemodialysis, and kidney transplantation.

There is a good deal of evidence to connect this human glomerulonephritis with the experimental glomerulonephritides caused by antibodies directed against the basement membrane,[72, 78] including the deposits seen on immuno-

Table 64. Goodpasture's Syndrome (Cases in Children)

Authors	Age at Onset, Sex	Pulmonary Manifestations	Renal Manifestations	Duration of Disease	Cause of Death	Renal Lesions at Autopsy
Soergel, and Sommers (1957)[77]	6 years, F	Hemoptysis Cough Hilar opacities	?	7 years	Massive pulmonary hemorrhage	"Acute focal glomerulonephritis"
O'Connel et al. (1964)[75]	8 years F	Hemoptysis Cough Perihilar opacities	Hematuria Proteinuria	1 year	Massive pulmonary hemorrhage	Segmental and focal necrotic glomerulonephritis
Maccioni et al. (1965)[74]	7 years F	Cough Hilar opacities 1 Episode of hemoptysis	Macroscopic hematuria Proteinuria Raised blood urea	1 month 1 week	Massive pulmonary hemorrhage	Advanced segmental glomerulonephritis with hypercellularity

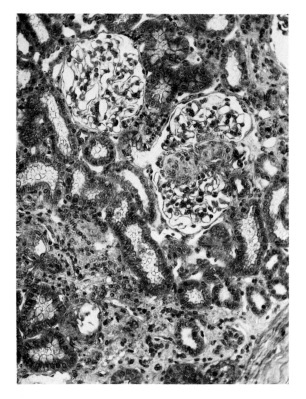

Figure 80. Goodpasture's syndrome. Appearance of segmental and focal glomerulonephritis. ×160.

fluorescence. The identifying characteristics of these deposits are their immuno-histochemical composition (IgG, B_1C-globulin) and their linear arrangement (Figure 81) along the basement membrane. Another characteristic feature is the presence of circulating anti-basement membrane antibodies.[69] Goodpasture's syndrome may be related to the rapidly progressive glomerulonephritis characterized by the presence of linear deposits on immunofluorescence and the finding of circulating anti-basement membrane antibodies.[73]

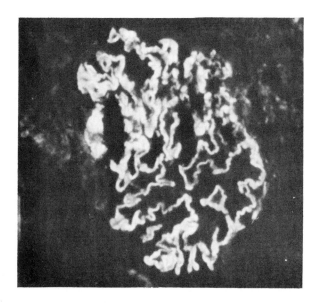

Figure 81. Immunofluorescence photograph showing linear deposits of IgG in a rapidly progressive glomerulonephritis without pulmonary disease. The patient had circulating anti-basement membrane antibodies. ×375.

Table 65. Shunt Nephritis (Personal Series)

Case	Age		Renal Signs			Histology
	At Insertion of Shunt (Months)	At Discovery of Renal Disease	Mode of Presentation	Symptomatology	C3 (mg./100 ml.)	
1	2	2 years 3 months	Edema	Nephrotic syndrome Hematuria	18	Membranoproliferative glomerulonephritis
2	2	1 year 8 months	Macroscopic hematuria	Proteinuria >1 g./24 hours Hematuria	25	Endocapillary and extracapillary glomerulonephritis
3	7	4 years 9 months	Routine urine examination	Proteinuria <1 g./24 hours Hematuria	76	Segmental and focal glomerulonephritis
4	1½	7 years 5 months	Routine urine examination	Proteinuria <1 g./24 hours Hematuria	90	Endocapillary and extracapillary glomerulonephritis

SHUNT NEPHRITIS

Septicemia, often caused by *Staphylococcus albus*, is a well recognized complication of ventriculo-atrial shunts in small children. The septicemia is secondary to infection from the material of the prosthesis, and it is manifested clinically by febrile attacks. After some months this disorder produces hypochromic anemia and hepatosplenomegaly.

Renal complications were first reported in 1965 by Black and associates,[79] and since then some 20 additional cases have been reported.[81-83] Immunofluorescence studies reveal fixation of various immune sera (anti-IgM, anti-IgG, and anti-B_1C-globulin) and of anti-*Staphylococcus albus* serum.[80] The lowered serum level of B_1C-globulin is strong evidence that the pathologic mechanism is immunologic. It is worth emphasizing that shunt nephritis is one of the rare examples of glomerulonephritis in which it has been possible to isolate the antigen entering into the composition of the soluble complexes, in this case the *Staphylococcus albus* growing on the intracardiac catheter. Antibiotic therapy alone is not effective, but removal of the infected material produces rapid cure of the septicemia and also of the nephropathy if this has been detected sufficiently early. Children who have been fitted with an intracardiac catheter should be followed carefully with a blood count and test for albuminuria every six months; at the slightest sign of septicemia, more detailed renal investigations as well as measurement of the serum B_1C-globulin, are indicated.

We have seen four cases of shunt nephritis in children who had been fitted with valves. The various clinical and histologic features are summarized in Table 65.

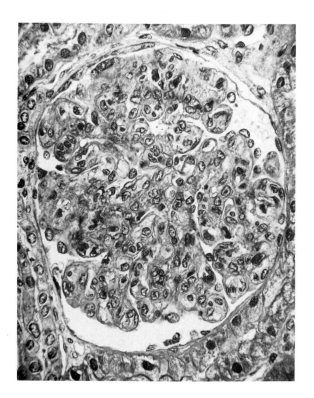

Figure 82. "Shunt" glomerulonephritis. Typical appearance of membranoproliferative glomerulonephritis with flaky appearance of the walls of the glomerular capillaries owing to the mesangial proliferation. ×295.

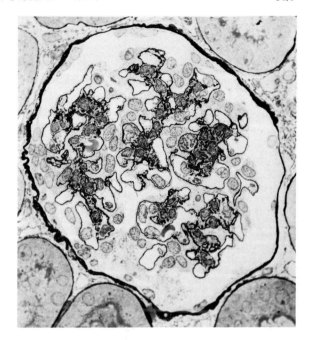

Figure 83. Ultrafine section illustrating "shunt" glomerulonephritis. After antibiotic therapy and removal of the prosthesis, the glomeruli returned to normal, with disappearance of the mesangial proliferation and the lesions of the glomerular capillary walls. (Same patient as Figure 82.) ×350.

Removal of the prosthetic material was followed by cure of the associated septicemic signs, return of the blood count and temperature to normal, and disappearance of the hepatosplenomegaly. Except for one child (case 2) who died of metabolic complications, the signs of renal disorder disappeared in a matter of weeks. In one case (case 1), renal biopsy eight months later showed that the deposits previously visible on immunofluorescence and electron microscopy had disappeared (Figures 82 and 83).

REFERENCES

RHEUMATOID PURPURA

1. Ayoub, E., and Hoyer, J.: Anaphylactoid purpura: streptococcal antibody titers and B_1C-globulin levels. J. Pediat. *75*:193, 1969.
2. Bariéty, J., Lagrue, G., Safar, M., Hesse, J. C., and Milliez, P.: Le syndrome néphrotique des "purpuras rhumatoïdes." Sem. Hôp. Paris *40*:1409, 1964.
3. Bariéty, J., and Druet, P.: Résultats de l'immunohistochimie de 589 biopsies rénales (transplantés exclus). Ann. Méd. Intern. *1*:63, 1971.
4. Berger, J., Yaneva, R., and Antoine, B.: Etude immunohistochimque des lésions glomérulaires. J. Urol. Néphrol. *75*:269, 1969.
5. Berger, J., Yaneva, H., and Hinglais, N.: Les glomérulonéphrites focales. *In* Actualités néphrologiquies de l'hôpital Necker. Paris, Flammarion, 1969, p. 141.
6. Berger, J.: IgA glomerular deposits in renal disease. Transplant. Proc. *1*:939, 1969.
7. Berger, J., Yaneva, H., and Hinglais, N.: Immunofluorescence des glomérulonéphrites. *In* Actualités néphrologiques de l'Hôpital Necker. Paris, Flammarion, 1971, p. 17.
8. Bernhardt, J. P., Chatelanat, F., and Veyrat, R.: Le syndrome de Schönlein-Henoch chez l'adulte: étude clinique de 16 cas, examen histologique du rein dans 7 cas. Schweiz. Med. Wschr. *37*:1228, 1966.
9. Coelho, A., Preto, V., and Almeida, F.: La nefropatia da purpura de Schönlein-Henoch. Bol. Clin. Hosp. Civ. Lisboa *32*:3, 1968.
10. Comellini, F., and Berni, M.: Rilievi clinico statisci sui casi di malattia di Schönlein-Henoch osservati nella nostra clinica negli ultimi dieci anni. Clin. Ped. (Bologna) *49*:672, 1967.

11. Conte, J., Mignon-Conte, M., Moreau, G., and Suc, J.: Les anti-inflammatoires ont-ils une efficacité réelle dans le traitement des néphropathies glomérulaires? *In* Actualités Néphrologiques de l'Hôpital Necker. Paris, Flammarion, 1970, p. 313.
12. Cream, J., Gumpel, J., and Peachey, R.: Schönlein-Henoch purpura in the adult. A study of 77 adults with anaphylactoid or Schönlein-Henoch purpura. Quart. J. Med., *39*:461, 1970.
13. Drummond, K., and Michael, A.: Immunopathologic studies of the cutaneous and renal manifestations of anaphylactoid purpura. J. Pediat. *69*:681, 1966.
14. Fillastre, J. P., Morel-Maroger, L., Ducroiset, B., and Richet, G.: Atteinte rénale du purpura rhumatoïde chez l'adulte. Etude de 20 biopsies rénales. Intérêt de l'examen glomérulaire en immunofluorescence. Presse Méd. *78*:2375, 1970.
15. Gary, N., Mazzara, J., and Holfelder, L.: The Schönlein-Henoch syndrome. Report of two patients with recurrent impairment of renal function. Ann. Intern. Med. *72*:229, 1970.
16. Gietka, M.: On the aetiology of Schönlein-Henoch syndrome. Ann. Paediat. *203*:145, 1964.
17. Giordano, J., and Cordone, G.: Sindrome di Schönlein-Henoch post vaccinica. Min. Pediat. *17*:59, 1965.
18. Goldbloom, R., and Drummond, K.: Anaphylactoid purpura with massive gastrointestinal hemorrhage and glomerulonephritis. An unusual case treated successfully with azathioprine. Amer. J. Dis. Child. *116*:97, 1968.
19. Gotoff, S., Fellers, F., Vawter, G., Janeway, C., and Rosen, F.: The B_1C-globulin in childhood nephrotic syndrome. Laboratory diagnosis of progressive glomerulonephritis. New Eng. J. Med. *273*:524, 1965.
20. Habib, R., and Levy, M.: Les néphropathies du purpura rhumatoïde chez l'enfant. Arch. franç. Pédiat. *29*:305, 1972.
21. Heptinstall, R.: Pathology of the Kidney. London, Churchill, 1966, p. 335.
22. Herdman, R., Hong, R., Michael, A., and Good, R.: Light chain distribution in immune deposits on glomeruli of kidneys in human renal disease. J. Clin. Invest. *46*:141, 1967.
23. Herdman, R., Edson, J., Pickering, R., Fish, A., Marker, S., and Good, R.: Anticoagulants in renal disease in children. Amer. J. Dis. Child. *119*:27, 1970.
24. Hughes, I., and Wenzi, J.: Anaphylactoid purpura nephritis in children. Data from a follow-up. Clin. Pediat. *8*:594, 1969.
25. Kobayashi, O., Kanasawa, M., and Kamiyama, T.: The anaphylactoid purpura nephritis in childhood. Acta Med. Biol. *13*:181, 1965.
26. Kuijten, R.: Nierbiopsie bij kindernen met glomerulopathieën. Thèse Méd., Amsterdam, G. Van Soest, Imprimeurs, 1969.
27. McCluskey, R.: Evidence for immunologic mechanism in several forms of human glomerular diseases. Bull. N.Y. Acad. Med. *46*:769, 1970.
28. Meadow, J. R., Glasgow, E. F., White, R. H. L., Moncrieff, M. W., and Cameron, J. S.: Schönlein-Henoch nephritis. Quart. J. Med. *41*:241, 1972.
29. Michael, A., Drummond, K., Vernier, R., and Good, R.: Immunological basis of renal disease. Pediat. Clin. N. Amer. *11*:685, 1964.
30. Michael, A., Vernier, R., Drummond, K., Levitt, J., Herdman, R., Fish, A., and Good, R.: Immunosuppressive therapy of chronic renal disease. New Eng. J. Med. *276*:817, 1967.
31. Mota, F., Garcia, R., and Gordillo, G.: Nefropatia de la purpura vascular aguda (correlacion clinico-pathologica i evolutiva en 26 casos). Bol. Med. Hosp. Infant (Mex.) *6*:957, 1968.
32. Ogg, C., Cameron, J., and White, R.: The C'3 component of complement (B_1C-globulin) in patients with heavy proteinuria. Lancet *1*:78, 1968.
33. Orsini, A., Pierron, H., and Perrimond, H.: Pronostic du purpura rhumatoïde de Schönlein-Henoch. A propos de 50 observations. Pédiatrie *22*:283, 1967.
34. Proesmans, W., and Habib, R.: Les glomérulonéphrites malignes (in press).
35. Royer, P., Habib, R., Mathieu, H., Vermeil, G., Gabilan, J., and Desprez, P.: Etude anatomo-clinique de 15 observations de néphropathies du purpura rhumatoïde. Ann. Pédiat. *39*:605, 1963.
36. Selye, H., and Tuchweber, B.: Experimental production of an anaphylactoid purpura. Proc. Soc. Exp. Biol. Med. *118*:680, 1965.
37. Shearn, M.: Mercaptopurine in the treatment of steroid resistant nephrotic syndrome. New Eng. J. Med. *273*:943, 1965.
38. Urizar, R., Michael, A., Sisson, S., and Vernier, R.: Anaphylactoid purpura. II. Immunofluorescent and electron microscopic studies of the glomerular lesions. Lab. Invest. *19*:437, 1968.
39. Urizar, R., and Herdman, R.: Anaphylactoid purpura. III. Early morphologic glomerular changes. Amer. J. Clin. Path. *5*:258, 1970.
40. Urizar, R., Schwartz, A., and Vernier, R.: Immunofluorescence microscopy and ultrastructural changes of kidney in experimental anaphylactoid purpura. Lab. Invest. *21*:77, 1969.
41. Vernier, R., Mauer, S., Fish, A., and Michael, A.: Les cellules mésangiales dans les glomérulonéphrites. *In* Actualités néphrologiques de l'Hôpital Necker. Paris, Flammarion, 1971, p. 37.

42. White, R., Cameron, J., and Trounce, J.: Immunosuppressive therapy in steroid-resistant proliferative glomerulonephritis accompanied by the nephrotic syndrome. Brit. Med. J. 2:853, 1966.

PERIARTERITIS NODOSA

43. Canet, J., Lancret, P., Pesnel, G., Fournier, J., and Lajouanine, P.: La périartérite noueuse du nourrisson. Ann. Pédiat. 47:604, 1964.
44. Dawson, J., Ball, J., and Platt, R.: The kidney in periarteritis. Quart. J. Med. 17:175, 1948.
45. Ducrot, H., Habib, R., and de Montera, H.: Les formes rénales de la périartérite noueuse. In Actualités Néphrologiques de l'Hôpital Necker. Paris, Flammarion, 1960, p. 185.
46. Habib, R.: Sur les aspects histologiques de la périartérite noueuse. Ann. Méd. 56:352, 1956.
47. Kaplan, M., Grumbach, R., and Signal, S.: Etude anatomoclinique d'une périartérite noueuse chez une enfant de 7 ans. Ann. Pédiat. 34:479, 1958.
48. Nuyts, J. P., Bombart, E., Debruxelles, P., Bombart, M., Gosselin, B., and Lacombe, A.: La périartérite noueuse (à propos de deux observations). Pédiatrie 24:984, 1969.
49. Pirani, C. L., and Managligod, J. R.: The kidney in collagen diseases: polyarteritis nodosa. In F. K. Mostofi and D. Smith, eds.: The Kidney. Baltimore, Williams & Wilkins, 1966.
50. Royer, P., Habib, R., and Mathieu, H.: Les néphropathies de la périartérite noueuse. In Problèmes actuels de néphrologie infantile. Paris, Flammarion, 1963, p. 93.
51. Rich, A. R., and Gregory, J. L.: The experimental demonstration that periarteritis nodosa is a manifestation of hypersensitivity. Bull. Johns Hopkins Hosp. 72:65, 1943.
52. Sorel, R., Bouissou, H., Dalous, A., Regnier, C., and Ghisolfi, J.: A propos de deux observations de périartérite noueuse. Arch. franç. Pédiat. 24:825, 1967.

SYSTEMIC LUPUS ERYTHEMATOSUS

53. Berger, J., Yaneva, H., and Hinglais, N.: Immunofluorescence des glomérulonéphrites. In Actualités Néphrologiques de l'Hôpital Necker. Paris, Flammarion, 1971, p. 17.
54. Baldwin, D. S., Lowenstein, J., Rothfield, N. F., Gallo, G., and McCluskey, R. T.: The clinical course of the proliferative and membranous forms of lupus nephritis. Ann. Intern. Med. 73:929, 1970.
55. Bariéty, J., and Milliez, P.: Inclusions d'aspect "viral" dans le rein de L.E.D. J. Urol. Néphrol. 76:106, 1970.
56. Cook, C. D., Wedgwood, J. P., Craig, J. M., Hartmann, J. R., and Janeway, C. A.: Systemic lupus erythematosus. Description of 37 cases in children. Pediatrics 26:570, 1960.
57. Estes, D., and Christian, C. L.: The natural history of systemic lupus erythematosus by prospective analysis. Medicine 50:85, 1971.
58. Gyorkey, F., Min, K. W., Sincovics, J. G., and Gyorkey, P.: Systemic lupus erythematosus and myxovirus. New Eng. J. Med. 280:333, 1969.
59. Hagge, W. W., Burne, E. G., and Stickler, G. B.: Treatment of systemic lupus erythematosus complicated by nephritis in childhood. Pediatrics 40:822, 1967.
60. Jacobs, J. C.: Systemic lupus erythematosus in childhood. Pediatrics 32:257, 1963.
61. Koffler, D., Agnello, V., Carr, R. I., and Kunkel, H. G.: Anti-DNA antibodies and renal lesions of patients with systemic lupus erythematosus. Transplant. Proc. 1:933, 1969.
62. Koffler, D., and Kunkel, H. G.: Mechanisms of renal injury in systemic lupus erythematosus. Amer. J. Med. 45:165, 1968.
63. Lambert, P. H., and Dixon, F. J.: Pathogenesis of the glomerulonephritis of NZB/W mice. J. Exp. Med. 45:165, 1968.
64. Meislin, A. G., and Rothfield, N.: Systemic lupus erythematosus in childhood. Pediatrics 42:37, 1968.
65. Méry, J. P., Sraer, J. D., Morel-Maroger, L., and Richet, G.: Les manifestations rénales du L.E.D. Rev. Méd. 12:27, 1971.
66. Morel-Maroger, L., Méry, J. P., Delrieu, F., and Richet, G.: Etude immuno-histochimique de 29 biopsies rénales faites au cours du L.E.D. K. Urol. Néphrol. 77:367, 1971.
67. Pollak, V. E., and Pirani, C. L.: Renal histologic findings in systemic lupus erythematosus. Proc. Mayo. Clin. 44:630, 1969.
68. Royer, P.: Le L.E.D. de l'enfant. Sem. Hôp. Paris 38:40, 1962.

GOODPASTURE'S SYNDROME

69. Bach, J. F., Dardenne, M., Hinglais, N., and Mathieu, P.: Rôle de l'immunité antimembrane basale dans les glomérulonéphrites humaines. In Actualités Néphrologiques de l'Hôpital Necker. Paris, Flammarion, 1972, p. 73.

70. Benoit, F., Rulon, Theil, G., Poolan, P., and Watteau, R.: Goodpasture's syndrome: a clinico-pathologic entity. Amer. J. Med. *37*:424, 1964.
71. Goodpasture, E.: The significance of certain pulmonary lesions in relation to the etiology of influenza. Amer. J. Med. Sci. *158*:863, 1919.
72. Lerner, R., Glassock, K., and Dixon, F.: The role of antiglomerular basement antibody in pathogenesis of human glomerulonephritis. J. Exp. Med. *126*:983, 1967.
73. Lewis, E., Cavallo, T., Harrington, J., and Cotran, R. S.: An immunopathologic study of rapidly progressive glomerulonephritis in the adult. Hum. Path. *2*:185, 1971.
74. Maccioni, A., Merrera, P., and Espinoza, J.: Hemorragia pulmonary nefritis. Rev. Chil. Pediat. *36*:216, 1965.
75. O'Connell, E. J., Dower, J., Burke, F., Brown, A., and McCaughey, W.: Pulmonary hemorrhage glomerulonephritis syndrome. Amer. J. Dis. Child. *108*:302, 1964.
76. Proskey, A., Weatherbee, L., Easterling, R., Greene, J., and Weller, J.: Goodpasture's syndrome. A report of five cases and review of the literature. Amer. J. Med. *48*:162, 1970.
77. Soergel, K., and Sommers, S.: Idiopathic pulmonary hemosiderosis and related syndromes. Amer. J. Med. *32*:499, 1962.
78. Steblay, R., and Rudofsky, V.: Autoimmune glomerulonephritis induced in sheep by injection of human lung and Freund's adjuvant. Science *160*:204, 1968.

SHUNT NEPHRITIS

79. Black, J. A., Challacombe, D. N., and Ockenden, B. G.: Nephrotic syndrome associated with bacteraemia after shunt operations for hydrocephalus. Lancet *2*:921, 1965.
80. Kaufman, D. B., and McIntosh, R.: The pathogenesis of the renal lesion in a patient with strepto-coccal disease, infected ventriculo-atrial shunt, cryoglobulinemia and nephritis. Amer. J. Med. *50*:262, 1971.
81. Lam, C. N., McNeish, A. S., and Gibson, A. A. M.: Nephrotic syndrome with complement deficiency and *Staphylococcus albus* bacteremia. Scot. Med. J. *14*:86, 1969.
82. Rames, L., Wise, B., Goodman, J. R., and Piel, C. F.: Renal disease with staphylococcus bac-teremia. A complication in ventriculoatrial shunts. J.A.M.A. *212*:1671, 1970.
83. Stickler, G. B., Shin, M. H., Burke, E. C., Holley, K. E., Miller, R. H., and Segar, W. E.: Diffuse glomerulonephritis associated with infected ventriculo-atrial shunt. New Eng. J. Med. *279*:1077, 1968.

Chapter Six

THE TREATMENT OF
GLOMERULAR DISEASE*

With the exception of treatment of nephrosis, there are few regularly effective therapeutic measures available to combat the glomerular nephropathies.

Although the control of certain symptomatic features such as edema and hypertension generally is possible, the course of the glomerulopathies is in the main unaffected by therapy. The effectiveness of treatment is all the more difficult to judge because many untreated cases recover spontaneously, and properly controlled clinical trials of treatment are still few in number. It is, in fact, very desirable that the prescription of certain drugs in the treatment of glomerular disease should form part of a national or even international study rather than the more usual practice of following the fashion of the moment.

NEPHROSIS

In this chapter, which is devoted to therapeutics, the term "nephrosis" includes those nephrotic syndromes associated with the presence of normal glomeruli on renal biopsy, whether all the glomeruli are normal, as is usually the case, or a few of the glomeruli present focal lesions. In this group, the clinico-pathologic correlation is such that renal biopsy is not always necessary to confirm the diagnosis when a frank nephrotic syndrome presents suddenly in a child aged 1 to 8 years, with no accompanying hematuria, hypertension, or renal insufficiency.

Under these circumstances, the diagnosis is sufficiently probable for the immediate introduction of steroid therapy. Disappearance of the proteinuria 10 to 15 days after starting this treatment is good evidence that the case is in fact a nephrotic syndrome with minimal glomerular lesions. The indication for renal biopsy is thus limited to cases in which the nephrotic syndrome is not pure at the outset and to cases resistant to steroid therapy.

Two types of treatment are currently used: steroids and immunodepressive drugs.

---

*This chapter was written in collaboration with C. Kleinknecht.

Steroid Therapy

This is always the first line of treatment. Preferably prednisone is used because none of the other steroids has been shown to be better, and they may have more serious side effects.

The initial dose is 2 mg./kg./day (with a maximum of 80 mg./day) given daily for one month. Depending on the effect of this treatment, two types of results may be distinguished.

Steroid Sensitivity

Eighty to 90 per cent of cases are sensitive to steroids. Treatment induces diuresis and the disappearance of the proteinuria in less than four weeks, or, more rarely, the nephrotic syndrome may disappear but a mild proteinuria persists. In these cases, steroid therapy is continued in an interrupted manner, with 2 mg./kg. being given as a single morning dose every second day for two months, and then decreasing the dosage by 0.5 mg./kg. every two weeks until treatment is stopped at the end of four and a half months. When treatment is stopped, two eventualities are possible – definitive cure or relapse. As a rule, the relapses, like the initial attack, are sensitive to steroid therapy. If the relapses are infrequent, they may be treated in the same fashion as the initial attack. Early relapse when treatment is discontinued or when the dose is diminished is fairly common, and the condition is then described as steroid-dependent, because proteinuria reappears within a few weeks of stopping steroid therapy. In these cases, maintenance of remission by steroid therapy requires permanent treatment, and this runs the risk of producing serious complications; in such cases, the use of immunodepressive agents w ll usually produce a prolonged remission.

Steroid Resistance

In 10 to 20 per cent of cases, the nephrotic syndrome persists after a month of continuous steroid therapy in adequate dosage, and then the treatment must be stopped. The chance of obtaining a remission by continuing the treatment for a longer period is poor, and there is an increasing risk of complications owing to the cumulative effect of prolonged steroid therapy and to a major persistent protein loss.

In this situation, recourse is usually had to the immunodepressive drugs. Some authors suggest that, before abandoning steroid therapy, ACTH should be tried for some days, and if this proves beneficial, the treatment should continue with interrupted steroid therapy of the type described above.

The use of steroids implies institution of a low-salt diet and careful monitoring of the blood pressure, of gastric tolerance, of psychic state, and the general condition of the patient. If signs of overdosage, with a Cushingoid appearance, set in rapidly, the treatment must be stopped before permanent damage is done. If these conditions are strictly observed, serious complications of the steroid treatment of the nephrotic syndrome should never occur. Such complications are nearly always linked to continuous dosage prolonged for more than two months. In addition to infectious complications, a special watch must be kept for peptic ulceration, severe osteoporosis with vertebral collapse, necrosis of the femoral head, cataract, myopathy, and psychiatric disorders. Prednisone in doses greater than 10 mg./m.^{2}/day interferes with growth, and, although the growth deficit generally is corrected when treatment is stopped, it is possible that, as a consequence of prolonged and repeated courses of treatment, the normal height may never be reached. Disorders associated with the cessation of steroid therapy should be prevented by very gradual reduction of dosage below the level of 0.5 mg./kg. after prolonged treatment. In the withdrawal period, any stress, such as surgery, trauma, or serious infection, is an indication for the administration of intramuscular hydrocortisone in doses of 100 to 200 mg./day.

Immunodepressive Drugs

The various reports of the use of immunodepressive drugs are difficult to analyze. In many series, there is no account of renal biopsy studies. In addition, the distinction between total and partial resistance to steroids is rarely made. The various treatments utilized differ in nature and duration and in their association with steroid therapy. There is a lack of properly controlled trials. Four studies of this type have been reported, and in two of these the immunodepressive drugs were given as the primary treatment, whereas steroids were given to the controls.[24] There was little difference in the number of remissions obtained, but the duration of remission was definitely longer in children treated with immunodepressive drugs.[6, 7, 9, 18, 19, 24, 25] A trial carried out by Barratt and Soothill[3] was confined to cases that had proved to be steroid-dependent. These authors found that the use of cyclophosphamide diminished the number of relapses after cessation of prednisone therapy.

An international study comparing the combination of azathioprine and prednisone with prednisone alone showed no appreciable difference between the two groups.[1]

Most authors have used the immunodepressive drugs in patients who were steroid-resistant or steroid-dependent. On the whole, the results agree.

In "steroid-dependent nephroses," immunodepressive drugs can produce complete remission for more than one year in 90 per cent of cases.

In "nephroses that are initially steroid-resistant," remission is obtained in approximately half of the cases. In our own experience, the percentage of complete remission is lower (only 12 of 61 cases, of which three in 33 had focal lesions), but our series does not include cases of partial steroid resistance. Although in steroid-dependent nephrotic syndromes, the results are identical at any stage of the disease, the immunodepressive drugs seem to be more effective if they are used in the early months; we had 12 complete remissions in 40 patients (30 per cent) treated during the first year, but no remission in 21 cases in which the treatment was instituted after one year.

The drugs most commonly used are azathioprine and the alkylating agents.

Azathioprine

Azathioprine (Imuran) appears to be less effective than the alkylating agents, especially in steroid-resistant nephrotic syndromes. In the long term, it predisposes to malignant disease, and it should not be used.

Alkylating Agents

Cyclophosphamide (Endoxan) is used extensively in the English-speaking countries and has been shown to be effective in the treatment of steroid-dependent nephrotic syndromes. The best-known side-effects are alopecia, which is very common but reversible, hemorrhagic cystitis, which may be avoided by an adequate fluid intake, and, most important of all, spermatic destruction with azoospermia that may prove permanent. This gonadal toxicity, which has been described in adults, has not yet been studied in children before the age of puberty; it seems to be linked to the duration of treatment. *Chlorambucil* (chloraminophene) has been used mainly in France; it is better tolerated in the early stages. Its action is slower than the action of cyclophosphamide. There are fewer studies of gonadal toxicity, but this remains a probable complication.

When these agents are used, a regular watch must be kept on the blood count, and treatment must be stopped if the polymorphonuclear leukocyte count drops below 2000/mm.[3] the lymphocyte count below 500/mm.[3] or the platelet count below 100,000/mm.[3] or if there is any intercurrent infection, either bacterial or viral.

In practice, cyclophosphamide in doses of 3 mg./kg./day or chlorambucil in doses of 0.2 mg./kg./day is used in steroid-dependent nephrotic syndromes, preferably in association with steroid therapy to induce rapid remission, or these agents may be used alone in steroid-resistant nephrotic syndromes. The drugs should not be given for more than six months, and throughout this period weekly hematologic review is necessary.

Indomethacin

Some authors advise treating the nephroses with indomethacin; little is known as yet about its efficacy, but it seems to be inferior to the steroids and immunodepressive agents. Further work with controlled trials is required to define the indications for the use of this drug in treating nephroses.

Symptomatic Treatment and Other Measures

Diet

Salt must be rigidly restricted, and the diet should include a liberal allowance of protein. There is no limitation of fluid intake unless there is hyponatremia or gross edema, neither is there a need to restrict the intake of fat. Once the edema has disappeared, if the blood pressure is normal, the salt restriction may be relaxed, although a certain limitation is imposed by steroid therapy.

Diuretics

Diuretics are not necessary unless there is gross edema, because steroid therapy will induce adequate diuresis in 10 to 15 days. Diuretics may, however, be useful in cases of severe edema with a urinary sodium output less than 1 mEq./day. Aldactone in doses of 10 mg./kg. gives the best results. The effect may not be apparent for four or five days. Diuresis in response to aldactone therapy may be accompanied by a considerable sodium loss, and this may require compensation. Sometimes the edema does not respond to aldactone, and the dosage may then be increased to 15 and later to 20 mg./kg., or hydrochlorothiazide may be given in doses of 1 mg./kg., or both may be given together. In principle, this combination of drugs should have the advantage of avoiding the risk of hyperkalemia. Aldactone may also be prescribed in combination with a more powerful diuretic, such as frusemide (1 mg./kg.) or ethacrynic acid (1 mg./kg.).

Infusion of Albumin

Virtually the only indication for albumin infusion is very gross edema resistant to all diuretics. In such cases, diuretics may regain their effect for a short period of time after restoration of the blood volume. It is usual to infuse 0.5 to 1 g./kg./day of human albumin (desalted if possible) for three or four days.

Antibiotics

Antibiotics have played an important part in improving the prognosis of the nephrotic syndrome. They should not be used prophylactically, but as soon as there is any evidence of infection, a suitable combination of antibiotics should be given without delay. However, when possible, material should be obtained first for sensitivity testing. Infection can cause temporary steroid resistance.

General Considerations

Mode of Life. The recurrent nature of nephrosis and the permanent uncertainty induced by relapses make it very desirable for the physician to have frequent discussion with the patient's family. The family should be alerted at the outset to the possibility of relapse, and they should also be told that the long-term prognosis is good in the majority of cases.

Hospitalization is not always necessary if the edema is mild, but it is generally desirable both for confirmation of the diagnosis and in order that treatment may be commenced under close supervision. Once treatment is established, hospitalization should be reduced to a minimum, and most children can be followed and treated as outpatients.

Bed rest is generally contraindicated except when there is gross edema, and then the patient should be kept in bed for only a short time. When the edema disappears, virtually normal activity is possible and desirable. Physical activity plays no part in the general evolution of the disease; in fact, its absence may even have unhappy psychologic consequences. Full-time schooling should be resumed as soon as possible. The only real risk in sending these children back to school is that they may come into contact with chickenpox, a disease that may prove serious during steroid therapy. If the child comes into contact with chickenpox, the prednisone dosage should be reduced to 0.25 or 0.5 mg./kg. and, if it is available, an injection of herpes globulin from a convalescent patient seems to be very effective. This risk of contagion can in no way be set against the loss of many years schooling, which may prove irreparable for certain children.

The question of vaccinations is often raised. Although it is possible to consider oral poliomyelitis and BCG vaccination during a remission after stopping all treatment with steroids or immunodepressive drugs, it is preferable to wait for three or four years after the last attack before vaccinating by injection.

Complicated Nephrotic Syndromes

There are many possible complications of the nephrotic syndrome (Table 66). In addition to the liability to infection, formerly a major cause of mortality in nephroses, the tendency to venous and even arterial *thromboses* should be emphasized. These thromboses represent a risk to life that has only recently been recognized. This risk is ample justification for the use of anticoagulants at the slightest sign of phlebitis in the limbs and particularly if there is deep venous thrombosis or pulmonary embolus (the diagnosis of both these conditions may be difficult). In such cases, continuous heparin therapy should be prescribed for two weeks, followed by oral anticoagulants if the thrombosis is proved.

Abdominal symptoms may cause serious difficulties in diagnosis. They may result from a simple "nephrotic crisis," in which abdominal pain and rapid swelling of the abdomen are due to the development of uncomplicated ascites. Abdominal complications may result from caval, mesenteric, or renal vein thrombosis, from peritonitis, perforated ulcer or even acute pancreatitis, which is a classic

Table 66. Extrarenal Complications of "Nephrosis" in Children
(665 Cases, 1957–1972)

Complications	Types		Number	Deaths
Infections	Septicemia Pulmonary infection Peritonitis Meningitis Cellulitis, abscess	9 11 4 1 28	53	4
Thromboembolism	Thrombosis of limb veins of renal veins of pulmonary arteries of cerebral arteries of renal arteries	18 6 18 3 1	36	3
Protein deficiency	Diarrhea Muscle wasting Osteoporosis Disorders of teeth and hair		19	4
Complications of steroid therapy	Osteoporosis Psychic disorders Acute adrenal failure	23 4 5	32	3
Abdominal disorders	Hepatitis Acute pancreatitis Attacks of pain	1 1	14	2
Various	Hyponatremia Collapse Encephalitis		14	1
Total			168	17

complication. The symptoms and signs of partial intestinal obstruction may be caused by severe potassium depletion. All of these possible complications must be recognized early and treated appropriately.

In steroid-resistant nephrotic syndromes, very difficult situations may sometimes give the impression of a therapeutic impasse. In these cases, in which serious urinary loss of protein persists and in which edema recurs very rapidly, the clinical picture is dominated by *protein denutrition* with cachexia and muscular wasting, often aggravated by steroid therapy, and there are often serious gastrointestinal disorders, including virtually total refusal of food, vomiting, and diarrhea. This situation generally develops in patients who have been maintained for many weeks or months on immunodepressive drugs, and it may be wise to suspend the use of these drugs in view of the risk to life. The essence of treatment is symptomatic. Adequate alimentation may have to be assured by continuous gastric or duodenal catheter, distributing the input equally over the 24 hours. This type of feeding should be begun very carefully, with small amounts of 25 to 30 calories/kg./day, gradually increasing over a period of 10 to 15 days to the normal caloric and protein requirements for the age of the child. Patiently pursued, this technique will restore the nutrition, sometimes with spectacular results. It is important at the same time to undertake reeducation of the muscles and joints, because the muscles may be atrophied and the joints stiffened, owing to the bedridden state, for which hospitalization and depression bear some responsibility.

Any deficiency in vitamins, calcium, or potassium should be corrected. Synthetic anabolic agents may be beneficial. In this situation, the child should return home as soon as possible.

"ACUTE POSTINFECTIVE" GLOMERULONEPHRITIS

Treatment for this condition is essentially symptomatic, because as yet there is no specific therapy of proved effectiveness.

General Measures

These consist essentially of a strict salt-free diet and rest in bed during the acute stage. Hospitalization is not always necessary if there is no evidence of cardiovascular overload or hypertension, provided that the condition is carefully reviewed every day during the acute phase. Clinical supervision should be directed particularly to any development of edema, and the patient's weight should be recorded daily. The cardiovascular status and blood pressure, as well as the urinary output, should be recorded several times a day. If there is oliguria, the blood urea nitrogen, serum creatinine, and plasma electrolytes should be measured early every day.

Antibiotics

After obtaining a throat swab, antibiotic therapy with oral or intramuscular penicillin (or with erythromycin in cases of penicillin allergy) should be commenced and continued for 10 days or until any infectious foci have been eradicated. There is little point in prolonging antibiotic treatment beyond two or three weeks, because in this disorder there is no indication for prolonged prophylactic antibiotic therapy.

Acute Cardiovascular Overload

In some cases in which the true diagnosis has not been recognized and the child continues to ingest salt, an acute cardiovascular overload may develop, with gallop rhythm on auscultation, x-ray evidence of cardiac enlargement, and, possibly, dyspnea with or without pulmonary edema. Urgent treatment is indicated. The first step is to give a diuretic such as frusemide intravenously in doses of 1 to 2 mg./kg.; this may be repeated at intervals of two or three hours, provided that the total dose in 24 hours is not more than 10 mg./kg. Hypotensive drugs such as reserpine and Aldomet may be useful. If signs of pulmonary edema are present and there has not been a very rapid response to treatment, peritoneal dialysis should be considered, using a hypertonic solution that will reduce the blood volume very effectively in one or two hours. In a situation of grave urgency, venesection may be necessary. Digitalis is not indicated and may even be dangerous.

Acute Renal Failure

In most cases, the oliguria is transient and the blood urea nitrogen level does not rise above 40 mg. per 100 ml., but there may be more prolonged oliguria in some cases, and then the general measures indicated in this situation should be applied (see page 352).

Hypertension

If the hypertension is moderate (diastolic pressure of 90 mm. Hg or less) and asymptomatic, rest and salt restriction generally are effective in rapidly restoring the blood pressure to normal. Hypotensive drugs (see page 412) are indicated if the diastolic pressure rises above 90 mm. Hg. Severe hypertension (diastolic pressure of 120 mm. Hg or more) is an indication for urgent measures, such as the use of intravenous diazoxide (10 mg./kg.) or peritoneal dialysis if there is evidence of vascular overload.

Indications for Renal Biopsy

In cases with endocapillary proliferation, there is usually rapid recovery, the oliguria lasts only a few days, and the blood urea nitrogen level and glomerular clearance return to normal in 10 to 15 days. The proteinuria disappears in a few weeks, and a nephrotic syndrome is rare.

In other words, the persistence of oliguria for more than a week, diminished glomerular clearance, or gross proteinuria persisting for more than 15 days may be regarded as indications for renal biopsy. In such cases, biopsy may reveal membranoproliferative glomerulonephritis or, even more important, endocapillary and extracapillary proliferation that may be indications for more specific therapy when the condition is diffuse (see page 338).

Convalescence—Return to Normal Activity

As soon as the edema disappears and the blood pressure has been controlled, bed rest is no longer necessary, and a progressive return to normal physical activity is possible. In most cases, the child can return to school four to six weeks after the onset of the disease. The persistence of urinary signs such as microscopic hematuria or mild proteinuria is not a contraindication to the resumption of virtually normal activity; the same can be said for a persistently high sedimentation rate, because this may last for several weeks without having any particular prognostic significance.

If justified by the local condition, the treatment of any focus of infection in sinuses, teeth, or tonsils is carried out under antibiotic protection. There is virtually no indication for tonsillectomy, and in any case the operation should not be performed until six or 12 months after the complete disappearance of all renal signs.

It is customary to wait for two years after the disappearance of symptoms before carrying out vaccination against diphtheria or tetanus. BCG and poliomyelitis vaccines can be given if special precautions are taken.

PROLONGED OR CHRONIC GLOMERULONEPHRITIS

Membranoproliferative and Lobular Glomerulonephritis

Immunodepressive drugs have been used for a considerable time in the treatment of glomerulonephritis, but only in recent years has certain evidence, such as the lowering of the C'3 fraction of complement or the fixation of immunoglobulin in the glomeruli, furnished a semblance of justification for this type of treatment in idiopathic membranoproliferative and lobular glomerulonephritis.

Although it is difficult to analyze and compare most of the reports in which mention is made of the treatment of this type of nephropathy, we have gathered in Table 67 data of a few series published since 1964. In these series, the type of treatment given and the results of treatment are clearly set out. This table shows how disappointing the results are. Steroid therapy appears to have been abandoned; certainly it carries definite risks and often aggravates preexisting hypertension in these patients. It has even been shown in a controlled trial that the mortality rate was greater with steroid treatment.[23] The immunodepressive drugs, or at least azathioprine and chlorambucil, seem capable in some cases of inducing remission or amelioration, but a cause-and-effect relationship is not established, because virtually the same percentage of remission and amelioration has been found in many patients who were given no treatment whatever (see

Table 67. Membranoproliferative and Lobular Glomerulonephritis: Treatment by Various Authors

Author	No Treatment				Steroids				Immunodepressive Drugs				
	Number	C.R.	I.R.	N.C.	Number	C.R.	I.R.	Failure	Drug	Number	C.R.	I.R.	Failure
Gotz et al. (1964)[8]					4	1	–	3					
Michael et al. (1967)[15]									A+P	6	1	1	4
Cameron (1968)					31	1	–	30					
Miller et al. (1967)[17]	4	2	2		3	–	–	3					
Lagrue (1970)									Ch/A	73	2	13	58
Habib (1972)	65	9	10	46	27	–	3	24	Ch	61	8	12	41
Total	69	11 (15%)	12	46	65	2 (3%)	3	60		140	11 (8%)	26	103

C.R.: Complete remission; I.R.: incomplete remission; N.C.: no change; A: azathioprine; P: prednisone; Ch: chlorambucil.

page 222). A controlled trial, conducted in Great Britain by the Medical Research Council, in which 67 cases treated with azathioprine and prednisone were compared with 67 untreated cases,[14] gave similar results. There was no significant difference in the progression of renal symptoms between the two groups of cases after six to 12 months' observation. The same result was obtained in two other studies.[4, 20]

In consequence, there would appear to be no indication for azathioprine or chlorambucil in membranoproliferative or lobular glomerulonephritis. The use of other immunodepressive agents, such as cyclophosphamide, or other types of drugs, such as indomethacin or heparin, is not justified at present except as part of a controlled therapeutic trial.

Extramembranous Glomerulonephritis

We are considering here only idiopathic extramembranous glomerulonephritis. Table 68 summarizes the therapeutic results obtained by various authors. The effect of treatment is very difficult to establish in this group in view of the absence of comparable control series, the possibility of spontaneous remission, the variability of the proteinuria from day to day, and the paucity of serial histologic studies.

The steroid therapy recommended by some authors coincided with complete remission in only 14 per cent of cases (29 of 209 cases gathered from 13 publications) (Table 68). In no case was the response to treatment frank, rapid, and reproducible, as in the nephroses; when remission did occur, it developed very slowly. Indeed, there have been some reports of aggravation of the proteinuria whenever steroid therapy was restarted.

The immunodepressive drugs would appear to be only a little more valu-

Table 68. Extramembranous Glomerulonephritis: Course With and Without Treatment According to Various Authors

I. STEROIDS

Author	Number	Complete Remission	Failure
Gotz (1964)	8	2	6
Rossi (1966)	60	3	57
Bariéty (1968)	14	1	13
Pollak (1968)	9	0	9
Ehrenreich (1968)	27	6	21
Rastogi (1969)	6	4	2
Ducrot (1969)	13	3	10
Farland (1969)	11	2	9
Miller (1969)	10	0	10
White (1970)	2	0	2
Horvath (1971)	13	0	13
Tsao (1971)	2	2	0
Habib (1972)	34	6	28
Totals	209	29 (14%)	180 (86%)

II. IMMUNODEPRESSIVE DRUGS

Author	Number	Complete Remission	Failure
Bariéty (1968)	17	6	11
(1971)	5	0	5
Tsao (1971)	2	2	0
Habib (1972)	31	8	23
Totals	55	16 (29%)	39 (71%)

III. UNTREATED

Author	Number	Complete Remission	Failure
Ehrenreich (1968)	16	2	14
Farland (1969)	9	1	8
White (1970)	2	1	1
Habib (1972)	37	19	18
Totals	64	23 (36%)	41 (64%)

able. In four publications, 16 complete remissions were noted in 55 patients, a 29 per cent "success" rate. The lesions were observed to disappear in two patients who had been in remission for many years after treatment with azathioprine.[2]

In fact, the incidence of spontaneous remission (23 of 64, or 36 per cent) is greater than that gained with therapy. Analysis of the reports reveals that the remissions occur after the same intervals, regardless of the treatment used, and remission is progressive whether the treatment is stopped or continued.

In summary, in view of this analysis and the generally favorable long-term prognosis in children with extramembranous glomerulonephritis, it is reasonable to eschew steroid therapy and immunodepressive agents in this nephropathy.

ENDOCAPILLARY AND EXTRACAPILLARY PROLIFERATIVE GLOMERULONEPHRITIS

The presence of epithelial crescents in more than 50 per cent of the glomeruli suggests that the condition will progress to terminal renal failure. This is virtually certain when more than 80 per cent of the glomeruli are affected (malignant glomerulonephritis or type III endocapillary and extracapillary proliferative glomerulonephritis).

The gravity of the condition justifies various attempts at treatment. Of the methods that are being tried, the combination of heparin and immunodepressive drugs seems to have given positive results in some cases. In fact, it is still difficult to assess the true effect of this type of treatment which, of necessity, must be instituted very early because of the rapid progression of the glomerular lesions to fibrosis.[13]

This is a difficult problem because the diagnosis of diffuse extracapillary proliferation can be made only on renal biopsy, which is practiced much too rarely in the first days of the disease. Consequently, very early renal biopsy is indicated in cases of acute glomerulonephritis with ominous signs, such as a nephrotic syndrome or renal insufficiency, even though moderate, persisting beyond the first week.

Whatever the histologic type of the nephropathy, it is obviously essential to use symptomatic treatment for any edema, hypertension, or renal insufficiency.

The patients must be kept under careful supervision, but their physical activity should not be limited. The object is to maintain a normal style of life because some of these nephropathies may pursue a prolonged course.

REFERENCES

1. Abramovicz, M., Barnett, H. L., Edelman, C. M. J., Greifer, I., Kobayashi, O., Arneil, G. C., Barron, B. A., Gordillo, G., Hallman, N., and Tiddens, H. D.: Controlled trial of azathioprine in children with nephrotic syndrome. Lancet 2:959, 1970.
2. Bariéty, J., Samarcq, P., Lagrue, G., Fritel, D., and Milliez, P.: Evolution ultrastructurale favourable de deux cas de glomérulonéphropathies primitives à dépôts extramembraneus diffus. Presse Méd. 76:2179, 1968.
3. Barratt, T. M., and Soothill, J. F.: Controlled trial of cyclophosphamide in steroid-sensitive relapsing nephrotic syndrome of childhood. Lancet 2:479, 1970.
4. Booth, J., and Aber, G. M.: Immunosuppressive therapy in adults with proliferative glomerulonephritis. Controlled trial. Lancet 2:1010, 1970.
5. Cameron, J. S., Glascow, E. F., Ogg, C. S., and White, R. H. R.: Membranoproliferative glomerulonephritis and persistent hypocomplementemia. Brit. Med. J. 4:714, 1970.

 6. Drummond, K. N., Hillman, D. H., Marchessault, J. H. V., and Feloman, W.: Cyclophosphamide in the nephrotic syndrome in childhood. Can. Med. Ass. J. 98:524, 1968.
 7. Etteldorf, J. N., Roy, S., Summitt, R. C., Sweeney, M. J., Wall, H. P., and Berton, W. M.: Cyclophosphamide in the treatment of idiopathic lipoid nephrosis. J. Pediat. 70:88, 1967.
 8. Gotz, J., McCaughey, W. T. E., and Womersley, R. A.: Steroids in treatment of the nephrotic syndrome in adults. Brit. Med. J. 1:351, 1964.
 9. Grushkin, C. M., Fine, R. N., Hevse, R. E., and Lieberman, E.: Cyclophosphamide therapy of idiopathic nephrosis. Calif. Med. 113:6, 1970.
10. Habib, R., Kleinknecht, C., and Gubler, M. C.: Extramembranous glomerulonephritis in children. J. Pediat. 82:754, 1973.
11. Pickering, R. J., Herdman, R. C., Michael, A. F., Vernier, R. L., Fish, A. J., Gewurz, H., and Good, R. A.: Chronic glomerulonephritis associated with low serum complement activity (chronic hypocomplementemic glomerulonephritis). Medicine 49:207, 1970.
12. Horvath, J. S., Johnson, J. R., and Horvath, D. G.: Prognosis in the nephrotic syndrome. A study based on renal biopsy findings. Med. J. Austr. 2:233, 1971.
13. Kincaid-Smith, P.: Coagulation and renal disease. Kidney Intern. 2:183, 1972.
14. Medical Research Council Working Party: Controlled trial of azathioprine and prednisone in chronic renal disease. Brit. Med. J. 2:239, 1971.
15. Michael, A. F., Vernier, R. C., Drummond, K. N., Levitt, J. I., Herman, R. C., Fish, A. J., and Good, R. A.: Immunosuppressive therapy of chronic renal disease. New Engl. J. Med. 276:817, 1967.
16. Michielsen, P., Verberckmoes, R., Desmet, V., and Hermerijckx, O.: Evolution histologique dans les glomérulonéphrites prolifératives diffuses traitées par l'indométhacine. J. Urol. Néphrol. 75:315, 1969.
17. Miller, R. B., Harrington, J. T., Ramos, C. P., Relman, A. S., and Schwartz, W. P.: Longterm results of steroid therapy in adults with idiopathic nephrotic syndrome. Amer. J. Med. 46:919, 1969.
18. Moncrieff, M. W., White, R. H. R., Ogg, C. S., and Cameron, J. S.: Cyclophosphamide therapy in the nephrotic syndrome in childhood. Brit. Med. J. 1:66, 1969.
19. Mongeau, J. G., and Robillard, J.: Etude de 32 cas de néphrose de l'enfant. Amélioration du pronostic par les médicaments immunodépresseurs. Union Méd. Canada 97:1, 1968.
20. Pollak, V. E., Rosen, S., Piravi, C. I., Muehrcke, R. C., and Kark, R. M.: Natural history of lipoid nephrosis and of membranous glomerulonephritis. Ann. Intern. Med. 69:1171, 1968.
21. Rastogi, S. P., Hart-Mercer, J., and Kerr, D. N. S.: Idiopathic membranous glomerulonephritis in adults: remission following steroid therapy. Quart. J. Med. 38:335, 1969.
22. Rose, C. A., and Black, D. A. K.: Controlled trial of steroid in the nephrotic syndrome. Quart. Med. J. 38:607, 1967.
23. Ross, E. J.: Effect of long term steroid therapy in adults. Proceedings of the Third International Congress of Nephrology, Washington, D.C., 1966. New York, S. Karger, 1967, pp. 108–116.
24. Tsao, Y. C., and Yeung, C. H.: Paired trial of cyclophosphamide and prednisone in children with nephrosis. Arch. Dis. Child. 46:327, 1971.
25. White, R. H. R., Glasgow, E. F., and Mills, R. J.: Clinicopathological study of nephrotic syndrome in children. Lancet 1:1353, 1970.

PART IV

Renal Failure and Hypertension

MICHEL BROYER

ACUTE RENAL FAILURE

Acute renal failure is defined by a collection of biochemical disorders linked to a temporary disturbance of renal clearance function and characterized essentially by a raised blood urea nitrogen level and disturbances of plasma water and electrolytes. This condition is generally the consequence of anuria or, more often, marked oliguria, with reduction of urine output below 250 ml./m.²/24 hours. In some cases, however, the urine output may be maintained even though the biochemical syndrome may be almost as severe. Acute renal failure of organic origin must be distinguished from functional renal failure, which is rapidly reversible after correction of the primary disorder, such as dehydration, hypotension, or severe acidosis.

Acute renal failure is much less common in children than in adults, and, even in very specialized hospital departments, it accounts for only a very small number of admissions.

ETIOLOGY

The causes of acute renal failure in children can be divided into three groups, glomerular and vascular diseases, acute tubular necrosis, and mechanical obstruction.

In a period of 15 years, we have treated 130 cases of acute renal failure in children (Table 69). Glomerular and vascular pathology accounted for 80 of the 130 cases. The most common cause was the hemolytic uremic syndrome (49 cases), and together with cortical necrosis (10 cases), it was the most serious cause. There were also 15 cases of glomerulonephritis and four cases of nephrotic syndrome presenting with anuria. Tubular disorders, often toxic, came a long way second to the glomerulopathies as a cause of acute renal failure, accounting for only 35 of the 130 cases. The 22 per cent mortality rate includes some cases from the early years of this period, and much better results can be expected with current methods of treatment.

Mechanical obstruction accounted for only 11 of the 130 cases, but nonetheless it is important because of the special therapeutic implications.

The majority of cases of acute renal failure due to cortical necrosis and to thrombotic microangiopathy occurred before the age of 2 years, whereas the acute tubular disorders were found chiefly in patients between the ages of 2 and 7 years, and the glomerulopathies that presented with anuria in patients between the ages of 3 and 15 years.

The vascular and glomerular causes have been described in other chapters,

343

Table 69. Etiology of 130 Cases of Acute Renal Failure in Children
(1955–1971)

	Number of Cases	Deaths
Hemolytic uremic syndrome	49	21
Cortical necrosis	10	5
Glomerulonephritis	15	4
Nephrotic syndrome	4	1
Renal vein thrombosis	2	1
Acute tubular disease:		
Toxic	14	3
Septicemia	1	–
Posttraumatic	3	1
Postdehydration	5	1
Origin unknown	4	2
Hyperuricemia	3	1
Postoperative	5	–
Nephroblastoma	3	1
Obstructive uropathy	2	–
Lithiasis	6	1
Unclassified	4	2
Total	130	44

and we shall confine ourselves in this chapter to consideration of the other etiologic varieties observed in our series of 130 cases (summarized in Table 69).

Acute Toxic Tubulopathy

Many toxic agents can cause acute renal failure (Table 70). In children, the responsible agent is nearly always a drug, notably an antibiotic or sulfonamide. It is obvious from Table 71 that, in our series, the antibacterial agents were responsible for two thirds of the cases in which a specific toxic origin was identified.

Sulfonamides — usually sulfadiazine or sulfamerazine — head the list. Often the drug had been given in excessive doses, but there were cases in which the dosage had been absolutely normal, and in these there may have been other factors involved, such as excessive concentration of the drug in the urine, a low urinary pH, or individual susceptibility. The prognosis of sulfonamide anuria is always good; diuresis returns between the second and fifth day, and it is rarely necessary to have recourse to dialysis. Hematuria and proteinuria may occur in the oliguric period.

Colimycin is also a common cause of acute renal failure, and in two of our cases this antibiotic had been given in doses of more than 100,000 units/kg. The oliguria may be prolonged and severe, and dialysis may be required.

Accidental poisoning with other substances is very much rarer in children, at least in our experience. We have seen only four such cases, mainly in the early years of the series; no doubt this accounts for the high mortality rate, because, with modern methods of treatment, such patients should not die of acute renal failure.

Table 70.   Principal Drugs and Poisons That Can Cause Acute Renal Failure

Organic compounds	Carbon tetrachloride
	Tetrachlorethylene
	Ethylene glycol and propylene glycol
	Diethylene glycol
	Oxalic acid
	Creosote
Metals	Arsenic
	Bismuth
	Boron
	Cadmium
	Copper
	Mercury
	Gold
	Lead
	Thallium
	Uranium
Antibiotics	Amphotericin
	Bacitracin
	Cephaloridine
	Colistin
	Kanamycin
	Neomycin
	Penicillins
	Polymyxin
	Sulfonamides
Various other drugs	Phenindione
	Iodized products used in radiology
	Dextrans
	Epsilon aminocaproic acid

Table 71.   Acute Toxic Tubular Necrosis: Summary of 14 Cases in Which the Source Was Identified

Toxic Agent	Number of Cases	Duration of Oliguria in Days (Mean and Extremes)	Maximum PUN* in mg./100 ml. (Mean and Extremes)	Extrarenal Purification	Result
Sulfonamide	8	3 (2–5)	90 (62–145)	None	8 Cured
Colimycin	2	8–10	75–150	1 Peritoneal dialysis	2 Cured
Arsenic	1	15	175	Exchange transfusion	Death
Creosote	1	5	250	Peritoneal dialysis	Death
Mercury	1	8	90	–	Septicemia; death
Carbon tetra-chloride	1	6	120	–	Cured

*PUN: Plasma urea nitrogen.

Acute Tubular Necrosis of Various Origins

This group includes a certain number of patients in whom acute renal failure presented with all the characteristics of an acute tubulopathy, although the precise cause could not always be determined. There are 13 such cases in our series, three post-traumatic, five secondary to acute dehydration, one as a complication of septicemia, and four unexplained.

Post-traumatic acute renal failure may result from shock but also from the liberation of myoglobin, which is toxic to the renal tubules. The trauma may also include damage to the renal parenchyma or kidney pedicle, or a perirenal hematoma. Difficult problems occur in the treatment of such patients, necessitating close collaboration between physician and surgeon. Acute dehydration may sometimes be followed by transient acute renal failure that must be distinguished from the functional renal insufficiency that is constantly found in dehydration states, but which is rapidly reversible on rehydration. Five of our patients fell into this category, and the oliguria did not last longer than three or four days, but one patient died of neurologic complications. Severe dehydration can also be complicated by cortical necrosis, and this produces a much more prolonged oliguria, with a grave prognosis, in contrast to the acute tubulopathy that is entirely reversible.

Septicemia, usually Gram-negative, is a classic cause of acute renal failure. This condition is probably more common than might appear from the solitary case in our series, which was one of pneumococcal septicemia complicated by peritonitis. The patient recovered after peritoneal dialysis.

Acute Hyperuricemic Nephropathy

This nephropathy occurs exclusively in children who have leukemia or a malignant condition that is treated by cytolytic drugs, and it is the consequence of extensive liberation of nucleoproteins from the lysed cells. The greater the tumor development, the greater is the likelihood of occurrence of the nephropathy, but the extent of tumor development is often difficult to estimate in the leukemias. Three of our four cases had considerable lymph node enlargement and hepatosplenomegaly; the remaining case (case 3) had bone disease clearly visible on x-ray (Table 72). It is important to emphasize the prophylactic measures designed to prevent the occurrence of acute renal failure as a complication of cytolytic therapy. These measures include a very high fluid intake, if necessary including intravenous infusion of an osmotically active solution, such as mannitol; alkalinization of the urine; administration of a diuretic such as Diamox or frusemide; and the prescription of allopurinol, which blocks the synthesis of uric acid at the stage of the more soluble oxypurines. If these measures should prove inadequate, it is important to recognize acute renal failure at an early stage so as to avoid overloading the circulation, especially with intravenous fluid. In principle, this type of acute renal failure has a good prognosis, but there is inadequate information about the long-term consequences. Three of our patients apparently were cured, without exhibiting any renal sequelae, but no biopsy was performed.

Table 72. Acute Renal Failure Due to Hyperuricemia*

Case Number	Disease	Chemotherapy	Allopurinol	Blood Uric Acid (mg./100 ml.)	Acute Renal Failure	Evolution of Renal Condition
1	Acute leukemia	Prednisone Rubidomycin (Daunomycin) Asparaginase	0	23.5	+ (anuria)	Death
2	Acute leukemia	Prednisone Cyclophosphamide Rubidomycin (Daunomycin)	600 mg./day	8.0–10.8	+ (diuresis maintained)	Cured
3	Hodgkin's disease	Prednisone Caryolysin Vincristine	0	14.8	+ (anuria)	Cured
4	Acute leukemia	Methotrexate	0	16.8	+ (anuria)	Cured

*All four patients were treated by peritoneal dialysis.

Urinary Tract Malformation

Apart from congenital malformations such as renal agenesis and bilateral multicystic kidney, which may be responsible for neonatal anuria, malformation of the urinary tract may cause obstructive anuria. The obstruction generally occurs at the pelviureteral junction or at the uterovesical junction and affects a solitary kidney. Our two cases included one of each of these two types. The anuria was complete, and examination revealed a tense mass extending from the loin into the abdomen that disappeared with spontaneous diuresis. The diagnosis is generally suggested by the palpation of a tumor mass of fluid consistency, and confirmation can be obtained by intravenous urography which gives a characteristic picture, especially on late films.

The treatment is surgical correction of the responsible abnormality, but preliminary nephrostomy may be necessary so that definitive surgery can be performed under better conditions.

Nephroblastoma was responsible for anuria in three patients in our series. Two of the cases resulted from obstruction caused by recurrent tumor in the remaining kidney, and both patients did well after radiotherapy and partial surgery. The third patient had postoperative anuria caused by ligature of the contralateral renal pedicle.

Calculous Anuria

Although rare, this must always be considered in a case of oliguria, especially if there is also hematuria and renal colic. A plain x-ray of the urinary tract is generally sufficient to confirm the diagnosis. There may be bilateral lithiasis or stone in a solitary kidney. The anuric episode is rarely the first symptom of the lithiasis. There is nearly always a previous history of hematuria, abdominal pain, or urinary infection. Treatment is surgical, with removal of the offending calculi after preliminary drainage with ureteric catheters. If the obstruction is removed early, the prognosis is excellent.

Four of our six patients had stone in a single kidney, and two had bilateral calculi. Two of these six cases involved cystine stones, and the remaining four magnesium-ammonium phosphate or calcium phosphate stones. Calculous anuria can occur at a very early age; in five of our six patients, it was found between 11 months and 5 years.

Acute Postoperative Renal Failure

This accounts for more than one third of cases of acute renal failure in adults, but it is much less common in children. Many factors may be involved, including cardiac disease, previous nephropathy or uropathy, operative shock, septicemic shock, transfusion errors, and nephrotoxic drugs (discussed previously). The renal failure may be aggravated by certain water and electrolyte disorders, such as extracellular dehydration, acidosis, and hypokalemia. These factors are responsible as a rule for rapidly reversible functional disorders. Not so rapidly reversible is the organic renal failure secondary to intracellular overhydration owing to excessive fluid intake, but even here the renal failure rarely lasts more than four of five days.

It is very important to diagnose acute renal failure at the earliest possible moment. The best guides are the composition of the urine and especially the urine osmolarity, the urine/plasma (U/P) ratio of urea, and the urinary sodium. An osmolarity below 350 mOsm./liter, a U/P urea ratio of less than 5, a urinary sodium level above 20 mEq./liter, better still, a Na/K ratio greater than 1 are all positive evidence in favor of organic renal failure that will not be relieved by correction of some water or electrolyte imbalance or metabolic disorder.

Postoperative renal failure is associated with intense catabolism, and dialysis is generally indicated. Dialysis should be early and frequent to provide the patient with the best chance of resisting infection and to facilitate wound healing. Peritoneal dialysis may be possible even after abdominal surgery unless intestine has been sutured, but it is more usual to use hemodialysis.

Our series included four patients with postoperative oliguria, and all four recovered. There was no clear-cut explanation in any of the cases, except for one patient who probably had acute glomerulonephritis, but who had been subjected to an unnecessary appendectomy because of abdominal pain.

Conclusion

The etiology of an acute renal failure is often very easy to diagnose on considering the history or associated signs. In other cases, the cause may not be so evident, and a certain number of routine investigations are needed.

After correcting any conditions that might cause functional renal failure, the possibility of mechanical obstruction should be excluded by a plain film and by intravenous urography with tomography; it is in fact possible to obtain interpretable pictures in acute renal failure by using 3 ml./kg. of Conray or 4 ml./kg. of Hypaque Sodium; the films may give an idea of the size of the kidneys and may reveal an obstructive uropathy or the small kidneys of chronic renal failure. The discovery of large kidneys is of little value in acute renal failure. Retrograde cystography is always possible and will clearly reveal certain malformations. Routine tests should include hematologic study for evidence of thrombotic microangiopathy (schizocytosis, reticulocytosis, thrombocytopenia) or of intravascular coagulation (a decrease in fibrinogen and factors V, VIII, and IX, presence of fibrin degradation products); in addition, infection should be excluded by repeated cultures of urine and blood.

Examination of the urine, whenever it is possible, is very important. As described previously, estimation of osmolarity and of urea, sodium, and potassium levels in the urine may give definite evidence of organic renal failure. The discovery of hematuria and proteinuria is evidence in favor of glomerular disease, but these signs are not absolutely specific. Further evidence suggesting glomerular disease is a Na/K ratio of less than 1, because this ratio is nearly always greater than 1 in tubular disease.

Serum protein estimation and electrophoresis may confirm the diagnosis of a nephrotic syndrome. The blood levels of the C'3 fraction of complement and of antistreptolysins may point to acute glomerulonephritis. The plasma uric acid level may reveal hyperuricemia.

Abnormalities in serum transaminases and coagulation factors, as well as hyperbilirubinemia, which indicate hepatic disease, may point to an infectious or toxic etiology. Samples of serum and urine should always be frozen and stored in case they are required later for toxicologic studies.

Renal biopsy may be indicated as a guide to prognosis if the renal failure continues for more than three or four weeks. It is essential in the glomerular diseases to determine the exact type and to follow the course of the disease. In general, renal biopsy is useful after the return of diuresis when the diagnosis remains doubtful or the course is atypical.

BIOCHEMICAL SYNDROME

There is nothing to distinguish the biochemical features of acute renal failure from those of chronic renal failure except possibly a question of degree in cases of total anuria or where there is intense catabolism. The cessation of kidney function disturbs water and salt homeostasis and is accompanied by the retention of nitrogenous waste products whose pathogenic role is certain though poorly understood.

Water Intoxication

This may occur if the patient is given too much fluid, either by mouth or intravenously. Increased weight or puffiness of the face may be suggestive, but these signs may be difficult to assess. The blood pressure may be elevated and there is sometimes edema of the ocular fundus. Nausea, vomiting, and clouding of consciousness may precede dangerous complications, such as convulsions and pulmonary edema. There are always hyponatremia and hypochloremia (sodium, 120 mEq./liter; chloride, 90 mEq./liter, and also hypoproteinemia.

Sodium Excess

Here again, this disorder is found only if the child continues to take salt food or drugs containing sodium, such as effervescent calcium, kayexalatate, sodium penicillin,* sodium bicarbonate, and intravenous infusions containing sodium.

Changes in weight and the presence of edema or simply puffiness are very valuable signs, but these are sometimes difficult to assess. Hypertension is common. The chief complications are cardiovascular, including pulmonary edema and asystole, but cerebral edema with convulsions may occur. There is no easily accessible biochemical index of this sodium excess. The plasma sodium and chloride levels are often normal or low. Measurements of the blood volume using labeled albumin or of the extracellular space using labeled bromine may provide proof of the diagnosis.

Hyperkalemia

Except for rare cases in which the potassium balance may be negative because of some gastrointestinal disorder, the plasma potassium tends to rise in renal failure. In the absence of any possibility of potassium excretion, account must be taken of dietary intake and especially of catabolism. Acidosis can also increase the plasma potassium levels. The chief risk of hyperkalemia is the threat of cardiac arrest. Electrocardiographic monitoring is the quickest and easiest method of detecting dangerous hyperkalemia. Hyperkalemia can also cause paresis or paralysis of voluntary and smooth muscles, with abolition of reflexes.

Metabolic Acidosis

As with potassium, hydrogen ion balance is positive in acute renal failure owing to nitrogen catabolism (1 g. protein $= 0.7$ mEq. H^+ ions), although vomiting may produce depletion of hydrogen ions. In most cases, the metabolic acidosis increases from day to day, with a progressive fall in the bicarbonate level. The pH remains normal because of respiratory compensation except in cases of severe acidosis or respiratory complications.

Hypocalcemia

Hypocalcemia occurs very early and is sometimes very marked in the course of acute renal failure. The mechanism of this disorder is not fully understood, but it is associated with the rise in blood phosphorus and magnesium levels. It

---

*1.7 mEq./1 million units.

should be noted that the acidosis provides a certain measure of protection against tetany, which occurs very rarely in acute renal failure. For this reason, care must be taken in compensating for the acidosis.

Accumulation of Nitrogenous Waste

Although it has long been known that urea is not toxic in the concentrations reached in renal failure, it is a fact that the rise in blood urea level goes hand in hand with a group of disorders that disappear after dialysis. These disorders include a hemorrhagic tendency and decreased resistance to infection. In cases of total anuria, the blood urea nitrogen level rises on average by 20 to 25 mg./100 ml./24 hours. The rate of rise may be much greater in the presence of fever or intense catabolism, or it may be less rapid if catabolism is inhibited by adequate caloric intake.

Hematologic Disorders

Anemia with relative erythroblastopenia and shortened red cell survival is observed during the course of acute renal failure. This anemia is reversible and recovers rapidly after the return of diuresis.

Period of Return of Diuresis

This stage formerly was feared because of the possibility that various complications caused by water and salt depletion might occur. Early and adequate dialysis has greatly diminished the risks of this period, risks that were associated with osmotic diuresis, in which a very high blood urea level may have played a considerable part. The most important features of this stage are the tendencies to lose sodium, to hypokalemia, and to acidosis.

Renal Failure with Continued Diuresis

Sometimes unrecognized, this form of acute renal failure is particularly common after surgery but can occur in other contexts. It may be detected by a U/P urea ratio of less than 10 (or often much lower), iso-osmolarity of the urine, and a urinary sodium level greater than 20 mEq./liter despite a low blood sodium level and no sodium intake. This last aspect may become very serious in a few very rare cases that develop a true salt-losing syndrome. With this sole exception, renal failure with continued diuresis involves the same disorders as total anuria.

TREATMENT

Many aspects of treatment must be considered, including the etiologic treatment of the condition responsible for the renal failure, clinical and laboratory surveillance of the anuric child, conservative treatment centered on diet and dialysis.

Etiologic Treatment

The etiologic treatment of the condition responsible for the acute renal failure has already been considered in the discussion of the principal causes.

Heparin is used in the hemolytic uremic syndrome and in certain glomerular nephropathies, although there is no definite proof of its efficacy. Heparin is indicated in renal vein thrombosis, in which case intravenous administration with a constant infusion pump is preferable to any other method. The renal failure does not affect the dosage, which should be adjusted according to the coagulation time. The average dose is of the order of 6 to 8 mg./kg./day.

Certain poisons may indicate the need for antidotes, such as dimercaprol (BAL) for poisoning with heavy metals (3 mg./kg. every 4 hours on the first day, every six hours the second day, and every 12 hours on the third day).

Dialysis may be needed urgently to remove poisons such as boron, ethylene glycol, and dextran.

Infection is an indication for broad-spectrum antibiotics that are not nephrotoxic, and dosage must be adjusted according to the excretion pattern of the particular antibiotic. Whenever possible, the plasma level of the antibiotics should be monitored to avoid a dangerous accumulation.

Hyperuricemia is treated with allopurinol. The uropathies and lithiases require surgery, either immediate if the condition of the child permits, or after dialysis or preliminary drainage if there is obstruction.

Clinical and Laboratory Surveillance of the Anuric Child

This must be very precise, and all quantitative data should be recorded on a flow sheet that is kept up-to-date every day.

The weight is recorded daily; it should fall gradually or remain stable. The daily urinary output is recorded, but an indwelling catheter should not be used, as it is a source of infection. Extrarenal losses, as from diarrhea and vomiting, are estimated as closely as possible each day. Several times a day the pulse and blood pressure are recorded. An electrocardiogram should be taken as often as may be indicated by the risk of hyperkalemia. A complete clinical examination once or twice a day should include assessments of the state of hydration, of the cardiac tolerance, and of the neurologic status. The plasma ionogram, the plasma urea nitrogen level, the serum calcium level, and the hematocrit should be estimated daily.

The anuric child should be got out of bed as soon as possible; a certain amount of activity is desirable because this makes the child easier to feed.

Conservative Medical Treatment

It should be emphasized at the outset that in many cases therapeutic errors are responsible for complications, even fatal complications. The most common error is excessive intravenous infusion after diagnosis of the renal failure. In most cases, such infusion is pointless, and any intravenous medication (such as heparin and antibiotics) can be given through a needle left in a vein* and flushed regularly with a heparin solution.

Anemia should be corrected cautiously and only if severe (hemoglobin less than 8 g./100 ml.). Transfusion may raise the serum potassium level, lower the ionized calcium (because of the citrate) and, most important of all, increase the blood volume to a dangerous degree. For these reasons, transfusion is best performed during dialysis, using packed red cells.

Hyperkalemia may be prevented or treated by oral or rectal administration of ion exchange resins in doses of 1 g./kg./day or more.

The hypocalcemia is difficult to correct. Vitamin D (10,000 to 20,000 units/day) and massive doses of oral calcium (500 to 1000 mg./m.^{2}) are useful. The intravenous route should not be used unless clinical manifestations of the hypocalcemia are present.

Hypotensive drugs may be needed to control the blood pressure. We generally use oral Nepresol (1 to 3 mg./kg./day) or oral α-methyldopa (10 to 20 mg./kg./day). Reserpine is a difficult drug to use in an anuric patient.

It is better to avoid digitalis, a drug that is rarely indicated in acute renal failure in children. An overloaded circulation is generally responsible for asystole, and the first line in treatment is dialysis. A further point is that the use of digitalis complicates the conduct of dialysis because the varying serum potassium levels during dialysis increase the cardiac toxicity of the digitalis.

In general terms, any drug that is not absolutely essential should be avoided. Barbiturates are particularly contraindicated but Valium may be useful in controlling convulsions.

Diet

Theoretical Basis of Diet or Parenteral Alimentation in Acute Renal Failure

The fluid intake should be calculated each day to replace fluid loss on a basis of 500 ml./m.^{2} or 20 ml./kg., which represents the insensible loss. To this must be added gastrointestinal losses, urine output, and a fluid supplement of 10 ml./kg./24 hours for every degree of body temperature above 37.5°C. in children with fever. An exact balance should take into account the endogenous water formed in cell catabolism, an amount that cannot be measured. Thus, in addition to the calculated amounts, it is necessary to pay attention to the state of hydration of the patient and to changes in weight; weight should fall gradually or remain stable. The calculated fluid allowance may have to be adjusted in the light of the clinical findings.

A similar calculation applies to electrolyte intake; in cases of total anuria and in the absence of vomiting or diarrhea, the administration of sodium and potassium should theoretically be reduced to zero. The blood ionogram is virtually useless in this matter, although hyponatremia is usually evidence of relative

---

*Butterfly, ® Abbott Laboratories, North Chicago, Ill. 60064.

overhydration and is an indication to reduce fluid intake. Hypokalemia rarely needs correction in acute renal failure in view of the probability that the blood potassium level will rise. In practice (except for a purely synthetic diet that is acceptable only to small infants or when given by catheter), in larger children it is impossible to avoid a sodium intake of the order of 0.5 mEq./kg./day and a potassium intake of the order of 1 mEq./kg./day.

The ideal caloric intake is between 60 and 100 cal./kg., according to age, essentially in the form of carbohydrate and fat. Protein (of animal origin) in amounts ranging from 0.5 to 0.8 g./kg./day may be given. Supplemental vitamins B and C are indicated.

Carrying Out Dietary Recommendations

This is much easier in small infants than in older children. Small infants tolerate synthetic preparations, such as those indicated in Table 73.

Table 73. Food Allowance for 24 hours for an Infant with Acute Renal Failure*

	Quantity (g.)	Protein (g.)	Fats (g.)	Carbo-hydrate (g.)	Water (ml.)	Potassium	Sodium	Calories
Hyperprotidine	4 g.	3.6	–	–	–	3.6 mg.	1.6 mg.	14
Oil	17 g.	–	17	–	–	–	–	153
Glucose	65 g.	–	–	65	–	–	–	260
Water	100 ml.	–	–	–	100	–	–	–
Total	150 ml.	3.6	17	65	100	3.6 mg.	1.6 mg.	427

*This food allowance is for an infant weighing 4 kg. with insensible water loss estimated at 80 ml., urine output at 30 ml., stools at 20 ml., and vomitus at 20 ml. This preparation must be mixed in an electric mixer or blender. It can be given by mouth or by gastric catheter in five doses of 30 ml.

Table 74. Dietary Allowance for 24 Hours for a Child Weighing 12 kg. with Estimated Loss of 400 ml./24 Hours

	Quantity (g.)	Protein (g.)	Carbo-hydrate (g.)	Fat (g.)	Water (ml.)	Potassium (mEq.)	Sodium (mEq.)	Calories
Iced drink:								
Fresh cream	50 g.	1	–	15 g.	35	1.6	0.6	139
Sugar	25 g.	–	25 g.	–	–	–	–	100
Glucose	25 g.	–	25 g.	–	–	–	–	100
Lemon juice	20 ml.	–	2 g.	–	20	0.6	–	8
Gruel:								
Creamed rice	40 g.	–	32 g.	–	5	–	–	128
Water	350 ml.	–	–	–	350	–	–	
Sugar	40 g.	–	40 g.	–	–	–	–	160
Glucose	40 g.	–	40 g.	–	–	–	–	160
Pennac	40 g.	8.8	20 g.	8.8	–	6	2	195
Butter	30 g.	–	–	25	5	–	0.1	225
Total		9.8 g.	184 g.	48.8 g.	415 ml.	8.2	2.7	1215

Table 75. Example of Dietary Allowance for a Child Weighing 30 kg. with Acute Renal Failure (Water Loss Estimated at 600 ml./24 hours)

	Quantity (g.)	Protein (g.)	Carbohydrate (g.)	Fat (g.)	Water (g.)	Sodium (mEq.)	Potassium (mEq.)	Calories
Morning								
Whole Pennac	10	2.2	5.0	2.2	–	0.49	2.60	48
Glucose (or sugar)	15	–	15	–	–	–	–	60
Weak coffee or tea	80	–	–	–	80	–	–	–
2 Aminex biscuits	28	0.2	22	2.0	2.0	0.3	0.2	106
Butter	20	–	–	16.8	4	0.08	–	154
Jam	40	–	30	–	10	0.2	0.1	120
Midday								
Rice	50	3.8	40	–	100	0.08	1.5	174
Meat	50	9	–	5	36	1.5	3.7	76
Butter	25	–	–	21	4	0.1	–	189
Snacks								
Glucose	15	–	15	–	–	–	–	60
Coffee or tea	80	–	–	–	80	–	–	–
1 Aminex biscuit	14	0.1	11	1.0	1.0	0.15	0.10	53
Butter	5	–	–	4.1	–	0.08	–	36
Jam	20	–	15.0	–	5	0.10	0.05	60
Evening								
Protein-free pasta	50	–	44.5	–	150	0.47	0.12	176
Swiss cheese	35	3.5	14	3.8	26	0.65	0.79	52
Fresh cream	10	0.3	0.4	3.0	6.2	0.07	0.15	29
Sugar	20	–	20.0	–	–	–	–	80
Butter	15	–	–	12.6	2.4	0.14	–	108
Ices								
Midday and evening (see Table 74) (half ration)	60	0.5	25	7.5	27.5	0.3	1.1	173
Total		19.6 (79% animal protein)	254.3	79.0	534	4.3	7.8	1750–1800
Caloric distribution		4%	56%	40%				58–60 kg.

Table 76.   Mixture for Gastric Catheter Feeding*

	Quantity (g.)	Protein (g.)	Fat (g.)	Carbo-hydrate (g.)	Water (ml.)	Sodium	Potassium	Calories
Hyperprotidine	10	9.6	–	–	–	–	–	38
Oil	50	–	50	–	–	–	–	450
Glucose	170 g.	–	–	170	–	–	–	680
Maizena	10	–	–	8	–	–	–	32
Water	430	–	–	–	400 (after cooking)	–	–	
Total	500 ml.	9.6	50	178	400		Traces	1200

*This mixture is for a child weighing 12 to 15 kg. whose water loss is estimated at 400 ml. It is given in five lots of 100 ml. evenly distributed over the 24 hours (first mix the dry foods, maizena, hyperprotidine, and glucose, then add the water and oil, heat until boiling, and blend in a mixer).

More elaborate dietary preparations are necessary in older children. An example is given in Table 74; iced drinks and soup prepared for 24 hours are stored in a refrigerator and offered to the child five to eight times a day. This caloric ration corresponds to the needs of a child weighing 12 kg. In fact, a child will rarely take all of this allowance, especially for several days running. This type of diet can nevertheless be very valuable in the first days of anuria. In children weighing more then 12 kg., the problem is the same as in adults. For example, an older child weighing 30 kg. whose water requirements are estimated at 600 ml./24 hours might be given the diet indicated in Table 75.

In some cases (unconsciousness, refusal of food), it may be necessary to give the daily ration by gastric catheter. This procedure seems to be tolerated better if a constant infusion pump is used. A sample mixture for catheter feeding is given in Table 76.

Dialysis

In the treatment of acute renal failure, dialysis may be needed urgently to combat an immediate threat to life or as a preventive measure to guard against lesser threats to life and to keep the anuric patient in the best possible condition until diuresis returns.

Urgent indications include a serum potassium level above 7 mEq./liter, a severe metabolic acidosis with a serum bicarbonate level below 10 mEq./liter, an acute water overload with convulsions and a plasma sodium level below 120 mEq./liter, or, more often, a water and salt overload with hypertension, pulmonary edema, and a gallop rhythm. All these indications are entirely independent of the level of plasma urea nitrogen or the urinary output. In some cases, it may be necessary to combine dialysis with artificial ventilation, in which case the latter is begun before the dialysis because respiratory embarrassment may prove to be the last straw for an exhausted patient.

In fact, everything possible should be done to avoid such situations and to practice dialysis in a preventive fashion—in general terms, to maintain the blood urea nitrogen below 100 or 150 mg./100 ml. This may involve one peritoneal dialysis every 48 hours or two hemodialyses of 6 to 8 hours per week.

The technique most commonly used is peritoneal dialysis (see page 378). Hemodialysis is used only if peritoneal dialysis is not possible because of a recent intestinal operation or because of the existence of an abdominal drain. Peritonitis is not an absolute contraindication to peritoneal dialysis.

The Stage of Recovery of Renal Function

In a properly treated patient, maintained in negative water balance, and in whom the blood urea nitrogen has not been allowed to rise above 100 mg./100 ml., the massive urinary output that used to occur in the recovery stage before the proper use of dialysis no longer is observed. The graph of the daily urine output and the composition of the urine (osmolarity, U/P urea ratio) indicate the degree of functional recovery and the possibility of allowing longer intervals between dialyses (or even of abandoning dialysis altogether), while at the same time progressively increasing the diet. These data will also indicate the need to compensate for any possible electrolyte deficit. The biochemical and clinical monitoring of the patient must be just as close in this stage as in the initial anuric stage.

Conclusion

In conclusion, the diagnosis and treatment of acute renal failure present a certain number of difficulties that are best resolved in a specialized department of pediatric nephrology linked with all the other services that may be involved, such as radiology, pediatric urology, and specialized histopathology. Only in this way can the maximum reduction in the mortality rate of acute renal failure be achieved, a rate that today, in children, should be nil.

REFERENCES

1. Meadow, S. R., Cameron, J. S., Ogg, C. S., and Saxton, H. M.: Children referred for acute dialysis. Arch. Dis. Child. 46:221, 1971.
2. Merrill, J. P.: Acute renal failure. J.A.M.A. 211:289, 1970.
3. Wrong, O.: Management of the acute uremic emergency. Brit. Med. Bull. 27:97, 1971.

Chapter Two

CHRONIC RENAL FAILURE

PATHOPHYSIOLOGY

A great deal of work has been devoted in recent years to the physiopathology of chronic renal failure. We propose to consider here only two particularly fertile series of investigations, the first concerning the function of residual nephrons and the second the very old problem of uremic toxicity.

Function

According to Bricker's hypothesis, residual renal function derives from the remaining healthy nephrons in a kidney parenchyma in which all the diseased nephrons have ceased to function. In support of this hypothesis, the classic experimental protocol of unilateral pyelonephritis provides two pieces of evidence. The first is that the ratio of the majority of tubular functions to glomerular filtration remains very similar in both the healthy and the diseased sides. This is true for these ratios: renal blood flow/GFR, urinary volume (Uv) NH_4/GFR, Uv TA/GFR, TmPAH/GFR, Tm glucose/GFR, Tm PO_4/GFR, Uv urate/GFR.[1, 2] In other words, the glomerulotubular balance is preserved in experimental chronic renal failure. The next evidence is the demonstration of the homogeneous character of the population of residual nephrons in the diseased kidney; this is well seen in the titration curves of glucose, in which the TmG is reached directly, with "splay."[1, 2] There are obvious dangers in extrapolating these experimental results to human pathology, and a certain amount of evidence exists against the residual nephron hypothesis, including microdissection studies of kidneys from patients with renal failure, the existence of a splay in glucose titrations performed in patients whose glomerular clearance is less than 15 ml./min.,[6] and the common finding of a proportionally greater diminution of TmPAH than of inulin clearance in patients in terminal uremia. But, in general, Bricker's hypothesis seems valid, at least when no more than a certain degree of renal failure, corresponding to a glomerular clearance of 15 ml./min., is involved.

Regardless of the homogeneity of the residual nephrons, it is interesting to note that these nephrons are capable of quite satisfactory regulation until a very advanced stage of renal failure is reached. For example, sodium excretion adapts to some extent to intake; the fraction excreted may reach 30 to 35 per cent of the amount filtered (Figure 84), whereas in healthy persons the excreted fraction stays about 0.5 per cent. In contrast, sodium restriction is not followed by a corresponding reduction in urinary sodium output. The response

358

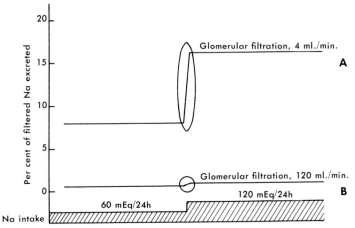

Figure 84. Modification of the excreted fraction of the sodium filtered after changing from a sodium intake of 60 mEq./day to 120 mEq./day. *A,* In a normal subject; *B,* in a patient with a glomerular filtration of 4 ml./min. (After Bricker and colleagues.)

of residual nephrons to parathormone is also to be emphasized. The tubular reabsorption of phosphate (TRP) is in fact lowered in proportion as renal failure progresses (Figure 85), parallel to the rising level of parathormone; conversely, diminished parathyroid activity elevates the TRP to a near normal level.[8]

In the area of acid-base balance, in addition to preservation of the Uv NH_4/GFR ratio, it may be recalled that the urinary pH is very often acid, around

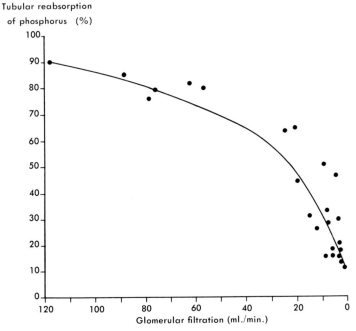

Figure 85. Changing tubular reabsorption of phosphorus with changes in glomerular filtration in chronic renal failure. (After Bricker and colleagues.)

5, in chronic uremia, which is good evidence of the adequate quality of the residual nephrons, as is the Tm of bicarbonates, which reaches levels higher than normal.[3, 7]

These functional features of the kidney in the stage of chronic uremia make it easier to understand the relative tolerance of renal failure and the fact that survival is possible to the point at which glomerular filtration is reduced to 3 or 4 per cent of its normal value.

Uremic Toxicity

Any discussion of the pathophysiology of renal failure would be incomplete without a comment on what is generally known as uremic toxicity. It has been known for a long time that the accumulation of urea probably plays no part in the symptomatology of chronic or terminal uremia. The blame has been placed on a number of substances — and the list is by no means complete — whose level in the blood rises parallel to the blood urea. These substances include certain organic acids, aliphatic amines such as dimethylamine and ethanolamine, phenols and their derivatives, indole compounds, guanidine and its derivatives guanidosuccinic acid and methylguanidine, and polypeptides with a molecular weight below 4000.[4] A correlation has already been established between the accumulation of some of these substances and particular enzyme or metabolic disturbances.[10] For example, guanidosuccinic acid inhibits transketolase and the enzyme activity that induces the formation of platelet factor 3 in the presence of ADP.[5]

A great deal remains to be learned about the pathophysiology of chronic uremia. In particular it is possible that defective growth in the uremic child in some part results from inhibitions at the subcellular level caused by the accumulation of some of the substances responsible for uremic toxicity.

INCIDENCE AND ETIOLOGY

When hemodialysis-transplantation programs were being developed, the first figures produced concerned the frequency of terminal renal failure in children, provisionally estimated to be in the region of one or two cases per million inhabitants per year.[14] In reality, there are no accurate statistics on this point. The same can be said for appraisals of various etiologic factors. The study presented in this chapter can add little to estimations of frequency but provides some interesting information about etiology.[13]

To determine the incidence of the different causes of renal failure in children, we have reviewed the records of all the patients admitted to the hospital or followed in the outpatient department of our service in the last 10 years. The only cases included were those children and adolescents under the age of 16 years whose creatinine clearance was permanently below 25 ml./min./1.73 m.^{2} and whose plasma urea nitrogen was 40 mg./100 ml. or more. We have found that 295 patients fulfill these requirements, and they can be divided almost equally into four groups according to causes (Table 77): the glomerular nephropathies, hereditary nephropathies, renal hypoplasia, and malformation of the urinary tract. Of the 295 patients, 193 are dead or are on a hemodialysis-transplantation program, 77 are alive and under regular surveillance, and 25 have been lost to follow-up.[12]

Table 77.　Causes of Chronic Renal Failure

Causes	Number of Cases	Percentage
Glomerular disease	71	24.1
Hereditary nephropathy	63	21.4
Renal hypoplasia	59	20
Malformation of urinary tract	62	21
Vascular nephropathy	29	9.8
Miscellaneous	11	3.7
Total	295	100

The number of cases reaching the stage of terminal renal failure is not the same in each of the etiologic groups. The glomerular diseases have the highest mortality rate. Table 78, which arranges the data in five-year age groups, gives the age at which the patients reached terminal renal failure. In this table it can be seen that the number of deaths is very similar in each five year age group, with a minimum occurring between the ages of 5 and 10 years and a maximum between the ages of 10 and 15 years. These figures are somewhat misleading because of changes in prognosis of certain diseases over the past 10 years; for example, nearly 50 per cent of the deaths between 0 and 5 years of age resulted from the hemolytic uremic syndrome, for which the mortality rate has dropped from 80 to 20 per cent with the development of new therapeutic methods.

Glomerular Nephropathy

Glomerular nephropathy is the chief cause of chronic renal failure and has the highest mortality rate at all age groups except the 0–5 year group, and even in this group a certain number of deaths from glomerular disease occur.

Table 78.　Age at Death or at Start of Maintenance Dialysis

	0–5 Years	5–10 Years	10–15 Years	15–20 Years	>20 Years	Total
Glomerular disease	6	12	23	19	5	65
Hereditary nephropathy	8	6	15	11	3	43
Renal hypoplasia	3	4	9	17	0	33
Urinary tract malformation	5	4	8	2	0	19
Vascular nephropathy	17	5	2	1	0	25
Miscellaneous	4	2	1	1	0	8
Total	43	33	58	51	8	193

Table 79.   Renal Failure Due to Glomerular Disease: Distribution of
Cases and Duration of Disease in the Different Histologic Types

Histologic Type	Number of Cases	Percentage	Number of Cases in Terminal Stage	Interval Between Onset of Renal Insufficiency and Terminal Failure
Segmental and focal hyalinization	16	22.5	15	1 year to 2 years 9 months
Systemic disease	14	19.7	14	1 month to 2 years
Membranoproliferative and lobular glomerulonephritis	10	14	8	4 months to 5 years 8 months
Endocapillary and extracapillary glomerulonephritis	9	12.6	7	1 month to 2 years
Nephrotic syndrome with minimal lesions	4	5.6	4*	1 month to 2 years*
Extramembranous glomerulonephritis	3	4.2	2	5 months to 3 years 4 months
Unclassifiable	8	11.2	8	
No histologic information	7	10.2	7	
Total	71	100	65	Average: 1 year 4 months

*One of these patients died of pulmonary artery thrombosis.

Of the different histologic types, the hyalinoses, systemic diseases, membranoproliferative glomerulonephritis, and endocapillary and extracapillary
glomerulonephritis are the most common causes (Table 79). There is on the
average an interval of four to five years between the onset of the disease and the
development of chronic renal failure, but once renal failure develops the progression to a terminal stage is much more rapid, usually one or two years.

Hereditary Nephropathies

These are an important cause of chronic renal failure in children, although
some are not seen until adult life. Nephronophthisis heads the list, followed by

Table 80.   Renal Failure Due to Hereditary Nephropathy:
Duration of Disease Related to Diagnosis

Diagnosis	Number of Cases	Percentage	Number of Cases in Terminal Stage	Interval Between Onset of Renal Insufficiency and Terminal Failure
Nephronophthisis	28	44.5	21	1 month to 5 years
Alport's syndrome	8	12.7	6	6 months to 4 years 4 months
Cystinosis	8	12.7	3	1 month to 3 years 8 months
Polycystic disease	6	9.6	4	3 months to 2 years 6 months
Oxalosis	5	8	5	4 months to 7 years
Congenital nephrotic syndrome	2	3.2	2	1 month to 3 months
Tubular acidosis	3	4.8	2	1 month to 8 years 6 months
Idiopathic hypokalemia	1	1.5	—	
Cystinuria	1	1.5	—	
Idiopathic hypercalcemia	1	1.5	—	
Total	63	100	43	Average: 1 year 10 months

Alport's syndrome and cystinosis, then by polycystic kidney and oxalosis (Table 80). Tubular acidosis is rarely involved. The only cases of congenital nephrotic syndrome in the list are in those patients who later died of renal failure.

The course follows the characteristic pattern of the disease, but once the stage of chronic renal failure is reached, except for the congenital nephrotic syndrome, the subsequent progression to terminal uremia is fairly uniform.

Renal Hypoplasia

Like the hereditary nephropathies, this group comprises causes of renal insufficiency that are relatively peculiar to childhood and adolescence. The most common forms are oligonephronic hypoplasia, segmental hypoplasia, and hypoplasia with dysplasia (Table 81). The course of the disease is generally slower than in other types of renal failure, and this is especially true of oligonephronic hypoplasia. The more rapid progression of segmental hypoplasia to a terminal stage is explained by the associated hypertension.

Malformations of the Urinary Tract

An important cause of chronic renal insufficiency, malformations of the urinary tract produce uropathies that progress to a terminal stage before the age of 20 years less often than the other groups. The most serious varieties are nearly always associated with renal hypoplasia and dysplasia, especially the obstructions of the lower urinary tract. Of the 62 patients with renal failure secondary to a malformation, 26 had massive bilateral reflux, 17 had urethral obstruction, 15 had bilateral megaureter without reflux, and four had various other anomalies.

Vascular Nephropathy

This is an etiologic group with a very high mortality rate that affected only young children in this series. The group included 18 cases of the hemolytic uremic syndrome, nine cases of cortical necrosis, one case of venous thrombosis, and one case of renal artery thrombosis.

It is difficult to speak of chronic renal failure in this context because the great majority of cases progress rapidly, in a matter of weeks, to death. In the

Table 81. Renal Failure Due to Hypoplasia: Distribution of Cases and Course in Relation to Type

Diagnosis	Number of Cases	Percentage	Number of Cases in Terminal Stage	Interval Between Onset of Renal Insufficiency and Terminal Failure
Oligonephronic hypoplasia	33	56	17	1 month to 10 years 8 months
Segmental hypoplasia	14	23.7	11	3 months to 5 years 6 months
Hypoplasia with dysplasia	9	15.3	2	5 months to 7 years
Poorly defined hypoplasia	3	5	3	1 month to 1 year 11 months
Total	59	100	33	Average: 3 years

future more prolonged survival times may be possible for this group owing to progress in the treatment of acute renal failure.

Conclusion

There are certain special features about the etiologic distribution of chronic renal failure in children, such as the incidence of hereditary nephropathy, of renal hypoplasia, and of vascular nephropathy, and the absence of interstitial nephropathy of infectious origin without associated malformation of the urinary tract. Certain causes, such as the hemolytic uremic syndrome and cortical necrosis, are peculiar to young children. Others, such as the hypoplasias and certain hereditary nephropathies, do not reach a terminal stage until the tenth or fifteenth year. However, after the age of five years, the glomerular diseases are the most important cause of renal failure with a consistently poor prognosis, in a proportion similar to that found in adults.

CLINICAL AND LABORATORY FEATURES

The clinical presentation, the laboratory findings, and the complications of chronic renal failure are the same in children as in adults. The special feature of chronic renal failure in children is that it occurs in an individual in the process of development, hence it affects maturation and growth, and these in turn affect the renal symptomatology. Furthermore, it is more common in children to find certain nephropathies originally presenting with signs of tubular disorder that may precede by a long time and modify the clinical features of overall renal failure.

Definition

It is difficult, if not impossible, to define the level of renal function below which one can speak of renal failure. Clinical symptoms may be almost completely absent, or at least not come to attention, until the stage of major terminal complications. Conversely, certain consequences of glomerular insufficiency, such as parathyroid stimulation, occur very early even when there is little retention of nitrogenous waste products.

It is convenient to distinguish three levels of renal insufficiency according to the degree of change in glomerular filtration. The first degree (glomerular clearance between 15 and 30 ml./min./1.73 m.^{2}) includes a potentiality for long-term complications that justifies regular surveillance and certain therapeutic measures. The second degree (glomerular clearance between 5 and 15 ml./min./1.73 m.^{2}) generally corresponds to the development of a concentration defect that marks a turning point in the course of the disease and requires additional restrictive measures. The third degree (glomerular clearance below 5 ml./min./1.73 m.^{2}), currently described as terminal renal failure, exposes the child to the risk of serious complications and makes it necessary for him to be treated by dialysis and transplantation.

In most cases of chronic renal failure in children, the loss of proximal tubular function parallels the failing glomerular filtration (see Chapter 1, Part

IV). However, this is not always so, and a glomerulotubular imbalance may be found. This imbalance is obviously important in the nephropathies such as cystinosis that primarily affect the tubules. In the extreme case of cystinosis, there is a chronic tubular insufficiency characterized by defective reabsorption of electrolytes, water, and various other substances, responsible for certain long-term complications. With reduction in glomerular filtration, the tubular symptomatology persists, but the urinary losses diminish progressively, and, in the terminal stage—counter to the initial situation—there may be deficient elimination of substances or elements that earlier had to be supplemented in this type of patient. Glomerulotubular balance is thus of fundamental importance in the nephropathies that affect the tubules, because of the progressive narrowing of the margin between the risks of deficiency and the risks of overloading.

Clinical Features

Chronic renal failure may be latent and may even reach the terminal stage before being recognized. It is, however, rare for this to happen without the development of some symptoms either of the causal disease or the renal failure syndrome.

Anorexia, a varying degree of polyuria-polydipsia, gastric disorders, and a certain pallor with a yellowish tint to the skin are usually seen as soon as the corrected glomerular filtration rate drops below 25 to 30 ml./min./1.73 m.^{2} The fact that growth is defective must be emphasized. It is well known that chronic renal failure affects development and may slow or even completely halt growth. In practice, it is difficult to predict the severity of the growth defect for a given level of renal failure. In other words, there is no close parallel between the growth defect and the fall in glomerular filtration rate; the growth defect is the consequence of a certain number of biologic abnormalities that are not all identified, and the degree and conjunction of these abnormalities vary from case to case. They are studied in Chapter 3, Part IV.

In adolescents, there is nearly always an apparent delay in pubertal development. In fact, in both the uremic and the normal child, puberty develops parallel to the bone age, which may lag behind the real age by several years if the renal insufficiency has been present for a long time. Hence, the retardation of puberty is only apparent and is in fact related to the delay in maturation.

General Evolutive Characteristics Peculiar to Children

There are some special features in the natural history of chronic renal failure in children. Although these are not constant, it is important, in appreciating the evolution of chronic nephropathy in children and the action of certain dietetic and therapeutic measures, to take into account the possibility of an apparent spontaneous improvement that may occur between six and 30 months, or conversely an apparent deterioration that is closely related to increase in weight, height, and surface area—that is to say, to excretory needs.

Spontaneous Improvement

It is not uncommon during the second or third year to find spontaneous improvement in a hitherto more serious nephropathy. There are many possible explanations. The most obvious, and this is seen very clearly in nephrogenic diabetes insipidus, is maturation of drinking habits and the development of an active thirst that makes it easier to compensate for the problems resulting from defective urine concentration. It is also possible that, when the nephropathy is partial, the normal or compensatory functional maturation of the intact nephrons may be responsible for a certain degree of true recovery in the early years of life.

Increased Excretory Needs

Conversely, it is much more certain that, in the presence of diseased kidneys, body growth is responsible for a gradual increase in the excretory needs of the organism. It is recognized that these needs increase with weight and surface area. Although the absolute renal insufficiency may continue to be the same in a nephropathy that remains in a constant state, there is increasing failure to meet the excretory requirements. Under these conditions, the renal insufficiency increases in terms of symptoms, a fact that is well demonstrated by clearance studies. The crude clearances remain the same while the clearances corrected for surface area diminish.

Biochemical Disorders

Nitrogen Retention

The rise in plasma urea nitrogen and plasma creatinine levels is used as a routine index of renal insufficiency. It should be noted, however, that in children there are often significant discrepancies between the plasma levels of these two substances. In particular, the plasma urea nitrogen level should be interpreted with caution. The plasma urea content is in fact the resultant of many factors, including the composition of the diet, the state of cell anabolism or catabolism, the functional environment of the kidney, the availability of water, and state of the kidney itself. The pathologic significance of nitrogen retention has already been considered (page 360).

Water Metabolism

In the initial stage of the renal insufficiency, the principal feature is the defect in concentration. This is more marked when the disease affects predominantly the tubulo-interstitial tissue (nephronophthisis, uropathy with chronic pyelonephritis), in which case it may be responsible for considerable polyuria-polydipsia. The development of a major defect in concentration marks a turning point in the course of the disease, because it implies a considerable reduction in the nephron mass and introduces the risk of water intoxication. Water intoxication is one of the most serious metabolic complications of chronic renal failure, being responsible for hypertension and pulmonary edema or neurologic disorders caused by cerebral edema. Fortunately, these complications can often be reversed by dialysis.

Sodium and Potassium Metabolism

Put very simply, it can be said that the greater the degree of chronic renal failure, the less able the kidney is to achieve rapid re-equilibration of water and electrolytes. This explains the tendency to hyperkalemia and also to sodium retention, which causes expansion of the extracellular fluid and hypertension.

This inability to restore the balance works also in the opposite direction, especially for sodium, whose fractional reabsorption is diminished to a greater or lesser degree in every type of chronic renal failure. For this reason, sodium intake must be within both limits of tolerance to avoid the risks of either overloading or excessive loss. Complications from excessive loss of sodium can be caused by ill-advised sodium restriction, leading to aggravation of the renal failure, with nausea, vomiting, loss of weight, elevation of plasma urea nitrogen level and plasma creatinine, hypochloremia, and hyponatremia. The earlier status can be restored by an appropriate intake of NaCl. Hyponatremia is not always evidence of sodium depletion; it may result from water intoxication and may camouflage sodium excess. Careful study of the recent course of the disease, of diet, and of changes in weight are very important in evaluating the condition of the uremic child.

It is important to remember that, when kidney function is depressed, the plasma potassium level is extremely sensitive to variations in dietary intake. Food rich in potassium can cause a very dangerous hyperkalemia, which often precipitates sudden death in uremic patients. Conversely, the careless use of ion exchange resins may cause hypokalemia.

Hydrogen Ion Metabolism

Here again, because of the reduction in nephron mass, the kidney has a very limited ability to maintain hydrogen ion balance. The daily dietary intake of hydrogen ions is of the order of 50 mEq./m.^{2} (0.7mEq. for every gram of protein). Thus there is, in chronic renal failure, a tendency to chronic metabolic acidosis that is controlled to some extent by the intracellular buffers, especially the bone buffers. Often a significant loss of bicarbonate in the urine occurs, and this may aggravate considerably the tendency to acidosis. We have been able to verify this point in several children with renal failure by titration of the bicarbonates, which revealed a very obvious lowering of the excretion threshold in direct proportion to the degree of tubular damage. On the other hand, patients with renal failure are not able to excrete an alkaline load, as is very evident during bicarbonate titration tests with Tm studies. With the same bicarbonate load, patients in renal failure remain alkalotic for much longer and their Tm of reabsorption is abnormally elevated, a situation that remains difficult to understand in the context of tubular physiology.[16]

Calcium, Phosphorus, and Magnesium Metabolism

The defect in phosphorus and calcium metabolism is probably one of the earliest disorders in chronic renal failure. The long-term result is an osteodystrophy, but in most cases this does not develop for five or 10 years. These facts are discussed further at a later stage. The blood phosphorus level is elevated in proportion to the decrease in the glomerular filtration rate. The blood calcium level may be normal, but in most cases it is low unless treated. The raised blood phosphorus is probably partly responsible for the low blood calcium level. The hypocalcemia may be very marked, as low as 5 or 6 mg./100 ml., especially in the terminal stages. It is generally very difficult to correct. There may be tetany or convulsions, but the hypocalcemia is usually latent, probably because of the protective role of the acidosis.

The serum magnesium is generally elevated in chronic renal failure, but there may be simultaneous magnesium depletion, especially in situations in which sodium loss occurs, and this may cause intense asthenia and neurologic disorders.[20]

Metabolic and Endocrine Disorders

The diminished tolerance of carbohydrate is attributed to a dialysable factor that inhibits the action of insulin.[19] The secretion of insulin itself is not affected by the renal failure.

Elevation of the plasma triglycerides with a diminished cholesterol level is frequently observed in uremic patients, and their serum is often milky.[15] This disorder has been reproduced in experimental animals by the use of methylguanidine. It is difficult to know what, if any, is the significance of these changes, and they do not appear to have any direct clinical effect.

Apart from the consequences of a very unbalanced diet and the general slowing of anabolism, there are no significant changes in protein metabolism. The total plasma proteins and the individual protein fractions may be affected by gross proteinuria, but any such effect is generally diminished by the onset of renal failure. On the other hand, the blood level of certain individual amino acids undergoes a virtually constant change in chronic renal failure: there are decreases in the amounts of alanine, ornithine, tyrosine, histidine, methionine, and leucine, and increases in the amounts of citrulline, proline, cysteine, phenylalanine, and aspartic acid.[17, 24]

No evidence has yet been produced of any gross change in hormone regulation. We have always found the protein-bound iodine (PBI) and the plasma cortisol levels to be normal in children with chronic renal failure. Growth hormone has been studied in greater depth. The adult with chronic renal failure is reported to have an elevated fasting level of growth hormone and possibly an abnormal regulation of secretion of the hormone, because a glucose load does not produce a rapid fall in the level of HGH, as it does in the normal subject.[23] In adults given a glucose load, there is never secondary elevation of the growth hormone level, although stress apparently continues to be an effective stimulant.[20]

In children, the response obtained after hypoglycemic stimulation seems to be greater when glomerular clearance is between 5 and 20 ml./min. than in patients with terminal renal failure maintained on hemodialysis. Certainly the growth hormone levels found in the latter group are higher than those found in hypophyseal dwarfism. Study of the peak physiologic secretion of growth hormone in the first two hours of sleep has revealed no difference between normal children and children with renal failure (Figure 86). Hence,

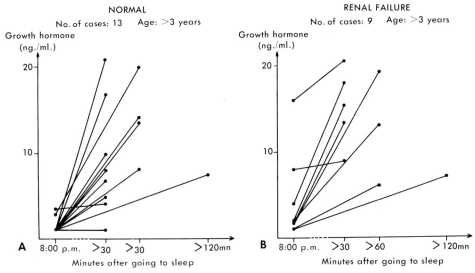

Figure 86. Peak secretion of growth hormone during the first hours of sleep. *A*, Normal children. *B*, Uremic children. The figures are comparable. The time is counted from the clinical onset of sleep; only the highest value of growth hormone has been plotted for each subject.

there is little evidence that defective growth is traceable to inadequate secretion of growth hormone.

Where the sex hormones are concerned, the plasma levels of LH and of FSH are within the limits of normal when viewed as a function of maturation age (Table 82). Plasma testosterone levels, on the other hand, are low in relation to the LH level,[18] as we have confirmed in several children.

Table 82. LH and FSH Values in Uremic Children Treated
by Maintenance Dialysis

Case Number	Sex	Real Age (years)	Bone Age (years)	Puberty Stage	LH‡ (mU./ml.)	FSH§ (mU./ml.)
1	F	5	3 years 6 months	P_1	3.75	2.5
2	F	10 years 9 months	7	P_1	3.0	3.3
3	F	11 years 11 months	8	P_1	7.5	4.6
4	F	11	10	P_1	3.5	2.3
5	F	14 years 9 months	10	P_2	8.5	4.1
6	F	11 years 6 months	10	P_2	5.75	2.8
7*	F	15 years 9 months	16	P_5	34.5	4.1
8	M	5	5	P_1	5	2.6
9	M	16 years 6 months	12 years 6 months	P_1	4.5	2.6
10	M	14 years 11 months	14 years 6 months	P_1	6.0	4.3
11†	M	13	10	P_2	3.25	2.3
12	M	13 years 6 months	13 years 6 months	P_2	6.25	3.6
13	M	16	13	P_2	12	3.6

*Ovulatory peak.
†Premature adrenarche.
‡LH is expressed in mU./ml. or 68/40 MRC.
§FSH is expressed in mU./ml. or 68/39 MRC.
Data courtesy of Dr. P. C. Sizonenko, Pediatric Clinic, Geneva, Switzerland.

Complications in the Terminal Stages

Anemia

This is a constant feature of renal failure and generally appears when glomerular clearance drops below 15 to 25 ml./min./1.73 m.² The degree of anemia varies from case to case, being particularly severe in nephronophthisis, for example. The anemia is normochromic or hypochromic and goes hand in hand with an erythroblastopenia. It is attributed to erythropoietin deficiency. Another factor in the etiology of anemia is chronic hemolysis, as shown by the significant shortening of red cell survival time. This hemolysis is of extracorpuscular origin. Other factors, such as folic acid deficiency associated with excessive dietary restriction and apparently accentuated by defective intestinal absorption, may also be involved. So far as is possible, the anemia of chronic renal failure should not be treated. Transfusions have only a transient effect, and moreover they have the disadvantage of inhibiting any remaining bone marrow activity.

Disorders of Hemostasis

These appear only in the terminal stage, when glomerular clearance is 5 ml./min. or less, and they may then be responsible for bleeding under the skin or mucous membranes or even for serious hemorrhage, especially from the gastrointestinal tract. This hemorrhagic tendency results from disordered platelet function. In severe uremia, platelet factor III is always diminished, as are platelet adhesiveness and ability to aggregate. The principal cause of these platelet defects is apparently the inhibitory action of guanidosuccinic acid. The disorders disappear after dialysis.

Gastric Disturbances

Anorexia, continuous nausea, and vomiting are constant features of terminal uremia. The classic uremic parotitis is now rare. These manifestations of uremic toxicity disappear after dialysis and may be controlled to some extent by a low-protein diet.

Hypertension

Hypertension is a common feature of terminal uremia. It generally results from an excessive positive water and sodium balance, but may also be due to excessive production of renin.

Uremic Pericarditis

This is a sinister complication and a harbinger of death unless the patient is treated by intensive dialysis. There is often intolerable precordial pain at the onset, but the condition may be latent. A pericardial friction rub is nearly always audible. Radiographic screening of the chest reveals an enlarged heart shadow with diminished cardiac movement. The electrocardiographic signs are less reliable.

The pathogenesis of this complication is not clear. It seems to be more common in cases in which there is hypertension, with a water and salt overload, and it develops parallel to the nitrogen retention.

Convulsions and EEG Changes

It seems that convulsive crises are particularly common in children suffering from terminal renal failure who are treated with maintenance hemodialysis.

We have found recurrent crises in a quarter of our patients. These attacks have always disappeared on treatment with phenobarbital and diazepam given between, and especially during, hemodialysis sessions. The EEG is abnormal in every patient with convulsions, but it is also abnormal in a large number of children who have never had a crisis. Definite changes in the EEG may be an indication for prophylactic treatment with phenobarbital.

Peripheral Nerve Disorders

These rarely occur as a complication of chronic uremia in children, although nerve conduction studies and electromyography do reveal electrical changes. The pathogenesis of uremic neuropathy is still poorly understood. Nutritional factors and the toxicity of certain nitrogenous residues are probably important. This neuropathy must be distinguished from the toxic polyneuritides to which these patients are prone, and drugs such as nitrofurantoin should not be used.

CONSERVATIVE TREATMENT

Conservative management comprises all the therapeutic measures, essentially dietetic, that are instituted at a certain stage of reduced glomerular filtration and in general before the stage of terminal renal failure, when the only worthwhile treatment is dialysis and transplantation.

The principles of this conservative treatment are the same whatever the cause of the renal failure. They are based on the need to diminish nitrogenous waste as far as possible and to maintain water, salt, and acid-base balances.

In children, the orientation of this conservative treatment has been changed significantly since the introduction of effective treatment for terminal renal failure. Because excretory needs are roughly proportional to body mass, there was formerly no point in encouraging growth in children with renal failure if this was considered from the simple viewpoint of length of survival. Nowadays, if there is any possibility that the child may ultimately be placed on a dialysis-transplantation program, it is important to achieve the best possible growth before the child goes on the program.

When necessary, it should be possible to achieve prolonged survival with very reduced kidney function by the use of a synthetic diet calculated exactly to provide only those elements that are strictly necessary.

Such a diet should include an adequate caloric intake in the form of carbohydrate and fat, essential amino acids in just the right amount for turnover and perhaps for growth, water and electrolyte intake corresponding exactly to the sum of renal and extrarenal losses, and also the essential vitamins and trace elements.

It is obviously impossible to maintain this type of diet for more than a few days, except perhaps in infants, but it should be possible at least to approach the ideal.

Caloric Requirements

There is evidence of the fundamental importance of adequate caloric intake if growth is to be maintained in a child with chronic renal failure.

Accurate calculation of food intake reveals a definite caloric deficiency in most patients with renal insufficiency, which stems from the anorexia, the gastric disorders, and the dietary restrictions imposed. Recent studies have shown that there is a definite relationship between restoration of growth and increased caloric intake in children treated by maintenance dialysis.[30]

The optimal needs, which vary with age, range from 55 to 110 calories/kg. (Table 83). The requirements are met by carbohydrates and fats, the former taken as glucose, sugar, jam, honey, protein-free bread, and high-calorie glucose polymers, and the fats as butter, oil, and fresh cream.

There is no limit to the amount of these products that may be taken, provided they do not contain more than the allotted amounts of mineral salts.

Protein Intake

It is very difficult in practice to limit protein intake to small amounts of essential amino acids for any length of time and, for this reason, various adaptations have been suggested and are currently used by adult patients.[26, 27] The protein intake is limited to 0.2 or 0.3 g./kg./day, and the only proteins used are animal proteins of high biological value with a well-balanced content of essential amino acids.

It is difficult to get patients to accept these diets that contain virtually no vegetables and no bread, although bread can be replaced by a substitute made of protein-free flour. Many authors stress the improved sense of well-being in patients who accept this type of diet, but there is still inadequate information on long-term and short-term benefits.

In children there is little information about the application of very low-protein diets. Such impressions as can be drawn from a few isolated cases treated in this way for one or two years are distinctly unfavorable because of the total cessation of growth. A further point is that it is even more difficult to get a diet of this type accepted by children than by adults. Thus, it seems preferable in practice to prescribe a less severe diet, providing 0.6 to 1.5 g./kg./day of protein, depending on age and the degree of renal insufficiency (Table 83), and at least 70 per cent of this protein should be animal protein.

Limitation of protein reduces the intake of hydrogen ions (7 mEq. for every 10 g. of protein), because the sulfated amino acids are the principal source of hydrogen ions.

The degree of renal failure below which it is desirable to introduce dietary limitation corresponds to a plasma urea nitrogen level of about 75 mg./100 ml., or a glomerular clearance in the region of 20 ml./min./1.73 m.^{2} With the introduction of a low-protein diet, the plasma urea nitrogen level decreases, but the creatinine level remains unchanged.

Table 83. Recommended Calorie and Protein Allowance in Children with Chronic Renal Failure

Age (years)	Weight (kg.)	Calories*		Proteins†								
				Glomerular Filtration (ml./min./1.73 m²)								
				20 to 40		10 to 20		10 to 5		<5	
		Cal./kg.	Cal./day	g./kg.	g./day†	g./kg.	g./day	g./kg.	g./day	g./kg.	g./day
0–2 months	4	120	480	2.2	8.8	1.7	6.8	1.5	6	1.3	5.2
2–6 months	7	110	770	2.0	14.0	1.6	11.2	1.4	9.8	1.2	8.4
6 months–1 year	9	100	900	1.8	16.2	1.4	13.6	1.2	10.8	1.0	9.0
1–2	12	91	1100	2.0	24	1.6	19	1.4	16	1.2	14
2–3	14	85	1200	1.7	24	1.3	19	1.1	16	1.0	14
3–4	16	87	1400	1.8	30	1.4	24	1.2	21	1.1	18
4–6	19	84	1600	1.5	30	1.2	24	1.0	21	0.9	18
6–8	23	86	2000	1.5	36	1.2	28	1.0	25	0.9	21
8–10	28	78	2200	1.4	40	1.1	32	0.9	28	0.8	24
Boys											
10–12	35	71	2500	1.3	45	1.0	36	0.9	31	0.7	27
12–14	43	62	2700	1.1	50	0.8	40	0.7	35	0.6	30
14–18	59	50	3000	1.0	60	0.8	48	0.7	42	0.6	36
Girls											
10–12	35	64	2250	1.4	50	1.1	40	0.9	35	0.8	30
12–14	44	52	2300	1.1	50	0.9	40	0.7	35	0.6	30
14–16	52	46	2400	1.0	55	0.8	44	0.7	37	0.6	33
16–18	54	42	2300	1.0	55	0.8	44	0.7	37	0.6	33

*According to M.R.C. recommendations for normal children.[29]
†These amounts relate to proteins of high biologic value, at least 70 per cent being of animal origin.

Water and Electrolytes

Depending on the degree of renal insufficiency and the etiology, water and electrolyte needs can vary greatly.

So long as there is no serious concentration defect, the child should be allowed to adjust his water intake according to his own thirst; this will depend in part on the osmotic load to be excreted and on the concentrating ability of the kidney. Excessive limitation of water intake leads to chronic dehydration and functional exacerbation of the renal failure.

When the renal insufficiency deteriorates to a glomerular clearance of 10 ml./min./1.73 m.^{2} or less, there is a risk of water intoxication, and fluid intake should be limited in proportion to the diminished urine output. Not more than 50 or 100 ml. of water should be taken at any one time, and the best guides are thirst and the weight chart, which is a very valuable diagnostic aid in this situation.

The problem of sodium intake must take into account two opposite phenomena. The first is the limitation of sodium excretion caused by severe renal failure with a progressive reduction in the number of functioning nephrons, and the second is the sodium loss — sometimes very considerable — that may occur in certain tubulo-interstitial diseases, and which exists in every case of severe renal failure if the patient is placed on a salt-free diet.

As a general rule, the diet of the uremic patient should include moderate sodium restriction (1 mEq./kg./day). More severe restriction may be needed if there is hypertension or obvious inflation of the extracellular fluid.

Conversely, more salt must be given to patients with a salt-losing tubulo-interstitial nephropathy, but the allowance will rarely be more than 5 or 6 mEq./kg./day. Even in this situation, care must be taken to avoid the risks of overload. In fact, in the terminal stages, the plasma urea nitrogen level may still be diminished by giving more salt but only at the cost of dangerous expansion of the extracellular fluid; therefore the plasma urea nitrogen level is of no value in deciding the amount of sodium that should be allowed.

Calculation of sodium intake must take into account certain drugs, some of which may contain unexpectedly large amounts of sodium — for example, effervescent calcium tablets* and sodium penicillin (1.7 mEq. per million units).

Hyperkalemia is a permanent threat in all cases of advanced renal failure. With a glomerular clearance greater than 10 ml./min./1.73 m.,^{2} all that is needed is to eliminate from the diet foods with a very high potassium content. With a glomerular clearance below 10 ml./min./1.73 m.,^{2} potassium intake should be limited to between 1.5 and 2 mEq./kg./day, and, in this regard, it is helpful to provide the parents with a table of potassium equivalents of various foods. If the plasma potassium level rises above 5.5 mEq./liter, an exchange resin should be prescribed in doses of 0.5 to 1 g./kg./day. One gram of resin removes 1 mEq. of potassium in exchange for 1 mEq. of sodium or calcium, depending on the type of resin. The blood potassium level must be monitored regularly and the dose of resin adjusted accordingly to avoid potassium depletion.

Acid-Base Balance

There is rarely any need for special therapy to control acid-base balance in the long-term treatment of chronic renal failure. Such treatment is needed only in special cases, such as obstructive uropathy with pyelonephritis or certain

---

*Calcium Forte Sandoz ®: 13 mEq. of Na per tablet.

chronic tubulo-interstitial diseases in which a buffer such as sodium bicarbonate is required in doses of 0.5 to 1 mEq/kg./day to compensate for a gross defect in the excretion of hydrogen ions or a loss of bicarbonate. But, in general, reduction of protein intake is enough to prevent the development of metabolic acidosis.

Calcium, Phosphorus, Vitamin D

Because of the limitation of dairy products, a calcium supplement is necessary. The amount of this supplement must take into account the defective intestinal absorption of calcium that occurs in all cases of renal failure. The current practice is to give a dose of the order of 500 to 1000 mg./m.^{2}/day of elemental calcium.

Vitamin D must also be given. The dose (5000 to 50,000 units/day) depends on the severity of the renal insufficiency and the presence of any bone lesions or serious hypocalcemia.

Although there is no definite evidence, it seems desirable to avoid a permanent elevation of the blood phosphorus levels by prescribing aluminum hydroxide. The dose is adapted to maintain the plasma phosphorus level between 4 and 5 mg./100 ml., but it is important to avoid phosphorus depletion, which may have serious consequences.[28] This prescription has the advantage of ensuring correction of the acidosis at the same time.

Hypertension

Hypertension may result from excess of water or salt or both, or from hyper-reninemia.

In the first instance, sodium and possibly even water must be restricted. In the second, hypotensive drugs such as α-methyldopa in doses of 10 to 20 mg./kg. are necessary. Larger doses of hypotensive agents may be required.

Contrary to the opinion that prevailed a few years ago, it is essential to treat hypertension even when the renal failure is advanced. Deterioration of kidney function is retarded by controlling the hypertension.[31]

Anemia

This is a constant feature of severe renal failure, but it is seldom obvious until the glomerular filtration rate falls below 10 ml./min./1.73 m.^{2} There is no effective treatment.

Iron should not be given unless there is proved iron deficiency. Vitamin B_{12} and folic acid are ineffective. Transfusion should be avoided; any benefit is only transient and any remaining bone marrow activity is depressed. Transfusion may even be dangerous, producing hyperkalemia and overloading the circulation in the short run, and running the risk of sensitization to histocompatibility (HLA) antigens that might imperil any subsequent kidney transplant in the long run. It is preferable to avoid transfusing any patient with renal failure if the hemoglobin level is 5 g./liter or more.

Drugs

It is essential to take the renal failure into account. The problem arises chiefly with certain antibiotics but also with some other drugs that are excreted mainly by the kidneys, so that there is a risk of reaching dangerous plasma levels. Table 84 gives a list of the principal drugs that are excreted by the kidneys and the time interval between standard doses as a function of the renal failure. This table is only a very approximate guide, and whenever it is necessary to prescribe drugs that could reach a dangerous plasma level, it is mandatory to measure the plasma levels of the drug every two or three days and alter the dosage accordingly, especially when the renal failure is advanced. Table 85 provides a list of drugs that must be avoided entirely in cases of renal failure.

The attitude to vaccination has changed in recent years. Chronic uremia is not in itself a contraindication and, in principle, in view of the prolonged survival that may be expected with dialysis and transplantation programs, vaccination should not be refused. Oral poliomyelitis vaccination and BCG are perfectly safe.

Although a certain prudence is indicated in the use of parenteral vaccinations in patients with glomerular disease (even though there is not at present the slightest proof of real danger), such vaccinations are completely safe in all other kidney disorders.

Table 84. Drugs Excreted Wholly or Partially by the Kidney
(Time Interval in Hours Between Two Standard Doses of the Drug)*†

	Glomerular Filtration			
	Normal	50–80 ml.	10–50 ml.	<10 ml.
Cephaloridine	6	6	12	24–36
Cephalothin*	6	6	6	8–12
Colistin	12	24	36–60	60–90
Gentamycin	8	12	24	48
Isoniazid*	8	8	12	24
Kanamycin	8	24	72	96
Lincomycin*	6	6	6	12
Penicillin G*	8	8	8	12
Synthetic Penicillins*	6	6	6	12
Streptomycin	12	24	72	96
Tetracycline*	6	12	48	72
Vancomycin	6	72	240	240
Aspirin*	4	4	6	12
Phenobarbital	8	8	12	24
Digoxin*	12	24	36	48
Digitoxin*	24	24	36	72
Allopurinol	8	8	12	24
Azathioprine	12	12	18	24
Methotrexate	24	24	36	48

*Asterisk marks those drugs that are excreted only partially.
†After Bennett, W. M., et al.: A practical guide to drug usage in adult patients with impaired renal function. J.A.M.A. 214:1468, 1970. Copyright 1968, American Medical Association.

Table 85. Drugs to be Avoided in Cases of Renal Failure
(Glomerular Filtration Rate Less Than 5 ml./min./1.73 m.²)*

Antimicrobial agents	Nitrofurantoin Mandelamine
Analgesic	Phenylbutazone
Diuretics	Mercurials Spironolactone Triamterene ⎫ Ethacrynic acid ⎬ if filtration rate is <10 ml./min./1.73 m.² Thiazide ⎭
Hypoglycemic agents	Chlorpropamide
Anti-gout	Probenecid

*After Bennett, W. M., *et al.:* A practical guide to drug usage in adult patients with impaired renal function. J.A.M.A. *214*:1468, 1970. Copyright 1968, American Medical Association.

General Considerations on the Mode of Life of the Uremic Child

The life style of the child with chronic renal failure should be as close to normal as possible. There is no reason to forbid physical exercise or swimming except in cases of hypertension, where a sudden exposure to cold or violent effort might cause a rise in blood pressure. School attendance should not be interrupted by unnecessary hospitalization. The laboratory supervision of a uremic child can be managed perfectly well on an outpatient basis at intervals depending on the degree of renal insufficiency. The object is not to deny the existence of the disease but to avoid any procedures that are not absolutely necessary or which might have an unfavorable psychological impact. The parents must be warned of the dangers of an excessively protective attitude.

When circumstances demand, the parents of a uremic child should be alerted to the fact that sooner or later conservative measures will no longer be adequate, but they should be told that when that stage comes, it may be possible to consider dialysis and transplantation. The child's own questions should be answered as accurately as possible.

Conclusion

Children with serious renal insufficiency may be maintained in an acceptable state, sometimes for many years, by ordinary conservative means, including dietetic measures and simple drug therapy. This is especially true in certain types of renal insufficiency resulting, for example, from renal hypoplasia or malformation of the urinary tract, conditions that may progress very slowly. Diet has a fundamental importance in this treatment and should be worked out very accurately, taking into account maximal tolerance and the minimal requirements for growth. Severe protein restriction is not suitable for children, who must receive an adequate caloric ration. Progress in this field will come from a better estimate of the minimal requirements for growth, and perhaps from the development of special foods that are adapted to the problems of renal insufficiency and yet are acceptable over long periods.

DIALYSIS AND KIDNEY TRANSPLANTATION

In children, two techniques of maintenance dialysis are used, peritoneal dialysis and hemodialysis.

Peritoneal dialysis is particularly valuable in infants and for certain special indications; it is being studied in many centers.[34] The use of maintenance hemodialysis is expanding rapidly and has been the subject of many reports in the United States[35, 36, 38, 41, 42] and Europe.[32, 33, 43, 44, 49] Several publications have been devoted to the pediatric problems of kidney transplantation.[37, 39, 40, 42, 45, 50] At the present time, maintenance hemodialysis and transplantation are linked in the treatment of chronic uremia and cannot be considered separately.

Indications and Contraindications for Treatment by Maintenance Hemodialysis and Transplantation

Indications

Maintenance hemodialysis becomes necessary when conservative treatment is no longer adequate, and in general this occurs when the blood urea nitrogen level is greater than 100 mg. per 100 ml. and the creatinine clearance below 5 ml./min./1.73 m.^{2} However, these figures must be verified repeatedly, and it must be shown that they are not the result of some possible functional deterioration, owing perhaps to sodium loss, dehydration, acidosis, or infection.

Contraindications

Malformations of the lower urinary tract, general diseases that might lead to reproduction of the nephropathy in the transplanted kidney, and encephalopathy have been regarded as basic contraindications, but, of these, only encephalopathy is a true contraindication. In fact, malformations of the lower urinary tract, such as vesical exstrophy, neurogenic bladder, or some untreatable abnormality of the urethra, no longer are absolute contraindications to transplantation. Kidney transplantation with diversion of the ureter to the skin by an ileal loop has been performed successfully. The risk that some general disease may affect the grafted kidney is never a contraindication to transplantation, because, at present, rejection phenomena cause graft destruction within a period of five years—that is to say, in general, before the reproduction of the causal disease in the graft would disturb its functioning. In the case of glomerulopathies of immune origin, there is reason to think that the immunodepressive and steroid therapy required to maintain the graft may to a greater or lesser extent prevent reproduction of the original disease in the grafted kidney. It is already clear that certain metabolic nephropathies can be treated satisfactorily by kidney transplantation. The only remaining medical contraindication, rightly or wrongly, is the presence of encephalopathy with mental retardation.

Transplantation technically is possible at any age, but success is very rare in patients under the age of 2 years. Hemodialysis in very small children is possible with modern equipment but, primarily because of vascular factors, the treatment of children weighing less than 10 kg. remains a doubtful proposition.

Technical Aspects of Maintenance Hemodialysis in Children

Our comments are based on experience with more than 2500 dialyses in 22 children, the youngest being 20 months old and weighing 8 kg.

Access to Vessels

The first problem is the need for continuous access to an artery and a vein.

Shunts.   Access to vessels may be achieved with Quinton-Scribner arteriovenous shunts.

The shunt is inserted under local or, more often, general, anesthesia. Usually the smallest size shunt designed for adults is used. In children weighing more than 20 kg., the cannulae are placed in the radial artery and in a superficial vein of the forearm, on the left side in right-handed children. In some cases, the cannulae are inserted into the posterior tibial artery and the short saphenous vein when it is no longer possible to use either forearm because repeated cannulation has used up all the vessels.[40] A shunt placed in the leg does not interfere with normal activity. In children weighing less than 13 to 15 kg., the cannulae are inserted in the brachial artery and cephalic vein or a deep vein of the upper arm because the vessels of the forearm are too small.

Fistulae.   An arteriovenous fistula can be created surgically in children by end-to-end anastomosis of the radial artery to a superficial vein in the forearm, and within a few weeks this will produce considerable dilatation of the superficial venous network into which two needles of fairly large caliber (16/10 to 18/10 mm.) can be inserted for each hemodialysis. In difficult cases, a saphenous vein graft can be used to provide a good subcutaneous fistula in the forearm, even in small children. Because of the high incidence of local complications with shunts we have created an arteriovenous fistula in nearly all the children, and shunts have gradually been abandoned in favor of fistulae.

Apparatus

Dialysis Machines.   In our department, three types of dialysis machines have been used: the two-layer Kiil, the pediatric Kiil, and the disposable, eight-layer Rhône-Poulenc kidney. Only the Rhône-Poulenc type is used at present, first because it is easy and quick to assemble, and second—but most important—because it permits adaptation of the volume of the blood sector to the weight of the child, a procedure that is difficult with machines of the Kiil type. Counting 100 ml. for the tubing and 35 ml. for each layer used, the volume of extracorporeal blood is easily adapted to the weight of the child with the Rhône-Poulenc machine. We have learned that this extracorporeal volume must not be more than 10 to 15 ml./kg. if acute anemia is to be avoided.

Dialysis Bath Fluid Generators.   The dialysis bath fluid is produced by individual generators that mix softened or, preferably, demineralized water with a commercially prepared concentrate. The final bath composition is sodium (132 mEq./liter), chloride (100.5 mEq./liter), potassium (1 to 2 mEq./liter), magnesium (1 mEq./liter), calcium (3.5 mEq./liter), and acetate (38 mEq./liter). The generators include a pump that can exercise a negative pressure of 0 to -250 mm. Hg on the blood sector; this negative pressure is regulated according to the desired amount of water to be extracted.

Heparinization

Clotting in the dialyzer is prevented by increasing the coagulation time to between 15 and 20 minutes. We normally use systemic heparinization, giving 40 mg. at the beginning and an additional 20 mg. every two hours in children weighing more than 20 kg. In smaller children, we give 30 mg. at the beginning and 15 mg. every two hours. In postoperative situations, we use a constant output pump to inject heparin at a rate of 3 to 16 mg./hour, with hourly estimation of coagulation time, which should be maintained at between 15 and 20 minutes by suitable adjustments of the pump.

Organization, Diet, Medication

After the first few dialysis sessions, the child returns home and resumes normal activity. Dialysis is performed two or three times a week, for 10 or 12 hours each time. The child generally comes to the dialysis center on his own, without need for special transport. The dialysis center functions 24 hours a day, so that some children can be dialyzed during the night.

A calculated diet is maintained in all cases providing 1 to 2.5 g./kg. of protein, depending on age. Sixty to 70 per cent of this protein should be of animal origin. The dietary sodium allowance (0.3 to 2 mEq./kg.) is calculated according to the urinary sodium output and the blood pressure. The potassium allowance (1 to 2 mEq./kg.) is calculated according to the urinary potassium output. The theoretical caloric requirement is of the order of 70 calories/kg. This diet is continued during dialysis sessions except when the child is allowed to take a normal meal during the first four hours of dialysis.

All the children are given a multiple vitamin mixture in double the physiologic dose to compensate for probable losses during dialysis. They are also given a calcium supplement to bring the total calcium intake to 450 to 1300 mg./day. In most cases, an ion exchange resin (sodium polystyrene sulfonate) should be given in doses sufficient to maintain the predialysis serum potassium level below 6 mEq./liter. Aluminum hydroxide is also given to keep the predialysis plasma phosphorus level below 7.0 mg./100 ml. A vitamin D supplement is generally given, even though a positive calcium balance during dialysis is ensured by a bath fluid calcium concentration of 3.5 mEq./liter. The vitamin D dosage depends on radiologic and biochemical criteria, but these parameters change slowly, so that accurate dosage is not possible to predict. In practice, we give 5000 to 10,000 units per day to patients with no radiologic abnormalities who have normal alkaline phosphatase levels. In the other cases, the vitamin D dosage is 16,000 to 20,000 units per day. 25-Hydroxycholecalciferol has also been used in doses of 900 to 5000 units per day.

Technical Results

Effective Clearance. Comparison of urea clearances in the three types of dialyzer reveals that for a given extracorporeal blood volume and a given blood flow rate, the best results are obtained with the Rhône-Poulenc dialyzer and the next best with the pediatric Kiil machine (Figure 87).

The mean blood urea level is 186 mg./100 ml. before dialysis and 42 mg./per 100 ml. after dialysis.

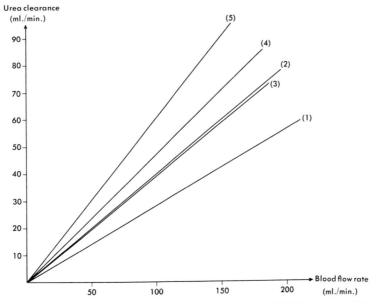

Figure 87. Dialysance of urea with the different types of artificial kidney used in children. (1) Single layer Kiil (250 ml.); (2) pediatric Kiil with two layers (220 ml.); (3) Rhône-Poulenc with four layers (140 ml.); (4) Rhône-Poulenc with six layers (210 ml.); (5) Rhône-Poulenc with eight layers (280 ml.).

Complications of Dialysis. A "disequilibrium syndrome" is very frequently seen in the first hours of dialysis, with headache, vomiting, and general malaise, symptoms that are due to cerebral edema caused by a high urea gradient between brain tissue and circulating blood. Ultrafiltration generally produces a weight loss of 1 to 2 kg. in each dialysis in children weighing more than 25 kg., and of 0.5 to 1 kg. in smaller children, a loss corresponding to the excess water and sodium retained between dialyses. Excessive ultrafiltration causes cramps and may even lead to collapse, but this is easily corrected by rapid infusion of normal saline. This type of accident can be avoided by hourly monitoring of the blood pressure. In areas in which hard water is common, defective function of the water softening apparatus may cause a "hard water syndrome," marked by headache, vomiting, and hypercalcemia.

Shunt Complications. These are common, especially thrombosis, which is usually due to angulation of the junction between the cannula and the vessel or to progressive sclerosis of the vessel. Sometimes the permeability of cannula and vessel can be restored by aspiration of clots, but in many cases the thrombosis is permanent, in which event recannulation is necessary. The cannulae may also have to be reinserted if there is skin infection with progressive necrosis that lays bare the cannulae. We have had two patients with septicemia of cutaneous origin, and they did not recover until the subcutaneous material was removed.

Progressive extrusion of the cannulae, hemorrhage, and local trauma are much rarer. Ligature of the brachial artery has not caused any problems. We have not found any significant cardiac enlargement owing to arteriovenous shunts, but the follow-up period is probably too short. In experience amounting to a total of 189 months, the mean life of the cannulae has been 5.4 months for arterial cannulae and 4.3 months for venous cannulae. Repeated cannulation in some cases has produced a situation in which all access to vessels by shunts seemed impossible, in which case we had recourse to subcutaneous fistulae. Arteriovenous fistulae have not given rise to any complication other than oozing of blood around the needles during dialysis, usually as a result of overheparinization. The majority of children are very happy to be rid of their shunt and the continued threat of repeated hospitalization for recannulation.

Results of Maintenance Dialysis

The clinical results have been good. The general condition was restored in 10 to 30 days. Signs of pericarditis, which were present in four children, disappeared rapidly. All the children were able to return to school. In experience totaling some 400 patient months, we have had two deaths. The few complications are recorded in Table 86.

Certain points require more detailed consideration.

Hypertension

The removal of fluid by hemodialysis has restored the blood pressure to normal in all but five cases. In one of these cases, the residual hypertension was controlled by hypotensive drugs. In the four other cases, bilateral nephrectomy was necessary to control the hypertension, and in these cases the blood pressure was restored to normal in periods varying from hours to three weeks. In fact, in these four patients, the blood pressure remained fairly unstable up to periods of six months or even a year after bilateral nephrectomy.

Anemia

A variable degree of anemia persists in all our patients. The principle of avoiding transfusion is applied strictly, but variable amounts of blood may have to be transfused to deal with acute anemia. Two of the children who have undergone bilateral nephrectomy have the most severe anemia. There may be other causative factors, such as blood loss in hemodialysis, which may be of the order of 10 to 15 ml. per session, or sometimes much more when using subcutaneous fistulae. An iron supplement is given when the serum iron level is low.

Table 86. Complications Observed in 400 Patient-Months of
Maintenance Dialysis Treatment in 24 Children

	Number of Cases	Deaths
Convulsions	6	—
Subdural hematoma	1	1
Attacks of pulmonary edema	5	1
Severe hyperkalemia	1	—
Secondary pericarditis	1	—
Septicemia	2	—
Hepatitis	5	—

Osteodystrophy

Four children had advanced osteodystrophy before commencing dialysis and two of them were bedridden. In one of these patients, administration of vitamin D_2 in doses of 12,000 units/day and hemodialysis produced a considerable improvement, and the child was able to walk after seven months. The other bedridden child was given 16,000 units of vitamin D_2 per day for a period of 10 months without benefit, but the radiologic abnormalities were reversed after two months' treatment with 25-hydroxycholecalciferol (25-OH-D_3) in the same dose; however, severe hypercalcemia persisted and had to be treated by parathyroidectomy. Study of bone biopsy material in our cases has shown remarkable improvement on treatment with 25-OH-D_3.

When no radiologic signs of osteodystrophy were present at the beginning of dialysis therapy, only one case occurred after 18 months of treatment in 11 children followed for more than one year and up to 26 months. No arterial calcification has been seen, but four patients developed corneal calcification. A girl with a serum calcium level of 8.8 mg./100 ml. and a serum phosphorus level of 10.4 mg./100 ml. had severe pruritus. The pruritus disappeared when the serum phosphorus was brought down to 6.0 mg./100 ml., with no change in the serum calcium, on treatment with aluminum hydroxide.

Growth

Growth is generally slowed on maintenance dialysis (Figures 88 and 89). However, the rate of growth varied considerably in the 11 children followed for more than one year. In two, the growth rate was virtually normal, in three it was moderate, in four very slight, and in two there was no growth at all. When the follow-up reaches 18 months to two years, it becomes clear that the growth defect is aggravated in four cases in five. This defect in growth does not result from hormone deficiency. Growth hormone has been estimated on many occasions under hypoglycemic stimulation and during peak physiologic secretion during sleep and has proved normal. The quality of dialysis is probably important, although we have not been able to establish any significant correlation between growth and the mean level of blood urea or creatinine before dialysis. There are, however, inverse correlations between the mean blood uric acid level before dialysis, the blood urea level after dialysis, and the amount of growth.

Caloric intake is probably important in the growth of uremic children.[48] We have investigated this subject, and our early results show a definite increase in growth rate in four of six children given caloric supplementation with polyglucose.

The osteodystrophy and the hyperparathyroidism that are always present in severe cases of renal dwarfism certainly play a significant part in the defective growth of children on maintenance dialysis. In two patients, we have found a very marked restoration of growth after parathyroidectomy.

Hyperuricemia and Acute Gout

Two children, aged 12 and 14 years, developed typical attacks of acute gout that responded to treatment with colchicine.

Although in both cases the hyperuricemia was considerable, it was compar-

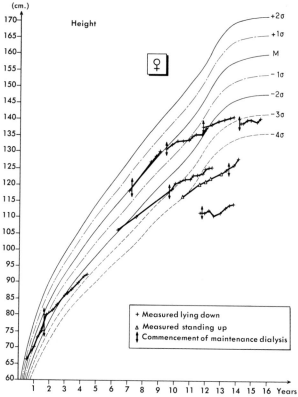

Figure 88. Rate of growth of girls on maintenance dialysis.

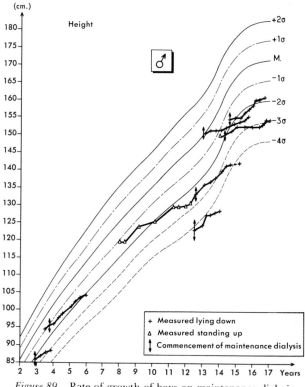

Figure 89. Rate of growth of boys on maintenance dialysis.

Table 87. Blood Uric Acid Levels in Chronic Uremia in
Children on Maintenance Dialysis

Case Number	Blood Uric Acid (mg./100 ml.) Before Hemodialysis	Blood Uric Acid (mg./100 ml.) (Minimum and Maximum Figures on Maintenance Dialysis)	Attacks of Gout
1	7.4	7.4–11.4	0
2	–	8.6–11.4	0
3	6.6	6.3–10.0	0
4	11.4	5.6–9.8	0
5	6.2	6.8–14.0	0
6	7.6	6.4–10.0	0
7	–	8.2–11.2	0
8	5.8	8.8–9.4	+
9	6.2	5.8–9.0	0
10	8.6	5.8–11.4	0
11	7.4	5.6–9.0	0
12	–	4.2–9.8	0
13	9.4	5.2–12.4	+
14	–	10.2–14.0	0
15	6.8	6.4–11.0	0
16	7.4	6.6–10.6	0
17	7.2	8.6–10.6	0
18	7.6	5.8–11.0	0
19	4.4	7.0–12.0	0
20	9.0	5.6–10.8	0
21	7.6	4.6–9.0	0
22	9.2	7.2–10.2	0

able to that observed in other patients who never developed any joint symptoms (Table 87).

Kidney Transplantation

Successful kidney transplantation remains the ultimate goal of treatment of children with terminal renal failure. Significant series of kidney transplantations in children have been reported by Starzl and colleagues,[50] Gonzalez and colleagues,[40] Potter and colleagues,[45] and Fine and colleagues.[37, 39]

It is technically possible to use an adult kidney if the children weigh more than 15 or 20 kg.[45] With the exception of some special points of surgical technique, kidney transplantation poses the same problems in children as in adults. Histocompatibility criteria, immunodepressive conditioning, and the natural history of the graft follow the same rules and are subject to the same complications as in adults.

The percentage of functioning kidneys varies with the type of kidney and the nature of the donor. Potter gives a figure of 50 per cent at one year with cadaver kidneys and 92 per cent at one year with kidneys from related living donors, a percentage that drops to 80 per cent at two years.

Fine had 73 per cent good results in 28 transplantations using related living donors and 63 per cent good results in 52 transplantations using cadaver kidneys.

In our small series, we have found no difference between cadaver kidneys and kidneys from living donors.

Transplantation does have a mortality rate greater than that for hemo-dialysis, but this rate is much lower than that for adults.

A fundamental point is the growth of children who have had transplan-tation. Growth is often inhibited completely by high doses of steroids and the im-possibility of interrupting steroid therapy. In cases in which it has been possible to stop prednisone administration or to keep the dose below 5 mg./m.²/day, normal growth has been restored so long as the bone maturation was such that growth was still possible. The possibility of growth appears to be very limited if bone age is more than 12 or 13 years.

Organizational Problems

The development of maintenance dialysis programs in children poses nu-merous organizational problems that have not been finally solved.

Even *the basic data* for discussion are not yet defined precisely. The first point concerns the number of children requiring such treatment. In Europe, and especially in France, there has been no epidemiologic survey of this sub-ject. An accurate study in California suggests that, each year, one to two children for every million inhabitants will enter a maintenance dialysis program.[45]

The second point is the *cost to the health budget* of the country. In France, we would assess the cost of hemodialysis in the region of $25,000 per year. Trans-plantation is less costly. It is probable that in the years to come the extension of these methods, improvements in apparatus, and the development of home dialysis will reduce the cost. Certainly the cost is no greater for children than for adults.

Another organizational problem concerns the *institutions* in which main-tenance hemodialysis for children should be developed. There are two possible solutions: the first is for already existing dialysis centers to take on the care of children, and the second is to develop specialized centers for children. In most countries, the first solution has been preferred, but many special centers for children have also been developed. Although it is necessary to maintain a great flexibility of organization, depending on availability of personnel, institu-tions, and money, it would seem that for technical, laboratory, and psychological reasons the preferable solution is to develop specialized centers for children. The development of research in many areas, such as (1) adaptation of apparatus to newborns and infants, (2) the problems posed by growth, osteodystrophy, and the special psychologic problems of children, and (3) the various social and educational problems of dialyzed children, may be handled more effectively by pediatricians than by practitioners whose patients are predominantly adults.

Conclusion

Children who have arrived at the stage of terminal renal failure can be maintained by the combination of hemodialysis and kidney transplantation. It is too early to assess the long-term results of this type of treatment. Experience so far affirms that the results in the short run are comparable to those ob-tained in adults and are sufficiently satisfactory to justify the investment needed for such therapy.

Many problems remain, problems that are especially important in children, such as effects on growth and on the development of personality, the possibility of social adaptation, the prospects for transplanted kidneys in hereditary disease, and the optimal time for transplantation.

SOCIOLOGICAL AND PSYCHOLOGIC PROBLEMS POSED BY CHRONIC RENAL INSUFFICIENCY IN CHILDREN*

Every chronic disease, in addition to its somatic aspects, poses the same sociologic and psychologic problems that are found in any process that progresses – or may eventually progress – inexorably to permanent invalidism or to a predictable end after a variable length of time. The socioeconomic and psychologic aspects have been studied extensively, but few such studies have been concerned with children afflicted with chronic disease.[52, 57] The principal studies have been in the field of tumors and leukemia.[51, 64] Little work has been done on the problems of the chronic nephropathies of children.[53]

Sociologic Problems

The cost to the state or to the individual of conservative treatment of moderate uremia, which varies with the treatment, the stage of uremia, and the country involved, ranges from $700 to $2500 per year. Placement on a maintenance dialysis program raises the cost to a figure in the region of $25,000 to $30,000 per year.

Hospitalization has unhappy economic, social and psychologic consequences. Every effort should be made to reduce these to a minimum. In this branch of pediatric practice, the organization of outpatient consultation and possibly of day hospitalization is essential.

The effects on the *family budget*, on the working life of father or mother, and on the schooling (e.g., the success of the studies) of brothers and sisters have not, to our knowledge, been studied systematically.

Three *sociologic problems* deserve further study in view of the considerably increased life expectancy provided by maintenance dialysis and transplantation; these are holidays, professional future, and marriage.

Since 1970 we have conducted an experiment in *summer vacations* at the seaside for children on maintenance dialysis, transporting several members of the medical team and some of the equipment to a children's hospital in Brittany. The children live with their families, in a hotel or in private houses, and come to the hospital twice a week for dialysis. The most interesting result has been the very valuable psychologic adjustment of both the children and their families.

The problem of *professional training* is being studied. At the present time children on maintenance dialysis or those who have had a kidney transplantation play games, go to school and attain skills just as normal children, the implicit goal being to encourage them to overcome or ignore their disease. If they are going to reach adult life, as some already have, it is necessary to identify the trades or professions that they can reasonably follow and to make it possible for these children to achieve their ultimate professional goals. There has not yet been a scientific study in this area.

---

*This section was written in collaboration with Dr. Ginette Raimbault.

The question of *marriage* has not yet arisen for any of our patients, but this question must be considered because sooner or later it will have to be answered.

Finally, there is the problem of *distant travel*. With the speed of modern air travel and the plurality of dialysis centers, it should be possible to arrange matters so that these patients are not inevitably chained to their own dialysis centers.

Psychologic Problems

The psychologic effects of chronic disease are inextricably linked to the somatic effects. The patient's personality adapts to the permanent physical assault according to his own psychologic makeup. When chronic disease strikes a child, the psychologic effects are made even more complex by the fact that the personality of the patient is still in the course of developing. We have investigated the problems of interrelationships, the development of communication, views of death, and the effects of a dialysis-transplantation program. Our studies have included tests derived from behavioral psychology, projective and design analysis tests, recordings of consultations, and also psychoanalytic studies.

The Child and His Disease[8]

Reactional Attitudes.   The child's reaction to his disease may be one of rejection or acceptance, but in every case there is an anxiety that may be either obvious or repressed, and also a desire to understand the cause of the trouble. Rejection is an effort at detachment from the disease, its causes and consequences. The child may dissociate himself from everything about his disease with the suggestion that this is the concern of others (his parents or doctors, for example). Alternatively, he may "reject" only specific features of his disease that are evidence of sickness—his kidneys, albuminuria, or blood pressure. Other children behave differently and assimilate the disease and its causes, progress, effects, and treatment. These reactional attitudes are always impregnated with anxiety. The anxiety may be diverted to another channel, such as physical or intellectual competition, or it may be manifested by fantasies of persecution, of abandonment, or of mutilation, or the anxiety may appear only in dreams or even in episodes of delirium. In a study on the "child's ideas about the origins of his disease," Nagy[56] described a certain number of stages by which the child arrives at an etiologic understanding of the disease. Our own studies of children with chronic disease have, on the contrary, demonstrated the existence at all ages of very elaborate etiologic hypotheses.

Body Image.   The phantasmagoria surrounding the disease is revealed in spectacular fashion in representations of body image that are especially useful in children between the ages of 5 and 12 years. The representation of the human body is not fully acquired until the age of 6 years. On the other hand, this mode of expression is either denied or devalued and rejected in different ways about the time of puberty. The representation can be regarded as a collection of signs to be deciphered like a code. The sick child's concept of his body image is always profoundly disturbed; this image is sometimes impossible to outline, even in older children, or it may be shattered by nonacceptance, or again it may be interpretative.

Relationship to Other Persons.   Apart from reactional attitudes and possible repercussions on the figuration and conception of the body image, the disease affects the interpersonal relationships of the child and those about him—his family and physicians. The physicians detect, objectivize and label the disease. Even when the child accepts his condition and its medical consequences, he finds himself trapped in a web of aggression and destruction. He identifies himself with an object, either persecuting or persecuted, but always a malign object, the cause of anxiety, irritation, and difficulties. In addition, the disease is responsible for the suffering of his parents, whether they accept it or dissociate themselves from it. He senses a danger of being disowned by his parents. In some children, the revolt against this imposed situation is expressed openly by character disorders or refusal of treatment, or it may be expressed more passively by inertia. Other children try to conciliate the adults on whom they depend.

The Child's View of Death.[10]   It is extremely important that anyone taking care of children in danger of death should understand the child's view of death. This has been defined for normal children by Nagy,[56] by Heuyer and colleagues,[54] and by Maurer,[55] for sick children by Solnit and Green,[64] and for leukemic children in particular by Alby and Bernard.[51] Children with chronic kidney disease that may prove fatal show evidence of a very early consciousness of death and of its integration in their destiny. The dominant fact is that from the age of 10 or 11 years, sick children reveal in their behavior or their comments a full understanding of their status and their probable death. It has become very obvious that the various images of death that the child may make in the course of his development are completely changed by his own experience of disease. He acquires, at a very early age, an understanding of life and death, of his own death, that very often renders him inaccessible to the adult who has not come through a similar experience.

The Attitude of the Mother to Her Child's Disease[9]

To what extent do mothers identify with the disease of their children and how do they describe it? A certain number of themes appears constantly in these descriptions. The mother very often describes psychologic symptoms in the child, such as changes in character, aggression, refusal of treatment, a complaisant attitude to the disease, and a deep need for affection. These symptoms are sometimes regarded as the cause and sometimes as the effect of the disease. A search for the cause appears in nearly every case; this search goes far beyond medical matters and always implicates primarily the mother-child relationship, nearly always in a context of guilt. A third theme is the repeated attempt to integrate the disease and its presumed cause into the individual's life history, either as a repetition of the problems that she had with her own mother, or as an echo of conjugal and sexual problems in a general context of failure.

The Attitude of the Physician to the Child and His Family

A number of hospital physicians agreed to be interviewed about their experience with children suffering from chronic kidney disease and with their parents. Where relationships are concerned, the difficulties of the physician appear predominant at the moment when relations are broken off. In some cases, this breaking off coincides with the end of the technical act; the dialogue had been accepted as a necessary prerequisite during the act, but it ended there. The technique of the examination may then become an end in itself and serve as a screen, sometimes quite consciously, for the difficulties of the physician in maintaining the confrontation with the patient. In this context, a problem may be stated only to be immediately denied or transferred to another person or another area. This process of denial may be found especially in physicians who have not been able to achieve a dialectic in their medical role, with its double function of aggression and empathy.

When the history of the patient and his family reflects a problem related to the personal history of the physician, he displays, in describing this privileged relationship, a vacillation between the respective demands of each one. The explicit demands of the family are interwoven with the implicit demands of the physician. This confrontation guides the behavior of the physician, determined by his personal feelings of culpability, his needs for reparation, and his combativity.

Lastly, obscurities may appear in a hitherto coherent account. Sometimes the physician will not talk about the basic problem, which is curtly avoided; words referring directly to the problem are no longer present and their place is taken by apparent digressions. Sometimes there is a complete dichotomy between the words spoken and the sentiments they express.

Analysis of the "Content of the Dialogue"

The relational problems surrounding the sick child rest on a "ternary" relationship of patient-family-physician, which is still poorly understood in comparison with the "binary" physician-patient relationship that is better known in adult medicine. From the foregoing analysis it is clear that what are commonly termed "psychologic problems of the sick child" do not constitute an entity in themselves but are the sum of the various modulations of the dialogue of the protagonists. The fundamental fact is that this dialogue is not an exchange between the child, his mother and the physician; it forms an indecipherable whole, what might be termed the "content of the dialogue." We have studied this by recording medical consultations on tape, and we have analyzed the tapes by psychologic and linguistic techniques.

The different problems and language of the three protagonists can be seen to unroll, oppose, break, amplify, interweave, or fade. The study is still in progress, but already it would appear that there are two fundamental elements.

The first is the initial consultation, in which what is said or left unsaid by the physician, and what is asked or hidden either implicity or explicitly by the child and his family, will profoundly affect the future "ternary" relationship. The questions the family asks in technical language are often related to deep emotional storms that are not explicitly expressed. By evoking these questions and taking the mystery out of them, the physician can rapidly enter into the "content of the dialogue."

The second notion is the existence of "key-words," gathering into a single dialogue the very different themes of the protagonists of the ternary relationship.[62] Close analysis reveals veritable structures and substructures of key-words that become organized in the content of the dialogue like certain notes or certain harmonies in a musical composition, key-words that have neither the same rational meaning nor the same emotional overtones for the child, the mother, or the physician.

Psychologic Changes During Maintenance Dialysis or After Transplantation[13]

The "artificial kidney" appears as a fourth element in the hitherto ternary relationship of parents-children-physicians. From the good or poor functioning of the machine there develops either an apparent adaptation of the child and his family, eliminating all problems, or, on the other hand, a loss—sometimes progressive, often sudden—of the defense mechanisms against anxiety, with manifestations of panic and despair. The physician appears as the intermediary between the patient and the machine, and he may be seen as the master or as the "emanation" of the machine, but he is as much tied to the machine as is the patient. This dependence of the entire group on an external element endowed with almost magical survival powers has the effect of strengthening the links between each of the members of the original group, but this collusion may run the risk of camouflaging the aggressivity of the sick group toward the medical group, with consequent depressive states of varying degree and duration.

The situation after kidney transplantation is variable. We have not seen any serious psychologic disturbances. About half of the children who have had transplants have reacted in positive fashion in surmounting their handicap in different degrees; in the other half the previous psychologic states have been confirmed.

Conclusion

It is obvious that there is still much to be learned in this field of pediatric nephrology. Much study of the epidemiologic, economic, and social problems is needed in most of the countries in which these problems may arise.

Little work has been done on the psychologic problems, and we have recorded here the early fragmentary results of our study on (1) the attitude of the child to his disease and the views of death that he is capable of elaborating; (2) the attitude of the mother to her child's disease; (3) the reactions of the physician; (4) the "content of the dialogue" elaborated in the course of the ternary child-mother-physician relationship, and the concept of "key-words" that assure this continuity; and (5) the psychologic problems that exist during maintenance dialysis and after kidney transplantation.

REFERENCES

PHYSIOPATHOLOGY

1. Bricker, N. S., Klahr, S., Lubowitz, H., and Rieselback, R. E.: Renal function in chronic renal disease. Medicine 44:263, 1965.
2. Bricker, N. S., Klahr, S., Lubowitz, H., and Slatopolsky, E.: The pathophysiology of renal insufficiency. On the functional transformations in the residual nephrons with advancing disease. Ped. Clin. N. Amer. 18:595, 1971.
3. Broyer, M., Proesmans, W., and Royer, P.: La titration des bicarbonates chez l'enfant normal et au cours de diverses néphropathies. Rev. Franç. Et. Clin. Biol. 14:556, 1969.
4. Hicks, J. M., Young, D. S., and Wootton, I. D. P.: Abnormal blood constituents in acute renal failure. Clin. Chim. Acta 7:623, 1962.

5. Horowith, H. I., Cohen, P. D., Martinez, P., and Papogoanou, M. D.: Defective ADP induced platelet factor 3 alteration in uremia. Blood *30*:331, 1967.
6. Bierelbach, R. E., Shankel, S. W., Slatopolsky, E., Lubowitz, H., and Bricker, N. S.: Glucose titration studies in patients with chronic progressive renal disease. J. Clin. Invest. *46*:157, 1967.
7. Slatopolsky, E., Hoffstein, P., Purkerson, M., and Bricker, N. S.: On the influence of extracellular fluid volume expansion and of uremia on bicarbonate reabsorption in man. J. Clin. Invest. *49*:988, 1970.
8. Slatopolsky, E., Hoffstein, P., Purkerson, M., and Bricker, N. S.: The control of phosphate excretion in uremic man. J. Clin. Invest. *47*:1868, 1968.
9. Symposium: Proceedings of the conference on the nutritional aspects of uremia. Amer. J. Clin. Nutr. *21*:349, 1968.
10. Teschan, P. E.: On the pathogenesis of uremia. Amer. J. Med. *47*:671, 1970.
11. Welt, L. G.: Symposium on uremia. Amer. J. Med *44*:653, 1968.

INCIDENCE AND ETIOLOGY

12. Habib, R., Broyer, M., and Benmaiz, H.: Chronic renal failure in children. Nephron *11*:209, 1973.
13. Legrain, M.: L'insuffisance rénale chronique; rappel des notions étiologiques et anatomiques. Rev. Prat. (Paris) *21*:2703, 1971.
14. Scharer, K.: Incidence and courses of chronic renal failure in childhood. Proc. Europ. Dialys. Transplant. Ass. 7:211, 1971.

CLINICAL AND LABORATORY SIGNS

15. Bagdade, J. D.: Lipemia, a sequela of chronic renal failure and hemodialysis. Amer. J. Clin. Nutr. *21*:426, 1968.
16. Broyer, M., Proesmans, W., and Royer, P.: La titration des bicarbonates chez l'enfant normal et au cours de diverses néphropathies. Rev. Franç. Et. Clin. Biol. *14*:556, 1969.
17. Condon, J. R., and Asatoor, A. M.: Amino acid metabolism in uraemic patients. Clin. Chim. Acta *32*:333, 1971.
18. Guevara, A., Viot, D., Hallberg, M. C., Zorn, E. M., Pohlman, C., and Wieland, R. G.: Serum gonadotrophin and testosterone levels in uremic males undergoing intermittent dialysis. Metabolism *18*:1062, 1969.
19. Hampter, C. L., Soeldner, J. S., Doak, P. B., and Merrill, J. P.: Effect of chronic renal failure and hemodialysis on carbohydrate metabolism. J. Clin. Invest. *45*:1719, 1966.
20. Lindsay, R. M., Webster, M. H. C., Duguid, W. P., and Kennedy, A. C.: Growth hormone secretion in the regular dialysis patient. Proc. Europ. Dialys. Transplant. Ass. *6*:157, 1969.
21. Lonergan, E. T., and Lange, K.: The use of a special protein-restricted diet in uremia and the mechanism of its effectiveness. Proceedings of the 3rd Annual Constructor's Conference of the Artificial Kidney. Program of the National Institute of Arthritis and Metabolic Diseases (in press).
22. Randall, R. E.: Magnesium metabolism in chronic renal disease. Ann. N. Y. Acad. Sci. *162*: 831, 1969.
23. Samaan, N. A., and Freeman, R. M.: Growth hormone levels in severe renal failure. Metabolism *19*:102, 1970.
24. Shear, L.: Selective alterations of tissue protein and amino acid metabolism in uremia. Proceedings of the 4th International Congress of Nephrology, Stockholm, 1969. Basel, Karger, 1970, Vol. 2, p. 233.

CONSERVATIVE TREATMENT

25. Bennett, W. M., Singer, I. S., and Coggins, C. H.: A practical guide to drug usage in adult patients with impaired renal function. J.A.M.A. *214*:1468, 1970.
26. Berlyne, G. M., Gaan, D., and Ginks, W. R.: Dietary treatment of chronic renal failure. Amer. J. Clin. Nutr. *21*:547, 1968.
27. Giovanetti, S., and Maggiore, Q.: A low protein diet with proteins of high biological value for severe chronic uremia. Lancet *1*:1000, 1961.
28. Lotz, M., Zisman, E., and Bartter, F. C.: Evidence for a phosphorus depletion syndrome in man. New Eng. J. Med. *278*:409, 1968.
29. Sebrell, W. H.: Recommended dietary allowances – 1968 revision. J. Amer. Diet. Ass. *54*:103, 1969.

30. Simmons, J. M., Wilson, C. J., Potter, D. E., and Holliday, M. A.: Relation of caloric deficiency to growth failure in children on hemodialysis and the growth response to caloric supplementation. New Eng. J. Med. *285*:653, 1971.

31. Vertes, V.: Hypertension in end stage renal disease. New Eng. J. Med. *280*:978, 1969.

DIALYSIS AND KIDNEY TRANSPLANTATION

32. Broyer, M., Loirat, C., Kleinknecht, C., Rappaport, R., and Raimbault, G.: Eighteen months' experience in child hemodialysis. Proc. Europ. Dialys. Transplant. Ass. 7:261, 1970.

33. Broyer, M.: L'hémodialyse chronique chez l'enfant (analyse des résultats). *In* Journées parisiennes de Pédiatrie. Paris, Flammarion, 1971, p. 273.

34. Feldman, W., Baliah, T., and Drummond, K. N.: Intermittent peritoneal dialysis in the management of chronic renal failure in children. Amer. J. Dis. Child. *116*:30, 1968.

35. Fine, R. N., de Palma, J. R., Lieberman, E., Donnell, G. N., Gordon, A., and Maxwell, M. H.: Extended hemodialysis in children with chronic renal failure. J. Pediat. *73*:706, 1968.

36. Fine, R. N., de Palma, J. R., Gordon, A., Maxwell, M. H., Grushkin, C. M., and Lieberman, E.: Hemodialysis in children. Proc. Europ. Dialys. Transplant. Ass. 6:149, 1969.

37. Fine, R. N., Korsch, B. M., Stiles, Q., Riddell, H., Edelbrock, H. H., Brennan, L. P., Grushkin, C. M., and Lieberman, E.: Renal homotransplantation in children. J. Pediat. *76*:347, 1970.

38. Fine, R. N., Korsch, B. M., Grushkin, C. M., and Lieberman, E.: Hemodialysis in children. Amer. J. Dis. Child. *119*:498, 1970.

39. Fine, R. N., Edelbrock, H. H., Brennan, L. P., Grushkin, C. M., Korsch, B. M., Riddell, H., Stiles, Q., and Lieberman, E.: Cadaveric renal transplantation in children. Lancet *1*:1087, 1971.

40. Gonzalez, L. L., Martin, L., West, C. D., Spitzer, R., and McEnery, P.: Renal homotransplantation in children. Arch. Surg. *101*:232, 1970.

41. Grushkin, C. M., Fine, R. N., and Stiles, Q.: Extended hemodialysis in an infant. Acta. Paediat. Scand. *59*:221, 1970.

42. Holliday, M. A., and Potter, D. E.: Treatment of chronic uremia in childhood. *In* I. Schulman *et al.*, eds.: Advances in Pediatrics. Volume 17. Chicago, Year Book Medical Publishers, 1970, p. 81.

43. Lindstedt, E., Lindergard, B., and Lindholm, T.: Arteriovenous fistula for hemodialysis in children. Acta Paediat. Scand. *60*:78, 1971.

44. Loirat, C.: L'hémodialyse chronique chez l'enfant (indications, contre-indications, aspects techniques). *In* Journées parisiennes de Pédiatrie. Paris, Flammarion, 1971, p. 261.

45. Potter, D., Belzer, F. O., Holliday, M. A., Kountz, S. L., Najarian, J. S., and Rames, L.: The treatment of chronic uremia in children. I. Transplantation. Pediatrics *45*:432, 1970.

46. Roberts, W. M., and Vanzyl, J. J. W.: Hemodialysis in children: technics of vascular shunts. S. Afr. Med. J. Suppl. *94*:9, 1968.

47. Royer, P.: Problèmes d'organisation posés par l'hémodialyse chronique chez l'enfant. *In* Journées parisiennes de Pédiatrie. Paris, Flammarion, 1971, p. 295.

48. Simmons, J. M., Wilson, C. J., Potter, D. E., and Holliday, M. A.: Relation of caloric deficiency to growth failure in children on hemodialysis and the growth response to caloric supplementation. New Eng. J. Med., *285*:653, 1971.

49. Shaldon, S., Shaldon, J., McInnes, J., MacDonald, H., and Oag, D.: Long-term maintenance domestic hemodialysis in children. Proc. Europ. Dialys. Transplant. Ass. 6:145, 1969.

50. Starzl, T. E., Marchioro, T. L., and Porter, K. A.: The role of organ transplantation in pediatrics. Ped. Clin. N. Amer. *13*:381, 1966.

SOCIOLOGIC AND PSYCHOLOGIC PROBLEMS

51. Alby, J. M., and Bernard, J.: Incidences psychologiques de la leucémie aiguë de l'enfant et de son traitement. Hyg. ment., *3*:241, 1956.

52. Balint, M.: The doctor, his patient and the illness. London, Pitman, 1957.

53. Korsch, B., and Barnett, H.: The physician, the family and the child with nephrosis. J. Pediat. *58*:707, 1961.

54. Heuyer, G., Levovici, S., and Giabicani, A.: Le sens de la mort chez l'enfant. Rev. Neuro-Psychiat. Infant. *3*:219, 1955.

55. Maurer, A.: Maturation of concept of death. Brit. J. Med. Psychol. *105*:75, 1964.

56. Nagy, M. H.: The child's view of death. J. Genet. Psychol. *73*:3, 1948.

57. Prugh, D. G.: Toward an understanding of psychosomatic concepts in relation to illness in children. *In* A. J. Solnit and S. A. Provence, eds.: Modern Perspectives in Child Development. New York, International Universities Press, 1963, p. 246.

58. Raimbault, G., and Royer, P.: L'enfant et son image de la maladie. Arch. franç. Pédiat. *24*:445, 1967.

59. Raimbault, G., and Royer, P.: La présentation par la mère de la maladie de son enfant. Arch. franç. Pédiat. 25:605, 1968.
60. Raimbault, G., and Royer, P.: Thématique de la mort chez l'enfant atteint de maladie chronique. Arch. franç. Pédiat. 26:1041, 1969.
61. Raimbault, G.: How do mother and child react to a child's illness? Clin. Pediat. 8:255, 1969.
62. Raimbault, G., Zygouris, R., and Royer, P.: Lithiase et/ou calcul. Arch. franç. Pédiat. 27:1005, 1970.
63. Raimbault, G.: Problèmes psychologiques posés par l'hémodialyse chronique en pédiatrie. *In* Journées parisiennes de Pédiatrie. Paris, Flammarion, 1971, p. 285.
64. Solnit, A. J., and Green, M.: The pediatric management of the dying child. *In* A. J. Solnit and S. A. Provence, eds.: Modern Perspectives in Child Development. New York, International Universities Press, 1963, p. 217.

Chapter Three

RENAL OSTEOPATHY

Bone tissue reacts to functional renal insufficiency the same way in children as in adults, but in children there are three special features: (1) The osteopathy appears more rapidly and with greater frequency because of the rapid rate of bone renewal (this rate is some 3 to 5 per cent per year in adults but may be as much as 50 per cent per year in the first years of life);[40] (2) apart from structural abnormalities, there are always disorders of bone development that slow the growth of the skeletal units in the long bones and the membrane bones, such as the lower jaw, and retard skeletal maturation;[19] and (3) the osteopathies seen in tubular insufficiency without uremia are nearly as common, especially in infants, as the uremic osteodystrophies. In a series of 149 children with chronic renal insufficiency, 41 had serious osteopathy, and 21 of these had global renal insufficiency, but 20 had only tubular insufficiency.[3]

DISORDERS OF DEVELOPMENT OF BONE TISSUE

Growth slows or stops. The maturation of epiphyseal and carpal "indicators" is retarded. The ratio of bone age to height age is in the region of 1. Puberty is delayed but occurs, as in normal children, at a bone age of 12 to 13 years.

The mechanism of the disorders of bone development, of growth, and of maturation that occur in the course of global or tubular renal insufficiency in children depends on many factors, including defective intake of calories and protein, acidosis or chronic hyperelectrolytemia, persistently negative calcium balance, and prolonged treatment with steroids and immunodepressive drugs. In some cases, the developmental defect is associated with structural abnormalities characteristic of osteodystrophy. Sometimes the developmental defect is isolated, and many special factors have been suggested.

Defective Development and Hypertension

When serious hypertension complicates a nephropathy or disease of the renal vessels and later is cured by medical or surgical means, the child's defective growth is corrected. We have called attention to this feature, without having been able to offer an explanation.[28] It is known that increased venous pressure and hypoxia induce limb growth, as is seen, for example, in unilateral venous malformations. Probably the rise in the arterial pressure has the opposite effect by modifying oxygenation or exchanges in the capillary loop.

395

Hormonal Activity

It is possible that endocrine disorders induced by the renal insufficiency may play a part in slowing skeletal development. Except in the nephrotic syndrome, there is no definite evidence of a disorder of thyroid function.[22] An interesting and little-known fact concerns adrenal function; histologic study of material obtained at bilateral adrenalectomy in 25 adults with chronic renal insufficiency has revealed a constant hyperplasia of the zona gomerulosa and the zona fasciculata.[41] We have not found any abnormal concentration of immunoreactive growth hormone in our patients after stimulation;[11] it seems that after a glucose load, uremic patients react paradoxically with a rise in the plasma level of immunoreactive growth hormone.[31, 43]

The Role of Hemodialysis

We have studied this problem in 11 children on maintenance dialysis. Growth was normal in two, fairly good in three, very poor in four, and nil in two. In the favorable cases, growth is particularly good in the months after the child is put on dialysis. The growth defect is related particularly to the presence of abnormalities of skeletal structure and to defective clearance. The role of inadequate caloric intake has been emphasized.[11] In favorable cases with resumption of bone development, we have found a discrepancy between the change in bone age as measured by Tanner's method and statural age, a discrepancy that varies with the chronologic age of the child.

OSTEOPATHIES OF CHRONIC TUBULAR INSUFFICIENCY

Serious bone abnormalities are seen in distal tubular acidosis, idiopathic hypercalciuria, the syndromes of Lowe and Fanconi, cystinosis, tyrosinosis, and Wilson's disease.[3] The clinical, radiologic, and histologic appearances are the same as in uremic osteopathy. We must emphasize the very early onset (in the first two years of life), the severity of the bone disorder, and the extreme predominance of osteoidosis with rickets and sometimes of osteomalacia with multiple fractures.

The principal factors involved in the skeletal abnormalities have already been considered. Predominant factors are (1) the negative calcium balance resulting at times from intestinal malabsorption but also from the common hypercalciuria, which may be as much as 10 or even 20 mg./kg./day; (2) the low serum phosphorus level, preeminently associated with a low tubular reabsorption of phosphate that may or may not be reduced by calcium perfusion; (3) the combination of the two foregoing factors; and (4) the positive hydrogen ion balance. Some patients develop secondary hyperparathyroidism, but there is a lack of information about parathyroid hormone levels in the serum.

Treatment varies. In distal tubular acidosis, correction by sodium or potassium bicarbonate regularizes the urinary calcium output, restores a positive calcium balance, and brings the tubular reabsorption of phosphate back to normal, all of which is sufficient to cure the osteopathy.[35] In certain tubular disease in which hypercalciuria is marked, a diet with a low sodium chloride content and possibly hydrochlorothiazide therapy in addition is useful. When the principal abnormality is lowering of the serum phosphate level and of the tubular reabsorption of phosphate, a daily supplement of 250 to 750 mg. of phosphorus with cholecalciferol in doses of 0.1 to 0.5 mg. per day is effective. 25-Hydroxycholecalciferol is also effective. In complex cases, as we found in a case of tyrosinosis, a very high phosphorus supplement will in addition lower the urinary calcium output so that high doses of cholecalciferol or its 25-hydroxylated derivative can be tolerated.

The development of uremia, as in the later stages of cystinosis, leads progressively to uremic osteodystrophy. In the transition stage, there may be temporary disappearance of the clinical and radiographic skeletal abnormalities.

UREMIC OSTEOPATHY

The abnormalities of skeletal structure seen in prolonged uremia are more common and more severe in children than in adults, no doubt because the clinical, radiologic, biochemical, and histologic expression of the disorders is magnified by growth and the much more rapid renewal of bone tissue.

Description

Clinical Features

Uremic osteopathy is seen particularly in children suffering from oligomeganephronia, nephrophthisis, chronic pyelonephritis, and, more rarely, chronic glomerular disease.[3] In most cases, it appears after several years of renal insufficiency. In some patients, it may be the presenting feature. The osteodystrophy may present with metaphyseal nodes, a rachitic rosary, genu valgum or varum, or coxa valga. In severe cases, bone pain is common, there is considerable deformity of the long bones, and invalidism is total; it is not uncommon to find slipping of the epiphyses of the knee, hip, and ankle.

Biochemical Changes

The most reliable sign is the elevated serum alkaline phosphatase level that may be two to six times the normal value. In most cases, the serum phosphorus level is more than 6 mg./100 ml. and may be as much 18 mg./100 ml.; the serum calcium level is between 6 and 8.5 mg./100 ml. Despite the low serum calcium content, tetany and convulsions are rare but can be provoked by alkalinizing therapy. The urinary calcium output is low, less than 0.5 mg./kg./24 hours. When the uremia is severe, serum magnesium and fluoride levels rise.[20] Many facts have now been established: (1) the serum calcium level may be normal or even elevated, the phosphorus level may remain normal, and there is no inverse correlation between these two parameters; (2) the plasma parathyroid hormone concentration rises early, when the glomerular filtration rate drops below 80 ml./min./1.73 m.^{2}, and before there is any change in other parameters; (3) the plasma concentration of stable vitamin D, in patients who have been given varying doses of this vitamin, is very high.

Radiographic Signs[32]

There is virtually always a diminution of bone density, with thinning of the cortex, poorly defined trabeculae, and clearly visible striae. The irregularity of the junction between diaphysis and epiphysis is similar to that seen in rickets, but the metaphysis is often asymmetrical and oblique. Many of the abnormalities resemble those seen in primary hyperparathyroidism, including marked subperiosteal bone resorption in the terminal phalanges, metacarpals, and lower extremity of radius and ulna, a loss of the lamina dura on the dental alveolae, and a ground-glass appearance of the cranial vault. Osteosclerosis is less common than in adults and is seen mainly at the base of the skull and in the vertebrae. These various appearances are generally associated, but there are cases with pure osteoporosis, rickets, or hyperparathyroid osteosis. Young children with moderate uremia usually have rickets or present mixed features. When the nephropathy is more prolonged and the uremia more severe, there is generally a mixed appearance or a picture of hyperparathyroid osteosis.[3] Subcutaneous and arterial metastatic calcification is less common than in adults. There is always retardation of bone growth, both in length and in thickness, and bone maturation is retarded.

Bone Morphology

In children, as in adults, bone biopsy from the iliac crest has provided material for a sequential analysis of the lesions; compared with the clinical and radiologic features, this material is very important for diagnosis, prognosis, and assessing the effect of treatment. The histologic lesions are clearly marked well before any radiologic changes or clinical signs appear. In addition to atrophy of the bone tissue, the lesions include excessive development of osteoid tissue and bone resorption, or a combination with varying proportions of these two lesions. Zones of osteosclerosis may be found.[42] An important point is that the mass of nonmineralized osteoid tissue is considerable, reaching as much as 3 kg. in adults; and the speed of osteon formation (about 50 to 80 days in adults) may be lengthened to as much as 1000 days in renal failure. Serial biopsies with tetracycline labeling have provided information about certain kinetic aspects of renal osteopathy and its response to treatment.[39]

Pathophysiology

Much is still unknown about the mechanisms that determine the structural abnormalities of bone tissue, including atrophy, diminished renewal rate, osteoidosis, and increased osteoclastic resorption and periosteocytic osteolysis. It is certain, however, that many factors are involved.

Positive Hydrogen Ion Balance

In chronic renal insufficiency, there is a lasting positive balance of hydrogen ions. This positive balance may or may not be revealed by a definite acidemia. It is often thought that this positive balance plays a negligible part in the onset of the abnormalities of structure and of skeletal development. This opinion is probably unjustified, especially if more attention is paid to the balance of hydrogen ions than to their extracellular concentration. It is true that the established facts are few: (1) the bone tissue has a diminished content of carbonate in uremic patients; (2) the administration of bicarbonate sometimes has no effect, but sometimes there is a partial effect on intestinal absorption and calcium balance in uremic children;[3] and (3) the effect of parathormone can be simulated by an acid overload in rats. This last effect is often attributed to stimulation of the parathyroid glands, but also occurs in parathyroidectomized animals.[16]

Raised Serum Phosphorus

Recent studies[37] on the control of phosphorus excretion in uremia have integrated this function with the theory of nephron reduction.[10] A fall in glomerular filtration rate from 120 to 25 ml./min./1.73 m.^{2} is compatible with maintenance of normal serum phosphorus levels because of the increased amount of phosphorus excreted per nephron under the influence of parathyroid hormone. The increased output of parathyroid hormone is thought to be secondary to a subtle effect of the serum phosphorus on the serum calcium, although the actual kinetics cannot be determined with present methods of measurement. In fact, the immunoreactive parathyroid hormone level rises when the glomerular filtration rate drops below 80 ml./min./1.73 m.^{2} When glomerular filtration falls below 25 ml./min./1.73 m.^{2}, this regulation of serum phosphorus is no longer possible, and the serum phosphorus level rises. Many details have been established. It is possible to induce hyperparathyroidism with a high-phosphorus diet. Continuous intravenous administration of sodium phosphate produces a drop in the serum calcium level in direct proportion to osteoblastic activity and/or significant bone resorption processes.[38] Lastly, in uremic patients, the lowering of serum phosphorus produced by oral aluminum hydroxide causes a rise in serum calcium, ionized calcium, and immunoreactive parathormone levels.[21] These facts suggest that a slight rise in serum phosphorus level may cause diminution in serum calcium level, stimulation of the parathyroid glands, and osteitis fibrosa. This theory fails to explain the considerable development of osteoid tissue. It also fails to explain why an excess of phosphate diminishes osteolysis and why phosphorus depletion increases bone resorption.[6] In rats, phosphorus depletion causes more intense osteoidosis and periosteocytic osteolysis in animals without parathyroids than in the intact animal, and the osteolysis is not inhibited by calcitonin.[29]

"Vitamin D Resistance"

Arguments in favor of an induction of resistance to vitamin D by renal failure have been advanced repeatedly.[18, 27, 39] These arguments include the considerable development of osteoid tissue, the disturbance of net intestinal absorption of calcium, the lowering of serum calcium level with secondary hyperparathyroidism, the high level of vitamin D activity in the plasma of uremic patients treated with large doses of the vitamin, and the success of treatment and prophylaxis with high doses of vitamin D.

The first difficulty concerns *intestinal absorption of calcium.* It is certain that, in uremic children, the percentage of net intestinal absorption of calcium is nearly always lowered and that the balance of stable calcium is insufficiently positive, nil, or negative.[3] It is also certain that the intestinal absorption of calcium depends partly on vitamin-dependent transport proteins and that this absorption is modulated according to the body's needs, possibly by an equilibrium in the intestinal cell of two cholecalciferol derivatives, one dihydroxylated at the 1 and 25 positions and the other dihydroxylated at positions 24 and 25.[8] There is no doubt that vitamin D in high doses increases the net intestinal absorption of calcium in renal insuffiiency. There are, however, many facets that raise problems. Accurate studies of the "true intestinal absorption" of calcium have shown that although in moderate uremia this absorption is inversely proportional to the blood urea concentration, in severe uremia, in contrast, the true absorption is normal or greater than normal.[34] The administration of high doses of various calcium salts (lactate, citrate, carbonate, and phosphate) produces a considerable increase in net intestinal absorption of calcium,[12] a fact that has been verified in children given calcium citrate.[3] In rats that have had five sixths of their kidney tissue removed, there is severe osteodystrophy without disturbance of intestinal absorption of calcium, demonstrating the possible dissociation of the intestinal disorder and the defect in mineralization of bone tissue.[14]

The second difficulty concerns the *role of vitamin D in bone tissue.*

One of the target organs of the active derivatives of cholecalciferol is bone tissue; in this site it liberates calcium by an unknown mechanism. This liberation of calcium from deep bone tissue might elevate the serum calcium level and place calcium at the disposal of the osteoid tissue for mineralization. It is conceded that vitamin D and parathormone are concerned in this action. 25-Hydroxycholecalciferol has no calcium-mobilizing effect in physiologic doses except in the presence of parathormone, but it does have a mobilizing effect in high doses, even in parathyroidectomized animals.[15] The important factor in renal failure is the abundance of unossified osteoid tissue despite the certain activity of parathormone on the bone tissue as revealed by the intense bone resorption.

Unfortunately, other direct actions of vitamin D on the skeleton have been suggested though not proved. On the one hand, there is indirect evidence that vitamin D may directly encourage the mineralization of osteoid tissue. On the other hand, vitamin D may act on the physiology of growth cartilage because injected, isotope-labeled cholecalciferol is rapidly and electively fixed in the chondrocytes and the proliferative zone.

The third difficulty concerns the *mechanism* of "vitamin D resistance." Two explanations have been proposed—the existence of inhibitors and abnormal metabolism of the vitamin. The list of inhibitors of the action of vitamin D on cartilage and bone tissue includes (1) high concentrations of pyrophosphates, (2) increased blood fluoride levels encouraging osteoidosis, (3) the presence of a toxin which, by inhibiting lysyloxidase, interferes with the transformation of soluble collagen into insoluble collagen, and (4) the existence of a serum peptide inhibiting the calcification of cartilage.

The disorder of vitamin D metabolism is not yet clear. In both rats and man, many disorders have been discovered that disappear after renal transplantation; these include defective 25-hydroxylation, the appearance of an excessive quantity of inactive water-soluble derivatives, and the nonphysiologic urinary loss of cholecalciferol and of its 25-hydroxylated derivative.[2] These abnormalities

Table 88. 1,25-Dihydroxycholecalciferol and Renal Osteodystrophy.*

Parameters	Patient	Days											
		−2	−1	0	1	2	3	4	5	6	7	8	9
Serum calcium (mg/100 ml.)	M.J.	5.4		5.0	5.5	6.6	6.3	6.4		5.9			5.8
	W.P.		7.8	8.0		9.6	9.7	10.0	10.6		10.8		8.7†
Serum phosphorus (mg/100 ml.)	M.J.	7.8		7.4				7.3					
	W.P.		5.0	4.4		3.3			3.9		4.0		8.6
Serum citrate (mg/100 ml.)	M.J.		0.89	2.05			1.04						
	W.P.		2.0						3.34				
1,25-Dihydroxycholecalciferol (μg/24 hours)		0	0	0	2 to 2.5	2 to 2.5	2 to 2.5	2 to 2.5	2 to 2.5	0	0	0	0

*In two of our patients suffering from renal osteodystrophy, the oral administration of 2 to 2.5 μg./24 hours of 1,25-dihydroxycholecalciferol produced a definite rise in the serum calcium levels (results of S. Balsan and M. Garabedian). This is comparable to the results obtained in adults by A. S. Brickman, J. W. Coburn, and A. W. Norman in three patients (New Eng. J. Med. 287:891, 1972).

†On the twentieth day.

are linked to the therapeutic results obtained with 25-hydroxycholecalciferol.[4] These facts have been established, but their interpretation is debated; they may be the consequence of previous loading with high doses of vitamin D and a high plasma level of the vitamin at the outset.[30]

It has been shown that the synthesis of 1,25-dihydroxycholecalciferol takes place in the kidney. The very important consequences of this fact in children on hemodialysis, whether binephrectomized or not, regarding vitamin D metabolism, the intestinal absorption of calcium, and the structure of bone tissue, are under study. Derivatives such as tachysterol or the *trans* forms of vitamin D, which do not require hydroxylation on carbon 1, are probably of great interest in this regard. Lastly, rapid cure of renal osteopathy has been obtained in adults and in children on our service with minimal doses of 1,25-dihydroxycholecalciferol (Table 88).

Low Serum Calcium

This is attributed to the hyperphosphatemia, to intestinal malabsorption of calcium, and to resistance of the deep bone tissue to the action of vitamin D or of its active metabolites. Although the urinary calcium level is low in renal insufficiency, the calcium output per 100 milliliters of glomerular filtrate is raised, possibly because of the acidosis and the increased sodium excretion per nephron; this is a possible cause of hypocalcemia before the onset of hyperphosphatemia.[13]

A problem is posed by the very frequent persistence of hypocalcemia (although in some cases the serum calcium level may be normal or elevated), despite a greater plasma concentration of immunoreactive parathyroid hormone. It has been suggested that "vitamin D resistance" may play a part because the action of the parathyroid hormone depends on the presence of vitamin D. The protective role of a high concentration of orthophosphate ions has been emphasized. In tissue cultures of the long bones of rat fetus, an increased concentration of phosphate in the medium inhibits the action of the parathyroid hormone on the mineral loss and on collagen resorption, whereas calcitonin inhibits only the mineral loss.[9]

Hyperparathyroidism

Whatever the primary process is, it has now been proved that there is a high level of immunoreactive parathyroid hormone in the serum at an early and moderate stage of renal insufficiency. The level is higher than in cases of primary parathyroid adenoma, no doubt linked to the diminished clearance of the parathyroid hormone. There is no correlation between the serum calcium and the immunoreactive parathyroid hormone levels, possibly owing to the lack of accurate measurement of the ionized fraction of calcium and to the part played by the magnesium concentration. These facts complement the well known observation that patients who die from uremia have hyperplasia of the parathyroids (and rarely adenoma).[19]

It is customary to distinguish between secondary hyperparathyroidism, that can be suppressed by calcium perfusion, and tertiary or autonomous hyperparathyroidism, that cannot be supressed.[17] In fact, these notions cannot be taken in too strict a sense. There is no morphologic difference in the parathyroid glands between the two groups, and the distinction depends on the total mass of parathyroid tissue.[7] From a practical point of view, the concept has been very helpful in explaining the occurrence, in uremic patients treated conservatively, of normal and elevated serum calcium levels and/or cases of osteitis fibrosa that are very resistant to treatment. The concept has led to the practice of subtotal parathyroidectomy and has also provided an explanation for certain facts observed on maintenance dialysis programs and after transplantation. Although there are divergences of opinion concerning the indications for subtotal parathyroidectomy, the operation is very effective; pruritus and gastrointestinal symptoms disappear in a matter of hours, bone pain in weeks, and metastatic calcification in two or three months, but vascular calcification disappears much more slowly.[43] Eight of our children on maintenance dialysis have been submitted to this surgery, with results varying from good to spectacular.[11]

Uremic Osteopathy, Maintenance Dialysis, and Kidney Transplantation

Hemodialysis

In children on maintenance hemodialysis, as in adults, improvement, stabilization, or aggravation of the preexisting osteopathy may occur. Sometimes bone abnormalities appear that previously were absent. The bone lesions of osteoidosis and intense resorption are very frequently accompanied by metastatic calcification in the cornea, in the soft tissues and arterial walls, especially in the coronary vessels, the cerebral vessels, and the main arteries of the limbs.

During dialysis, the serum concentration of calcium, phosphate, magnesium and fluoride is influenced by the concentration of these minerals in the dialysate. The ionized calcium of the serum is often stable during dialysis, although the total calcium is more variable.[36] In the long run, parathyroid activity and the development of secondary or tertiary hyperparathyroidism depend on three factors that are easily controlled.

1. The calcium concentration of the bath should reach 7 mg./100 ml. to ensure a positive calcium balance, and it may even need to be as much as 8 mg./100 ml. to obtain complete inhibition of parathyroid activity and so maintain a constant appearance in bone biopsies.[24]

2. The concentration of magnesium in the dialysate is usually 1.4 mEq./liter. If it is lowered to 0.5 mEq./liter, the serum parathyroid hormone level rises from 0.84 to 1.84 ng./ml., and if it is raised to 2.5 mEq./liter, the serum parathyroid hormone level falls from 2.41 to 1.93 ng./ml.[33]

3. The dialysate does not contain phosphate, and the intestinal absorption of phosphorus can be limited by giving the patient oral aluminum hydroxide. The objective is to maintain the serum phosphorus in the region of 5 mg./100 ml. Phosphorus depletion owing to overtreatment leads to various complications, including nonmineralization of osteoid tissue and increased periosteocytic osteolysis, even in the absence of any parathyroid hyperactivity.[29]

Two other factors may be significant. The dialysate fluoride concentration is important because of the role of this mineral in encouraging osteoid formation. Osteoid formation is nine times greater in biopsies when the dialysate fluoride concentration is 50 μM./liter than when the concentration is only 5 μM./liter. A low fluoride concentration is obtained by treating the water with a deionizer, not with a water softener.[24] The role of heparin must also be considered. Heparin is a calcium chelator and encourages resorption of bone tissue in culture. Heparin has a hypercalcemic effect in thyroparathyroidectomized kittens.[25] In maintenance hemodialysis, the heparin mobilizes bone calcium and phosphate.[26]

Kidney Transplantation

After successful kidney transplantation, the serum levels of calcium, phosphorus, magnesium, and alkaline phosphatase return to normal. The serum parathyroid hormone level drops rapidly for six days and then decreases more slowly.[1] Sensitivity to vitamin D is restored. The bone lesions are repaired.

Sometimes, however, there is hypercalcemia after transplantation. The mechanism is complicated and may include involvement of certain thiazide diuretics, the influence of phosphorus depletion owing to overdosage with aluminum hydroxide, the continued action of high doses of vitamin D given before surgery and stored in the body, the mobilization of metastatic calcium deposits,[23] and the unmasking of tertiary hyperparathyroidism, which may require treatment by subtotal parathyroidectomy.

Treatment

The *curative treatment* of uremic osteopathy in children is well established. Acidosis is corrected accurately and, if it is very high, the serum phosphorus level is reduced to the region of 5 mg./100 ml. by dietetic measures and the regular administration of aluminum hydroxide. Then cholecalciferol is given in doses of 0.10 to 1.0 mg./day, as well as a calcium supplement in doses of 500 to 1000 mg./day. Ergosterol or especially tachysterol may be substituted for the cholecalciferol. With this treatment there is clinical and radiologic improvement, the blood calcium level rises, and the serum phosphorus and alkaline phosphatase levels drop without aggravation of the renal insufficiency. Excessive dosage may cause hypercalcemia and reversible aggravation of the uremia.[3, 18, 39]

There is little information about the effect of 25-hydroxycholecalciferol (25-OH-D_3) in treating the renal osteopathy of children. In six children aged 10 to 17 years, who had glomerular filtration rates below 10 ml./min./1.73 m.[2], repeated bone biopsies have been performed before and after two months of treatment with 25-OH-D_3. In three of the children the lesions were predominantly osteomalacia, and in three they were predominantly osteitis fibrosa. One child in each group had received no previous treatment; two in each group had been given vitamin D, with very inadequate results. The daily dose of 25-OH-D_3 was between 2500 and 12,000 units, always less than the dose of vitamin D previously given. The treatment was clearly effective clinically, radiographically, and histologically, with disappearance of the osteomalacia, the osteitis fibrosa, and the large osteoblasts[4] (Figure 90).

25-Hydroxycholecalciferol seems to be more effective than cholecalciferol

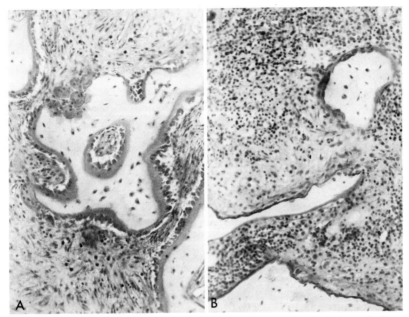

Figure 90. Renal osteopathy. Appearance of bone tissue (iliac crest biopsy) before (*A*) and after (*B*) two months' treatment with 25-hydroxycholecalciferol. Before treatment there is marked osteitis fibrosa: the medullary cavities are invaded by the fibrous tissue, and the trabeculae, formed mainly of fibrous bone, are covered with osteoid (in grey) and large osteoblasts, or they are eroded by osteoclasts (at the top left of *A*). After treatment, there is very much less medullary fibrosis and far fewer osteoblasts; there is also less osteoid and fewer osteoclasts. (Sections not decalcified, basic fuchsin stain, ×245.)

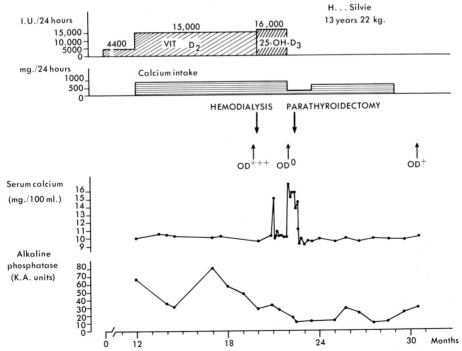

Figure 91. Severe renal osteodystrophy treated by vitamin D, 25-OH-D₃, and parathyroidectomy.

in treating the bone lesions. However, in two patients it caused severe hypercalcemia. In one of these two cases, the hypercalcemia resolved after seven to 10 days of treatment with injections of purified pig calcitonin[5] in doses of 150 M.R.C. units/day/1.73 m.², whereas parathyroidectomy was necessary in the other case (Figure 91).

The prophylactic treatment of uremic osteopathy in children consists in the administration of 0.1 to 0.2 mg./day of cholecalciferol and 250 to 500 mg. of calcium in addition to the normal dietary intake. Hypercalciuria and hypercalcemia should be avoided by checking the urinary calcium and serum calcium every two or three months. This treatment will prevent the onset of osteopathy in the majority of cases of chronic renal insufficiency.[3]

CONCLUSION

Delayed development and lesions in the bone tissue are common in chronic global renal insufficiency and in certain cases of tubular insufficiency in children. From a practical viewpoint, it is essential to look for a renal cause in every case of dwarfism and in every osteopathy resistant to vitamin D.

Considerable progress has been made in the prevention and the treatment of these abnormalities, particularly with the use of cholecalciferol or its derivatives, and of tachysterol, calcium, and phosphate chelators.

There is still considerable uncertainty about the pathophysiology of these disorders, and they are being studied extensively. There are also many problems to be resolved concerning terminal renal failure, including secondary or tertiary hyperparathyroidism, the indications for parathyroidectomy, and the effects of maintenance dialysis and transplantation on growth and skeletal development.

REFERENCES

1. Arnaud, C. D., Johnson, M. J., Fournier, A., and Goldsmith, R. S.: Parathyroid function following renal transplantation in man. Clin. Res. *18*:450, 1970.
2. Avioli, L. V., Birge, S., Lee, S. W., and Slatopolsky, E.: The metabolic fate of vitamin D₃-³H in chronic renal falure. J. Clin. Invest. *47*:2239, 1968.
3. Balsan, S., Royer, P., and Mathieu, H.: Les rachitismes et les fibroostéoclasies des insuffisances rénales de l'enfant. Arch. franç. Pédiat. *23*:769, 1966.
4. Balsan, S., and Witmer, G.: Treatment of renal osteodystrophy with 25-hydroxycholecalciferol. *In* Second International Symposium of Pediatric Nephrology. Paris, Sandoz, 1971, p. 108.
5. Balsan, S., and Jehanne, J.: Effets d'une calcitonine-retard purifiée d'origine porcine chez l'enfant. International Congress of Pediatrics, Veinna, August 29 to September 4, 1971, pp. 135–140.
6. Baykink, D., Wergedal, J., and Stauffer, M.: Formation, mineralization and resorption of bone in hypophosphatemic rats. J. Clin. Invest. *50*:2519, 1971.
7. Black, W. C., Slatopolsky, E., Elkan, I., and Hoffstein, P.: Parathyroid morphology in suppressible and nonsuppressible renal hyperparathyroidism. J. Lab. Invest. *23*:497, 1970.
8. Boyle, L. T., Gray, R. W., and Deluca, H. F.: Regulation by calcium in *in vivo* synthesis of 1,25-dihydroxycholecalciferol and 21,25-dihydroxycholecalciferol. Proc. Nat. Acad. Sci. U.S.A. *68*:2131, 1971.
9. Brand, J. S., and Raisz, L. G.: Effects of thyrocalcitonin and phosphate ion on the parathyroid hormone stimulated resorption of bone. Endocrinology *90*:479, 1972.
10. Bricker, N. S.: Renal osteodystrophy. J.A.M.A. *211*:97, 1970.
11. Broyer, M.: L'hémodialyse chronique chez l'enfant. *In* Journées parisiennes de Pédiatrie. Paris, Flammarion, 1971, p. 273.

12. Clarkson, E. M., Durrand, C., Philipps, M. E., Gower, P. E., Jewkes, R. F., and de Wardener, H. E.: The effect of high intake of calcium and phosphate in normal subjects and patients with chronic renal failure. Clin. Sci. 39:693, 1970.

13. Cochran, M., and Nordin, B. E. C.: The causes of hypocalcaemia in chronic renal failure. Clin. Sci. 40:305, 1971.

14. Cuisinier-Gleizes, P., and Debove, F.: Ostéodystrophie rénale chez le rat. In Second International Symposium of Pediatric Nephrology. Paris, Sandoz, 1971, p. 109.

15. Cuisinier-Gleizes, P., Delorme, A., Dulac, H., and Mathieu, H.: Parathyroid glands and bone mobilization by 25-hydroxycholecalciferol. Res. Europ. Et. Clin. Biol. 17:903, 1972.

16. Cuisinier-Gleizes, P., Mathieu, M., and Royer, P.: Effet d'une surcharge acide sur l'équilibre phosphocalcique du rat parathyroïdéctomisé et du rat normal. Rev. Franç. Et. Clin. Biol. 12:566, 1967.

17. Davies, D. R., Dent, C. E., and Watson, L.: Tertiary hyperparathyroidism. Brit. Med. J. 3:395, 1968.

18. Dent, C. E., Harper, C. M., and Philpot, G. R.: The treatment of renal glomerular osteodystrophy. Quart. J. Med. 30:1, 1961.

19. Fourman, R., and Royer, P.: Calcium Metabolism and the Bone. 2nd Ed. Philadelphia, F. A. Davis, 1968.

20. Fournier, A., Bordier, P., Weil, B., Safar, M., and Idatte, J. M.: Physiopathologie de l'ostéodystrophie rénale. Presse Méd. 79:2017, 2291, 1971.

21. Fournier, A. E., Johnson, W. J., Taves, D. R., Beabout, J. W., Arnaud, C. D., and Goldsmith, R. S.: Etiology of hyperparathyroidism and bone disease during chronic hemodialysis. J. Clin. Invest. 50:592, 1971.

22. Frankhauser, S., Zeyer, J., Huber, D., and Reubi, F.: Le retentissement de l'insuffisance rénale sur l'appareil endocrinien et plus spécialement sur la fonction thyroïdienne. J. Urol. Néphrol. 73:767, 1967.

23. Hornum, I.: Posttransplant hypercalcemia due to mobilization of metastatic calcifications. Acta. Med. Scand. 189:199, 1971.

24. Jowsey, J., Johnson, W. J., Taves, D. R., and Kelly, P. J.: Effects of dialysate calcium and fluoride on bone disease during regular hemodialysis. J. Lab. Clin. Med. 70:204, 1972.

25. Jowsey, J., Adams, P., and Schlein, A. P.: Calcium in response to heparin administration. Calc. Tiss. Res. 6:249, 1970.

26. Korz, R.: Heparin-induzierte mobilisation von Calcium und anorganischem Phosphat im Zusammenhang mit extrossären Verkalkungen bei chronischer Hämodialyse. Klin. Wschr. 49:684, 1971.

27. Liu, S. H., and Chu, H. I.: Studies of calcium and phosphorus metabolism with special reference to pathogenesis and effects of dihydrotachysterol (AT 10) and iron. Medicine (Baltimore) 22:103, 1943.

28. Marie, J., Royer, P., Gabilan, J. C., and Vandevoorde, J.: Le traitement médical de l'hypertension artérielle permanente chez l'enfant. Ann. Pédiat. (Paris) 4:251, 1965.

29. Mathieu, H., Cuisinier-Gleizes, P., George, A., and Guiliana, C.: Résorption osseuse par privation de phosphore chez le rat. C. R. Acad. Sci. (Paris) 272:3180, 1971.

30. Mawer, E. B., Lumb, G. A., Schaefer, K., and Stanbury, S. W.: The metabolism of isotopically labeled vitamin D_3 in man: the influence of the stage of vitamin D nutrition. Clin. Sci. 40: 39, 1971.

31. Orskov, H., and Christensen, N. J.: Growth hormone in uremia. Scand. J. Clin. Lab. Invest. 27:51, 1971.

32. Parsons, L. G.: Bone changes occurring in renal and celiac infantilism and their relationship to rickets. Arch. Dis. Child. 2:198, 1927.

33. Pletka, P., Bernstein, D. S., Hampers, C. L., Merrill, J. P., and Sherwood, L. M.: Effects of magnesium on parathyroid hormone secretion during chronic haemodialysis. Lancet 2:462, 1971.

34. Recker, R. R., and Saville, P. D.: Calcium absorption in renal failure. Its relationship to blood urea nitrogen, dietary calcium. J. Lab. Clin. Med. 78:380, 1971.

35. Royer, P., and Broyer, M.: L'acidose rénale au cours des tubulopathies congénitales. In Actualités néphrologiques de l'Hôpital Necker. Paris, Flammarion, 1967, p. 73.

36. Sachs, C., Bourdeau, A. M., Broyer, M., and Balsan, S.: Le calcium ionisé au cours de l'hémodialyse dans l'insuffisance rénale chronique. Ann. Biol. Clin. 28:137, 1970.

37. Slatopolsky, E., Robson, A. M., Elkan, I., and Bricker, N. S.: Control of phosphate excretion in uremic man. J. Clin. Invest. 47:1865, 1968.

38. Stamp, T. C. B.: The hypocalcemic effect of intravenous phosphate administration. Clin. Sci. 40:55, 1971.

39. Stanbury, S. W.: Bone disease in uremia. Amer. J. Med. 44:714, 1968.

40. Steendijk, R.: Metabolic bone disease in children. Clin. Orthop. Rel. Res. 77:247, 1971.

41. Trabucco, A. E., Marquez, F. J., and Borzon, R. J.: Adrenalectomy in cases of severe renal sclerosis. J. Urol. *101*:426, 1969.
42. Vaughan, J. M.: The physiology of bone. Oxford, Clarendon Press, 1970.
43. Wilson, R. E., Hampers, C. L., Bernstein, D. S., Johnson, J. W., and Merrill, J. P.: Subtotal parathyroidectomy in chronic renal failure. Ann. Surg. *174*:640, 1971.
For recent additional information, see:
a. Brickman, A. S., Coburn, J. W., and Norman, A. W.: Use of 1,25-dihydroxycholecalciferol in uremic man. New Eng. J. Med. *287*:891, 1972.
b. Slatopolsky, J., Calgar, S., Gradowska, L., Canterbury, J., Reiss, E., and Bricker, N. S.: On the prevention of secondary hyperparathyroidism in experimental chronic renal disease using "proportional reduction" of dietary phosphorus intake. Kidney Intern. *2*:147, 1972.

Chapter Four

HYPERTENSION OF RENAL ORIGIN

More than 80 per cent of cases of hypertension in children are secondary to an abnormality of the parenchyma or of the vascular pedicle of the kidney.[4, 11] The most frequent nonrenal causes are coarctation of the aorta, pheochromocytoma, lead poisoning, and primary hyperaldosteronism. Hypertension can also occur as a complication of certain neurologic disorders, such as dysautonomy, acrodynia, and the polyradiculoneuritides, or certain abnormalities of adrenal hormone synthesis, including 11β-hydroxylation and 17-hydroxylation, or certain metabolic disorders, such as hypercapnia. Idiopathic or essential hypertension is rare in childhood and is not seen until adolescence.[1, 10, 12]

The mechanisms of the hypertensions of renal origin are still poorly understood. There is no proof of the existence of renoprival hypertension in man. Two major mechanisms seem to play important parts: excessive retention of sodium or water, or both, and inappropriate function of the renin-angiotensin-aldosterone system. There is still much to be learned, but, from a practical point of view, the hypertension of the acute nephropathies (owing largely to hypervolemia) can be distinguished both from the hypertension of terminal uremia, which is principally due to water intoxication, and from the renovascular hypertensions, in which hyperreninemia is the most important factor. These distinctions are somewhat artificial, but they help to clarify the problems of diagnosis, prognosis, and treatment.

CLINICAL FEATURES

Normal Blood Pressure

The measurement of blood pressure in children and especially in infants requires great patience. It should be performed after a meal, when the child is quiet and relaxed, and must be repeated several times before any conclusion can be drawn. It is quite common to find a high blood pressure in the first one or two days after admission to hospital, but the pressure often returns to normal when the child becomes acclimatized to his new environment. The methods most commonly used are the method of palpation or auscultation and the "flush" method. The arm band must be adapted to the size of the child and should cover the upper two thirds of the upper arm. There are significant individual variations from the normal, and these variations are more accentuated in the first year of life and be-

409

tween the ages of 10 and 15 years. In our experience, the figures, expressed in millimeters of mercury, vary slightly with age.

	Systolic Pressure	Diastolic Pressure
0–1 year	90 ± 20	?
1–5 years	100 ± 10	60
5–10 years	110 ± 10	70
10–15 years	120 ± 20	70

A diastolic pressure above 80 mm. Hg is pathologic at any age.

Presenting Signs

Hypertension may be discovered at routine examination — for example, in a child with some urinary disorder, such as proteinuria or hematuria. It may be revealed by signs which include, in order of incidence, headache, violent abdominal pain, polyuria-polydipsia, visual disorders, and certain neurologic disorders, sometimes unexpected ones such as repeated facial palsy. Lastly, hypertension may be discovered on the occasion of some cerebral or cardiac complication, such as blindness, coma, convulsions, and pulmonary edema. In children, two particular features should be emphasized. The first is the rapid and intense wasting characteristic of badly tolerated hypertension. The second is the slowing or cessation of growth, amounting even to dwarfism, that is produced by chronic hypertension; successful treatment of the hypertension restores the growth and any growth deficit is corrected (Figure 92).

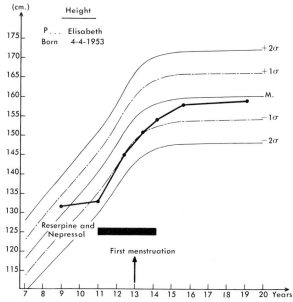

Figure 92. Growth curve after control of hypertension in a patient with segmental hypoplasia treated by hypotensive drugs.

Secondary Nephroangiosclerosis

Every serious hypertension not only damages the retinal and cerebral vessels but also produces secondary nephroangiosclerosis. The kidney lesions include necrosis of the afferent arteriole and segmental hyalinization of the glomerulus. In principle, the arteriolar lesion is reversible while the glomerular lesion is irreversible, thus adding a new nephropathy to the original disease. Appreciation of the degree of nephroangiosclerosis is very important for prognosis. It seems that in children the nephroangiosclerosis can more often be reversed with control of the hypertension than it can in adults.

HYPERTENSION IN ACUTE NEPHROPATHY

Glomerulonephritis of Acute Onset

Postinfectious glomerulonephritis of acute onset, in particular with diffuse endocapillary proliferation (see page 271), is very often accompanied by hypertension in the initial stages. This hypertension is the cause of the only complications that may threaten life at this stage, cardiac failure with pulmonary edema and hypertensive encephalopathy. The most important factor in this hypertension is without any doubt the hypervolemia owing to retention of water and salt and possibly also vasoconstriction in certain vascular beds.

Treatment is remarkably effective; apart from rest in bed, it includes three measures: (1) Restriction of water and sodium is adequate treatment in moderate cases. (2) Antihypertensive drugs are indicated when the blood pressure is greater than 140/90 mm. Hg after 12 hours of bed rest and of water and salt restriction. Dihydralazine (Nepresol) is given in doses of 1 mg./kg./day together with reserpine (0.1 mg./kg./day) until the blood pressure falls to normal. If this treatment is ineffective, methyldopa (Aldomet) can be given in doses of 10 to 20 mg./kg./day either orally or intravenously. (3) Peritoneal dialysis may be required urgently in cases of pulmonary edema or hypertensive encephalopathy with an obvious water overload. In urgent cases, we have had remarkable results from the intravenous injection of diazoxide.

Special Cases

Three types of acute nephropathy pose particular problems.

Hemodialysis or peritoneal dialysis is indicated for the relief of hypertension associated with acute renal failure and oliguria, cases in which the hypertension results from water intoxication.

In the nephrotic syndrome with minimal glomerular lesions, hypertension may be found at the onset of edema before any treatment is given. This is an indication for diuretics (spironolactone) and possibly for hypotensive drugs. Steroid therapy is contraindicated until the blood pressure is restored to normal. The mechanism of the hypertension in these cases is not understood, but it may be traceable to secondary hyperaldosteronism.

Finally, the hemolytic and uremic syndrome is very often complicated in the acute stage by hypertension. This hypertension is associated with a very high blood renin level. Specific treatment for acute glomerulonephritis is often effective, but sometimes it is insufficient.

HYPERTENSION AND CHRONIC UREMIA

Advanced Chronic Uremia

Every chronic glomerular disease with severe renal failure may be accompanied by hypertension when the glomerular filtration rate drops below 10 to 15 ml./min./1.73 m.^{2} This hypertension may be controllable by hypotensive drugs (Nepresol, reserpine, Aldomet) in association with a diuretic such as frusemide or Aldactone. The thiazide diuretics must be given with prudence in cases of renal failure. A low-sodium diet should be prescribed with very careful supervision in order to avoid sodium loss and consequent aggravation of the renal failure. In 24 cases of moderate renal failure, we have had five failures and 19 satisfactory responses, marked by regression of the retinopathy, stabilization or even improvement of renal function, and return of growth.[6]

When the renal failure arrives at a terminal stage (clearance $\leq$ 5 ml./min/ 1.73 m.^{2}) these measures are generally insufficient. When the child is placed on maintenance dialysis, the blood pressure often improves or returns to normal when the hypertension is the result of excess of water or sodium or both. An elevated blood pressure persisting after several months of treatment is an indication for bilateral nephrectomy; if the symptoms are threatening, the surgery may be indicated after only a few weeks on dialysis. In these cases, there is a rise in the plasma renin level, sometimes a very considerable one, and surgery generally cures the hypertension in spectacular fashion.

Special Cases

Three types of nephropathy in childhood are accompanied very early by hypertension at a stage at which the uremia is moderate and there is no water intoxication. These are the congenital polycystic diseases running a prolonged course, the hypercalcemic kidney, and the bilateral and symmetric forms of segmental hypoplasia of the kidney. The hypertension in these cases is generally sensitive to hypotensive drugs and to a low-sodium diet, but specific therapeutic measures may be indicated.

RENAL VASCULAR HYPERTENSION

Definition

"Renal vascular hypertension in childhood" is used to designate severe, lasting hypertension secondary to lesions that diminish the blood flow and/or the pulsatility of the kidney, whether it results from abnormality of the renal vascular pedicle, from severe obstructive lesions of the larger intrarenal vessels, or from perirenal compression. It is now known that these various causes lead to hyperreninemia.[2, 3, 12] Renal vascular hypertension is related to the experimental models of Goldblatt (constriction of the renal artery) and Page (perinephritis produced by wrapping the kidney in cellophane). They must be considered in detail because of the great possibility of surgical cure.

Table 89. Causes of Renal Vascular Hypertension in Children

1. *Abnormalities of vascular pedicle*
    - *a.* Extrinsic pressure (adrenal and renal tumors; ganglioneuroma)
    - *b.* Arterial lesions
      Congenital stenoses and aneurysms
      Thromboses
      Arteritis
      Fibromuscular hyperplasia
    - *c.* Venous lesions (thromboses; tumors)

2. *Abnormalities of intrarenal arteries*
    - *a.* Aneurysms of branches of the renal artery
    - *b.* Periarteritis nodosa (macroscopic form)
    - *c.* Segmental hypoplasia
    - *d.* Diffuse calcifying arteriopathy and the arteriopathy of hypercalcemia (?)
    - *e.* Thrombotic microangiopathy of kidney (hemolytic uremic syndrome)

3. *Perirenal abnormalities*
    - *a.* Sclerolipomatous perinephritis
    - *b.* Perirenal hematoma (hemophilia, periarteritis, renal biopsy, trauma)

4. *Various*
    - *a.* Sudden ureteral obstruction (acute hydronephrosis)
    - *b.* Cysts and polycystic disease of the kidney (vascular compression, intracystic tension?)

Causes

The causes of renal vascular hypertension in children are listed in Table 89. Most of them are considered in other chapters. Although it is regarded as a classic cause, we have not seen a case of hypertension secondary to unilateral chronic pyelonephritis. In this chapter we shall consider only the abnormalities of the renal vascular pedicle.

Pedicle and Perirenal Abnormalities

The data of the 15 cases in our series are set out schematically in Table 90.

Clinical Features. In our experience, the condition has been discovered at ages varying from 18 months to 16 years. The systolic blood pressure is generally greater than 180 or 200 mm. of mercury. Left ventricular failure, moderate renal insufficiency, or proteinuria was found in half of the cases. Hypertensive retinopathy was seen in two thirds of the cases.

There are only two features that are somewhat peculiar to hypertension stemming from an abnormality of the vascular pedicle. The first is a bruit heard in the subdiaphragmatic region but we have found such a bruit on only one occasion. The second is the discovery of phacomatosis either in the patient or in his family. The most common is neurofibromatosis, and we found this on three occasions. It should, however, be noted that neurofibromatosis can cause hypertension by various mechanisms in addition to vascular malformation with specific lesions (Figure 93), including extrinsic compression of the renal pedicle by a ganglioneuroma or the development of a pheochromocytoma.

Table 90. Causes and Course of 15 Cases of Hypertension Due to Renal Vascular Abnormality

Case	Diagnosis	Age (years)	Treatment	Results
	Simple Vascular Abnormalities			
1	Aneurysm of branch of right renal artery	7 years 6 months	Polar nephrectomy	Cure
2	Aneurysm of left renal artery	8	Nephrectomy	Cure
3	Arteriovenous aneurysm of right renal pedicle	6 years 6 months	Nephrectomy	Cure
4	Fibromuscular hyperplasia of right renal artery	1 year 10 months	Arterial reconstruction	Cure
5	Recanalized thrombosis of left renal artery	2	Arterial reconstruction	Cure
6	Thrombosis of right renal artery	13	Nephrectomy	Cure
7	Fibromuscular hypoplasia of left renal artery	12	Arterial reconstruction	Cure
	Unclassified Abnormalities			
8	Venous thrombosis in small dysplastic kidney	1 year 6 months	Nephrectomy	Cure
9	Venous thrombosis in small kidney containing calculi	16	Nephrectomy	Failure
	Multiple Vascular Abnormalities			
10	Abnormality of abdominal aorta and stenosis of right renal artery	11	Arterial reconstruction	Failure
11	Stenosis of right and left renal arteries and of superior mesenteric artery. Aneurysm of mesenteric artery		Nephrectomy on most affected side	Partial failure
12	Multiple stenoses of the branches of both renal arteries and of the lumbar and other arteries. Thrombosis of right external iliac artery, absence of radial pulse	2	Hypotensive drugs	Good control of blood pressure
13	Multiple aneurysms of branches of both renal arteries and abnormality of aorta (neurofibromatosis)	9 months	Hypotensive drugs	Good control of blood pressure
14	Aneurysms of right renal artery. Stenosis of left renal artery. Stenosis of aorta (neurofibromatosis)	2 years 6 months	Right nephrectomy	Temporary success
15	Thrombosis of left renal artery. Abnormality of aorta (neurofibromatosis)	11	Left nephrectomy	Failure

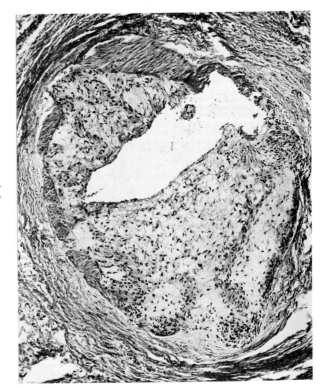

Figure 93. Lesions of neurofibromatosis in a renal artery in a hypertensive child. ×25.

Investigation.   We no longer use tests involving separation of the urine from the two kidneys.

RADIOGRAPHY.   Radiographic study is very important. It includes a plain radiograph, urography, and arteriography.

A plain radiograph without preparation may demonstrate abnormalities in the size and shape of the kidneys and sometimes reveals a calcified aneurysm of the renal artery at the level of the second lumbar vertebra.

Intravenous urography gives information about both morphology and function. One kidney may be radiologically silent, a kidney may be small, or there may be loss of substance at one pole, and it is important to note whether or not the contralateral kidney is hypertrophied. Films are taken at 30 seconds and at one, two, and three minutes, and a note is made of any asymmetry in the nephrographic and pyelographic stages. Differences in tonality have some significance. The diagnosis may be evident on intravenous urography. A great disparity in size, notches on the lateral borders, and a swallow-tail appearance of the calyces suggest segmental hypoplasia; delay in appearance of the contrast medium with greater concentration of the medium on the same side but without any major discrepancy in size suggests an abnormality of the renal pedicle.

Renal arteriography often solves the problem. It is essential to perform this in every case in which renal vascular hypertension is suspected, and it can be performed even in small children, from the age of 12 or 18 months. The arteriographic stage provides information about abnormalities of caliber, of contour, and of continuity of the aorta and its major branches. Localized stenosis may be difficult to see, whereas poststenotic dilatation is obvious. Aberrant arteries and anomalies of the aorta or regional arteries may be disclosed. The nephrogram stage reveals the size of the kidney, its contour, and the homogeneity of its vascularization (Figure 94).

RENIN ESTIMATION.   Measurement of plasma renin by a biologic or radio-immunologic method is very valuable in cases of renovascular hypertension. Elevation of the renin level in the peripheral venous blood is inconstant. Sampling from the vena cava or renal veins is much more helpful but is not without the risk of causing secondary thrombosis. Response to taking an upright posture or to other stimuli may be significant. It has been established in adults that there is a good correlation between surgical cure and the results obtained with these two last techniques.

ISOTOPE STUDIES.   A method complementary to the radiologic studies consists in the use of a radioactive isotope of mercury in the form of the chloride or of chlormerodrin (Neohydrin). The renal scintiscan is of little value compared with renal arteriography, but the comparative fixation of the mercury on the two sides is of significance. This provides a test of separate renal function without ureteral catheterization and allows an estimate of the degree of compensatory hyperfixation in the contralateral kidney in strictly unilateral diseases.[9] This method is of particular value in cases of hypertension due to some abnormality of the renal parenchyma.

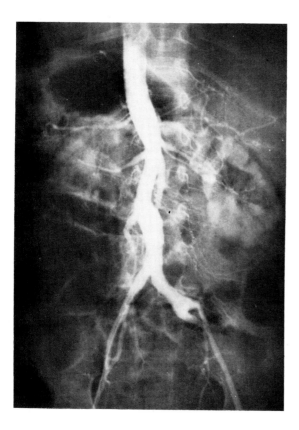

Figure 94.   Arteriography in a patient with hypertension who had multiple vascular abnormalities (von Recklinghausen's neurofibromatosis).

Treatment and General Prognosis

When a precise diagnosis has been made, it is necessary to assess the possibility of surgical cure. The presence of a vascular lesion in a child, especially if it is unilateral, is nearly always an indication for surgery. Two solutions are possible when the lesion is unilateral: nephrectomy or vascular repair. Although theoretically repair is preferable, it is not always possible in practice despite advances in surgical technique. Nephrectomy is always necessary for renal atrophy secondary to thrombosis of the main artery and also when disease affects the smaller branches of the renal arteries. Partial nephrectomy sometimes is a possible solution. In bilateral vascular disease, the indications are more difficult to assess, and it may be prudent to try medical treatment before attempting surgical repair on one side at a time.

In our 15 patients, the results were generally good (Table 90), except when removal of a small kidney left the patient with vascular lesions or nephroangiosclerosis in the contralateral kidney. With hindsight, a poor prognosis was indicated from the beginning; apart from the bilateral character of certain anomalies, there were major proteinuria and significant disturbance of renal function. These latter symptoms, indicating nephroangiosclerosis, should not in themselves be regarded as a contraindication to surgery if there are good indications for operating.

Conclusion

In children, at least 80 per cent of cases of hypertension are secondary to disease in the kidney parenchyma or in the renal vascular pedicle. The hypertension may be latent, manifest, or malignant. Sometimes the hypertension appears in a child with obvious acute or chronic kidney disease and is discovered by routine blood pressure measurement; sometimes hypertension is the presenting symptom of a previously unrecognized renal disease, in particular segmental hypoplasia of the kidney and abnormalities of the pedicle. The hypertension may itself present serious threats to growth, nutrition, and vision, and to the cardiac and central nervous systems. It may be responsible for deterioration of the state of the kidney by provoking secondary arteriolar and glomerular lesions of nephroangiosclerosis. It should be possible to achieve a satisfactory reduction of blood pressure by appropriate treatment in most cases.

The mechanism of the disorder in any particular case may be obvious, as with hypervolemia, water intoxication and disordered function of the renin-angiotensin-aldosterone system, but often the mechanism is far from clear, and further study is required. There is still a lack of information about the effects of the long-term use of hypotensive drugs, the long-term prognosis of reconstructive surgery of the renal vessels in very young children, the regulation of blood pressure in children who have had bilateral nephrectomy, and the late consequences of nephroangiosclerosis resulting from serious hypertension.

REFERENCES

1. Caliguiri, L. A., Shapiro, A. P., and Holliday, M. A.: Clinical improvement in chronic renal hypertension in children. Pediatrics 5:758, 1963.
2. Favre, R.: Hypertension arterielle et son traitement chirurgical chez l'enfant. Helv. Paediat. Acta 22:54, 1967.

3. Guntheroth, W. G., Howry, C. L., and Ansell, J. S.: Renal hypertension: a review. Pediatrics *31*:767, 1963.
4. Loogie, J. M. H.: Hypertension in children and adolescents. I. Causes and diagnostic studies. J. Pediat. *74*:331, 1969.
5. Marchal, C., and Sapelier, P.: Hypertension artérielle, sténose de l'artère rénale et phéochromocytome. Méd. Infant. *74*:341, 1967.
6. Marie, J., Royer, P., Gabilan, J. C., and Vandewoorde, J.: Le traitement médical de l'hypertension artérielle permanente de l'enfant. Ann. Pédiat. *41*:251, 1965.
7. Mathieu, H., Habib, R., l'Hirondel, J., Leveque, B., and Royer, P.: Hyperaldostéronisme chronique de l'enfant, secondaire à une hypertension artérielle par anomalie rénale unilatérale. Arch. franç. Pédiat. *23*:101, 1966.
8. Matsaniotis, N., Bastis-Maounis, B., and Balas, P.: Traumatic renal hypertension corrected by nephrectomy in a child. Helv. Paediat. Acta *21*:438, 1966.
9. Raynaud, C., Schoutens, A., and Royer, P.: Intérêt de la mesure du taux de la fixation rénale du Hg dans l'étude de l'hypertrophie rénale compensatrice chez l'homme. Néphron *5*:300, 1968.
10. Rosenheim, M. L.: Hypertension in childhood. Proc. Roy. Soc. Med *54*:1093, 1961.
11. Royer, P.: Physiopathologie des hypertensions artérielles de l'enfant. Path. Biol. *7*:1513, 1959.
12. Royer, P.: L'hypertension artérielle rénovasculaire chez l'enfant. Päd. Fortbildungskurse. Basel, Karger, 1970, p. 63.
13. Sakai, T., and Kokubun, Y.: Renal artery stenosis with secondary hyperaldosteronism. Acta Paediat. Jap. *8*:13, 1966.
14. Winer, B. M., Lubre, W. F., Simon, M., and Williams, J. A.: Renin in the diagnosis of renovascular hypertension. Activity in renal and peripheral vein plasma. J.A.M.A. *202*:121, 1967.

APPENDIX

MICHEL BROYER

MEASUREMENT OF GLOMERULAR CLEARANCE

A large number of techniques for measuring glomerular clearance is possible. Those most commonly used are:

1. Endogenous creatinine clearance.
2. Clearance of exogenous substances such as inulin, with accurate collection of urine.
3. Plasma clearance of substances such as labeled EDTA, without collection or urine.

There are various difficulties in the application of all three techniques in children. Endogenous creatinine clearance may be objected to on theoretical grounds, but it is the simplest method and the method most often used. Inulin clearance is the reference method, but it is a difficult technique, especially in small children; it is generally reserved for accurate physiologic studies. The plasma clearances are much easier to carry out and are reliable; they should be adopted as the routine method for the future.

Endogenous Creatinine Clearance

Three conditions are necessary if this technique is to have the reliability that it often lacks. These are:

1. Accurate *24 hour* collection of urine is mandatory.
2. The biochemical estimation should be done by an automated method.
3. Exogenous creatinine should be excluded by putting the patient on a meat-free diet for two or three days before the test.

Under these conditions, we have found no significant difference between creatinine clearance and inulin clearance in 41 children in whom glomerular filtration was estimated simultaneously by several techniques. Some authors have suggested that the 24 hour creatinine clearance should be estimated on three occasions and that the average of the three results should be taken as the correct figure. In our hands, this technique applied to 25 children gave results that did not differ significantly from those obtained in a single test. It is essential to collect urine over a 24 hour period, since a shorter collection period gives results that differ significantly from inulin clearance.

It is recognized that in cases of renal insufficiency, the creatinine clearance provides an overestimate of glomerular filtration owing to the relative increase of tubular secretion of creatinine. The ratio of creatinine clearance to inulin clearance may reach 1.5, 2, or even more when glomerular filtration drops below 10 ml./min. In the small number of cases with renal insufficiency that we have studied, we have generally found the ratio of creatinine clearance to inulin clearance to be greater than 1, but the ratio varies to such a degree that it is impossible to introduce any routine coefficient of correction.

Inulin Clearance

Inulin, a hexose (mainly fructose) polymer, has a molecular weight in the region of 5200. It is one of the most widely used reference indicators of glomerular function because in theory this substance is not metabolized, reabsorbed, or secreted by the tubule.

The classic technique of inulin clearance was defined by Homer Smith. It consists in establishing a fixed plasma level by continuous injection and, when this level is attained, taking accurate samples of urine by a bladder catheter at the same time as plasma samples are taken, so that the clearance can be established according to the formula:

$$C = \frac{UV}{P}$$

The inulin must be very pure. In many cases commercial inulin contains variable amounts of metabolizable fructose, which constitute a source of serious error.

Preparation of the Subject

Fructose must be excluded from the diet for 12 hours immediately preceding the test. In small children premedication with diazepam and phenobarbital may be given one hour before the test. A Foley catheter is placed in the bladder with the usual aseptic precautions, and the urine collected when the catheter is passed is kept to act as a control (U_0). Using local analgesia, a suitable cannula is placed in a forearm vein for blood sampling. In small children a needle mounted on a siliconed catheter* may be used, and the size of the needle depends on the largest available veins. Once in place, the needle is kept patent by a slow perfusion of heparinized saline.

A second needle is placed in a vein of the other arm for injection of the inulin.

Dosage and Preparation of Solutions

To obtain a plasma level of 25 mg./100 ml., an initial dose of 60 mg./kg. is injected rapidly at time 0, followed by a maintenance dose injected by a pump.

This maintenance dose is calculated as a function of the state of glomerular filtration; in the absence of evident renal insufficiency, it is estimated to be 70 ml./min./m.² In cases with renal insufficiency, the creatinine clearance may be used to estimate the probable glomerular filtration rate. The formula for cal-

---

*Butterfly, ® Abbott Laboratories, North Chicago, Ill. 60064.

culating the maintenance dose is:

$$0.25 \text{ mg.} \times \text{GFR (ml./min.)} \times \text{duration of test (minutes)}$$

For example, for a normal child with a body surface area of 1 m.², the dose would be:

$$0.25 \text{ mg.} \times 70 \text{ ml./min.} \times 180 \text{ min.} = 3150 \text{ mg.}$$

The maintenance dose is dissolved in a 5 per cent glucose solution, and the total volume is calculated as a function of the output chosen for pump injection; in general, 2 to 3 ml./min. The bottle containing the maintenance dose must be shaken frequently to avoid sedimentation. The time required for stabilization of the plasma level is of the order of 45 minutes to one hour.

Taking the Samples

At time 0, before injection of the inulin, blood and urine samples are taken for control determinations.

The actual test begins one hour after beginning the injection of the maintenance dose. It is usual to work over four periods of 15 minutes, accurately timed. In each of these periods, the urine is collected and also two blood samples, one each at the beginning and end of each period, are taken.

The urine must be collected with great accuracy, and in order to recover all the urine produced in the given period, the bladder must be rinsed with distilled water and air. The rinsing must be done with strict asepsis, using sterile 50 ml. syringes. The volume of rinsing fluid depends on the size of the child and the urinary output:

If the volume of urine collected is less than 10 ml., rinse three times with 50 ml. of distilled water and then twice with 50 ml. of air.

If the volume collected is between 10 and 80 ml., rinse twice with 50 ml. of distilled water and twice with 50 ml. of air.

If the volume is greater than 80 ml., rinse only twice with 50 ml. of air.

During the rinsing procedure, the child is asked to strain as at stool.

Calculation

The clearance is calculated for each collection period according to the formula:

$$\frac{\text{In}_{U_1} \times V_{U_1}}{\left(\dfrac{\text{In}_{P_1} + \text{In}_{P_2}}{2}\right) \times T_{\text{min.}}}$$

where In_{U_1} = concentration of inulin in the urine (U_1)

In_{P_1} = concentration of inulin in the plasma (P_1)

In_{P_2} = concentration of inulin in the plasma (P_2)

V_{U_1} = volume of the sample of urine U_1

$T_{\text{min.}}$ = duration of period of collection of urine U_1

An average can then be taken of four or five collection periods.

Plasma Clearance of ^{51}Cr EDTA

Principle

^{51}Cr EDTA is a purely glomerular indicator. Its plasma clearance is thus theoretically equivalent to glomerular filtration. This plasma clearance is easily determined from the graph of decrease of ^{51}Cr EDTA in the plasma after injection of a known dose of the substance.

Dose

The dose is 1 to 2 μc./kg., but not more than a total of 50 μc.

In calculating this dose, account is taken of the half-life of ^{51}Cr, which is 28 days. The correction factor required to determine the activity on the day of the test is shown in Table 91.

Preparation of the Dose

After calculating the dose according to the activity of the solution on the day of the test, the corresponding volume of ^{51}Cr EDTA solution is taken up with a disposable insulin syringe and placed in a sterile wide flask of the penicillin type (P). This flask has been previously weighed and its weight (P_0) noted. Five milliliters of isotonic glucose solution may now be added to the flask. Next, 0.5 ml. is taken from the flask P, using an insulin syringe, and placed in a graduated 50 ml. flask (F) that has previously been weighed (p_0). This flask (F) is

Table 91. Correction Factors for Calculating Dosage of ^{51}Cr EDTA

Correction Factor	Time Elapsed (days)
1	1
0.995	2
0.992	3
0.93	4
0.885	5
0.86	6
0.84	7
0.82	8
0.80	9
0.78	10
0.76	11
0.745	12
0.725	13
0.705	14
0.69	15
0.675	16
0.655	17
0.63	18
0.625	19
0.610	20

weighed again (p_1) to provide an accurate measurement of the amount of solution transferred from P to F. After adjusting the volume of the graduated flask F to 50 ml., an accurate dilution of the solution injected into the patient is available. The dilution titer is:

$$\frac{p_1 - p_0}{50}$$

The flask P is weighed again (P_1). All is now ready for injection of the dose. The content of flask P is taken up in a 10 ml. syringe, with great care not to lose a drop of the fluid. The injection is made through a scalp needle previously set in place and kept clear with a glucose solution. The syringe itself is rinsed twice with 5 ml. of fluid from flask P, which is weighed again after these operations (P_2).

The actual dose injected can be calculated from the dilution prepared in the graduated flask F. If the activity of this dilution is I for 1 ml., the dose is:

$$I \times \frac{p_1 - p_0}{50} \times (P_1 - P_0) - (P_2 - P_0) \times R$$

R represents the activity of the rinsing solution collected from flask P.

Blood Sampling

Blood samples may be taken from a siliconed needle placed in a forearm vein or via a suitable cannula. When the ^{51}Cr EDTA is injected, timing with a stopwatch is begun, and 2 ml. samples of blood are taken at 5, 10, 15, 20, 30, 45, 60, 80, 100, and 120 minutes. The time corresponding to the center point of each sampling period is noted accurately.

Counting

The blood samples are centrifuged and 1 ml. of plasma from each sample is transferred to a hemolysis tube. Counting is then performed with a scintillation counter previously set for the energy level of ^{51}Cr.

Calculation of the Clearance

The results of the count are used to plot a graph of disappearance (Figure 95), which is the sum of two decreasing exponentials; it is easy to trace the two lines corresponding to these two exponentials on semilogarithmic paper.

The clearance is then given by the formula:

$$Clearance = \frac{dose \times \lambda1 \times \lambda2}{a_1\lambda2 + a_2\lambda1}$$

where a_1 and a_2 are the ordinates at the origin of the two exponentials, and $\lambda1$ and $\lambda2$ are the slopes of the two exponentials (λ can be determined graphi-

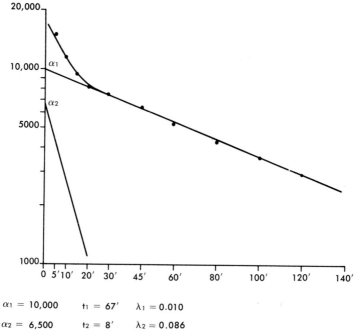

$$\alpha_1 = 10,000 \qquad t_1 = 67' \qquad \lambda_1 = 0.010$$

$$\alpha_2 = 6,500 \qquad t_2 = 8' \qquad \lambda_2 = 0.086$$

Figure 95. Graph of decreasing plasma level of ^{51}Cr after and injection of EDTA ^{51}Cr. The curve can be broken down into two decreasing exponentials α_1 and α_2 whose ordinates lie at the origin of the exponentials. λ_1 and λ_2 are the respective slopes.

cally by measuring the time necessary for disappearance of half of the substance):

$$\lambda = \frac{\log 2}{t} = \frac{0.693}{t}$$

CLEARANCE OF PAH

Clearance of PAH provides an estimate of renal plasma flow, because at a concentration of 2.0 mg./100 ml., the PAH is completely extracted from the arterial blood in one passage through the kidney. This is not true in the newborn, in whom the extraction level is only 60 to 80 per cent.

The technique is the same as for inulin clearance, and both clearances are generally measured at the same time.

Dose Required

Priming dose: 8 mg./kg.
Maintenance dose: $0.02 \times GFR \times 5 \times t$
where GFR = glomerular filtration rate in ml./min.
        t = the duration of the test

Calculation

As for all clearance techniques at a constant plasma level:

$$\text{clearance} = \frac{UV}{P}$$

TmPAH

This test of proximal tubular function is generally carried out at the same time as the inulin clearance and after measuring PAH clearance.

The TmPAH, or maximal excretion of PAH, can be determined only if the plasma concentration of PAH is 40 mg./100 ml. or more.

In practice, after determining PAH clearance, which is done at a very low plasma level of PAH, a second priming dose of 160 mg./kg. PAH is injected, followed by a maintenance dose calculated according to the formula:

$$(\text{supposed TmPAH} + \text{GFR} \times 0.4 \times 0.8)\ t$$

where the supposed Tm is 80 mg./min. for a GFR of 120 ml.;

GFR is expressed in ml./min.;

0.4 represents the plasma level of PAH;

0.8 is the filtrable fraction of PAH, which is only 80 per cent;

t = duration of the test in minutes: 45 minutes for equilibration and then three periods of 15 minutes each.

The maintenance dose is prepared in advance in a flask to which inulin is added for the simultaneous determination of glomerular filtration (see page 420), and isotonic glucose solution is used to bring the volume up to that required for the predetermined injection rate (2 to 3 ml./min.).

It must be remembered that the PAH is given as the sodium salt and that the Tm test represents a considerable sodium load. Rapid injection of the priming dose of PAH may cause unpleasant symptoms, including a warm flush, tingling, and malaise, but these reactions are transient.

The blood and urine samples are taken exactly as for inulin clearance (see page 420).

Calculations

$$\text{Tm} = \text{PAH excreted} - \text{PAH filtered}$$
$$\text{Tm} = UV_{PAH} - (P_{PAH} \times 0.8 \times \text{GFR})$$

U = the concentration of PAH in the urine
V = the volume of urine per minute
P_{PAH} = the plasma concentration of PAH
0.8 = the filtrable fraction of PAH
GFR = glomerular filtration expressed in ml./min. and determined simultaneously by inulin

The average of three periods is generally taken.

Tm GLUCOSE

The principle of measuring the Tm of glucose consists in raising the blood glucose level to the point at which the tubular cells reach their maximal capacity to reabsorb glucose. From this point, the amount of glucose excreted rises parallel to the amount filtered because the amount reabsorbed is constant. This maximal level is reached with a blood glucose level at or above 400 mg./100 ml., and it is normally 350 to 400 mg./min./1.73 m.^{2}

To determine the Tm glucose, one must measure the glomerular filtration simultaneously by the inulin or radioactive indicator technique.

Technique

1. A Foley catheter is placed in the bladder for accurate collection of urine and the initial urine (U_0) is collected.
2. A cannula or needle for blood sampling is placed in a vein. The control sample (S_0) is taken.
3. Through an intravenous cannula in a different limb, the priming dose of the chosen glomerular indicator is injected, and the maintenance dose is then injected by a pump for 45 minutes.
4. After this equilibration period, 800 mg./kg. of 30 per cent glucose solution is injected rapidly without interrupting the administration of the maintenance dose of the glomerular indicator, and this is followed by the maintenance dose of glucose, 3.6 ml./min./m.^{2} of a 20 per cent solution. Flasks containing adequate amounts of the maintenance dose of glucose and the glomerular indicator are prepared in advance.
5. After a second 15 minute equilibration period, the urine is collected over 10 to 15 periods that are accurately measured with a stopwatch. The beginning and end of each period corresponds to the end of bladder rinsing with sterile water followed by air. Blood samples are taken at the beginning and end of each period. The test is usually continued for four or five periods.
6. At the end of the last period of TmG measurement, the 20 per cent glucose solution is replaced by 5 per cent glucose solution so as to obtain a falling blood sugar in order to determine the "splay." Again the test is continued for three or four periods.

Taking the Samples

Blood: On each occasion, two specimens are required:
    1. 2 ml. of blood for measurement of the glomerular indicator.
    2. 1 ml. of blood for measurement of the blood sugar. This specimen should be collected over sodium fluoride and immediately centrifuged cold to separate the cells and plasma as quickly as possible. The plasma samples are subsequently kept in a refrigerator until the measurement is carried out, with a delay of not more than two or three hours.

Urine: All the urine from each period is collected with the rinsing water in a single container of adequate volume. The containers are carefully stoppered and kept in a refrigerator.

Special Precautions

If the child has a urine concentration defect, it is important to give enough water to compensate for the osmotic diuresis.

The test must not be carried out in hypokalemic children because of the danger of sudden death.

Care must be taken not to cause dangerous hypervolemia in children with hypertension or severe renal failure.

Calculation

The following determinations are made for each period:

TmG = filtered glucose − excreted glucose
Filtered glucose = blood sugar (mg./ml.) × GFR (ml./min.)
Excreted glucose = glycosuria × V ml./min.

It must be remembered that one cannot speak of Tm unless the blood sugar is greater than 400 mg./100 ml.

The average Tm must be calculated for a minimum of three of four periods.

BICARBONATE TITRATION

The object of this test is to estimate the tubular reabsorption of bicarbonate as a function of the plasma bicarbonate level and hence to determine two important parameters in acid-base regulation: the threshold, which is to say the plasma bicarbonate level at which bicarbonate appears in the urine, and the Tm, which is expressed in relation to the glomerular filtration.

To determine the threshold, it is necessary to begin the test with the patient in a state of acidosis, either natural or induced by an acid load (NH_4Cl, methionine, or arginine chlorhydrate).

The test is conducted like any clearance technique: after light premedication, an indwelling balloon catheter is placed in the bladder, a cannula is inserted in a vein for blood sampling, and a needle is placed in a vein in another limb for perfusion of the solution.

The glomerular filtration should be estimated at the same time and the indicator generally chosen is inulin. After verifying that the plasma bicarbonate level is no greater than 15 mEq./liter, the bicarbonate perfusion is begun. The concentration of the perfusate and the rate of perfusion are calculated to raise the blood bicarbonate level by 1 or 1.5 mEq./hour.

As soon as the urine pH reaches 7.5, indicating a significant bicarbonate concentration, the speed of bicarbonate perfusion should be doubled.

The urine is collected during successive 30 minute periods, with a blood sample taken at the beginning and end of each period.

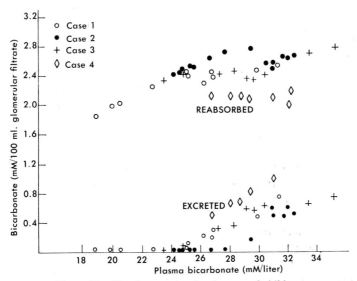

Figure 96.   Bicarbonate titration in normal children.

The pH, HCO_3, inulin, sodium, and potassium in the urine, and the inulin, pH, and HCO_3 in the blood are estimated.

Calculations

The urinary HCO_3 is calculated from the total CO_2 by using the following equations:

$$pH = pK + \log \frac{HCO_3}{H_2CO_3}$$
$$HCO_3 + H_2CO_3 = \text{total } CO_2$$

The pK is calculated from the equation $pK = 6.33 - 0.5\sqrt{Na + K}$, where Na and K are expressed in Eq./liter.

If the glomerular filtration is known, it is easy to determine the amount of bicarbonate filtered and the amount reabsorbed is calculated by subtracting the amount excreted in the urine. The titration graph can then be constructed (see Figure 96).

Precautions

There are several risks in this test, including:
1. Significant sodium overload and hypervolemia.
2. Hypokalemia.
3. Tetany owing to alkalosis.

Close supervision is thus required throughout the test.

SHORT ACIDIFICATION TEST

The object of an acidification test is to estimate changes in pH and hydrogen ion excretion in the urine in a condition of relative metabolic acidosis.

Many substances may be used to provide the acid load, including NH_4Cl or methionine given by mouth, and arginine chlorhydrate given intravenously. Whatever substance is employed, the excretion of hydrogen ions in the urine depends only on the fall in plasma bicarbonate.

The test described here employs intravenous arginine chlorhydrate. A dose of 150 mM/m.^{2} of a commercial solution of arginine chlorhydrate at a strength of 240 mM/liter is given intravenously over a four hour period.

The urine is collected directly into a clean laboratory specimen bottle every hour from the third to the eighth hour. This provides six urine specimens in which the pH, the titratable acidity, the ammonium, and possibly also the bicarbonate levels are estimated.

The plasma constants of acid-base balance—pH, HCO_3, and P_{CO_2}—must be determined both before and two hours after the end of the perfusion.

The test is valid only if the plasma bicarbonate level falls below 19 or 20 mEq./liter.

The urinary excretion of hydrogen ions can be expressed as output (μEq./min./m.^{2}), and the highest output is taken to be the most significant. The total amount excreted in eight hours can also be considered.

The results obtained in 50 children ranging in age from three months to 15 years are given in Figures 97 and 98.

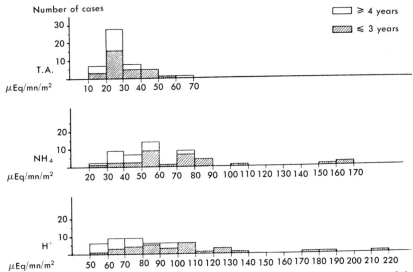

Figure 97. Distribution of maximum hydrogen ion output, ammonium output, and titratable acidity (T.A.) in 50 normal children after acid loading with arginine chlorhydrate.

Precautions

The infusion of arginine chlorhydrate causes osmotic diuresis and this may lead to dehydration if there is a serious defect in urine concentration; in such cases, the solution must be diluted and the child should be given plenty to drink; there is no point in giving an acid load if the patient is already acidotic; if the plasma bicarbonate level is 17 or 18 mEq./liter or less, it is necessary only to study the spontaneous output of hydrogen ions.

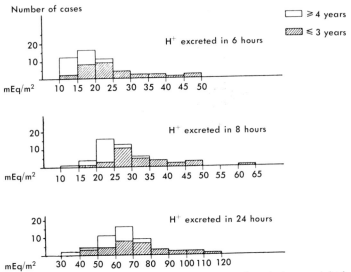

Figure 98. Distribution of excretion of hydrogen ions after six hours, eight hours, and 24 hours in 50 normal children given an acid load with arginine chlorhydrate.

SODIUM CONSERVATION TEST

The protocol of this test is very simple, but the diet must be strictly controlled. The actual test is preceded by a period of five days during which the patient is restricted to a fixed sodium intake, with the amount depending on the age of the child.

After this preliminary period, sodium restriction is begun, and the total 24 hour intake should be in the region of 0.3 mEq./kg./day. This must be estimated as accurately as possible. The sodium restriction is continued for six days.

Weight and blood pressure are recorded several times a day. All the urine passed in each 24 hour period is collected for electrolyte estimations.

The tetrahydroaldosterone can also be measured before and on the sixth day of sodium restriction. The plasma sodium, chloride, and osmolarity are also measured.

In normal children, the sodium output in the urine is always, in our experience, less than the intake after the third day of sodium restriction (Figure 99).

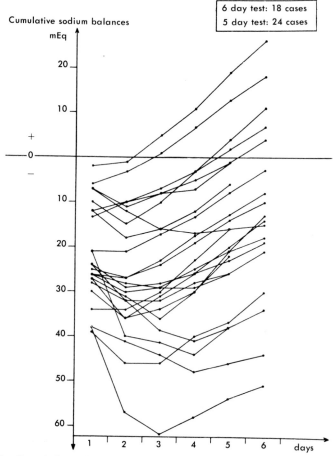

Figure 99. Cumulative sodium balances on a low-sodium diet in normal children. Before the test, the sodium intake is 2 mEq/kg./24 hours; during the five or six days of the test the sodium intake is 0.3 mEq/kg./24 hours. It can be seen that the "sodium loss" ceases by the fourth day at the latest.

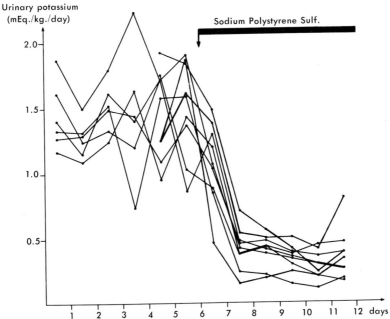

Figure 100.   Urinary potassium excretion in normal children given 1 g./kg. of sodium polystyrene sulfonate (Kayexalatate) from 6 onwards.

POTASSIUM CONSERVATION TEST

The principle is the same as that of the sodium conservation test but dietary restriction is replaced by the administration of an ion exchange resin such as sodium polystyrene sulfonate (Resonium A).

The actual test is preceded by a five day observation period during which the diet is carefully calculated to provide a fixed and known amount of potassium, about 3 or 4 mEq./kg./day. Administration of the resin is then begun in doses of 1 g./kg./day divided into two daily doses.

All the urine passed in each 24 hour period is collected for electrolyte determinations, and the plasma potassium, sodium, and bicarbonate levels are measured.

The test may be interpreted by comparing the response with that of six normal children whose urine potassium level always fell below 0.5 mEq./kg./day after the first or second day of the test (Figure 100).

URINE CONCENTRATION TEST WITH WATER RESTRICTION

In Continent Children Without Gross Polyuria

No fluid or food with a high fluid content, such as fruit, is allowed after 5 P.M.

The child is asked to empty his bladder at 4 A.M. the following morning, and this urine is discarded. Urine is then collected at 8 A.M. in a clean, stoppered container and taken immediately to the laboratory for measurement of specific gravity and osmolarity. The urine must not be left near a radiator.

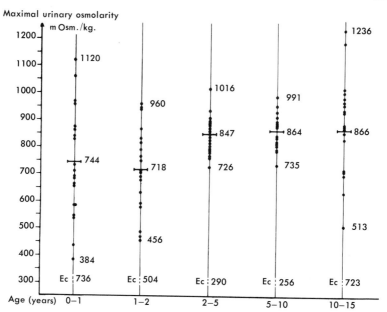

Figure 101. Urinary osmolarity in 100 normal children given no liquids for 12 hours. Distribution according to age.

If the child is unable to pass urine at 8 A.M., the test may be prolonged a further two or three hours under strict supervision, and the child must take no fluid during this time.

Infants and Incontinent Children

The principle for these patients is the same, but the urine must be collected by some device such as a plastic attachment. Urine collected up to 4 A.M. is discarded. From then until 8 A.M., or later if the child has not passed urine, each micturition must be noted and the urine placed in separate containers.

In infants, the last two feeds should be prepared with the usual quantity of dried milk, but with only half the usual amount of water.

Patients with Gross Polyuria

It is better to begin the test in the morning, so that any possible complications are quickly detected. Close supervision is essential. The blood pressure is recorded every hour, and weight and body temperature are recorded every two hours. The test must be stopped if there is any significant change in these parameters.

The results for normal children are shown in Figure 101.

SELECTIVITY OF PROTEINURIA

Proteinuria is described as being very selective if clearance of proteins of high molecular is slight but clearance of proteins of low molecular weight is increased. Conversely, in nonselective proteinuria, the clearance of high molecular weight proteins approaches that of the low molecular weight proteins.

Methods that determine the selectivity of proteinuria by determining the clearance of a large number of proteins are very complex and unsuited to routine examination. The simplified technique described by Cameron and Blandford, which is termed the *selectivity index*, is much more widely used.

In this technique, the clearance of only two proteins is measured: a low molecular weight protein, transferrin (T), and a high molecular weight protein, IgG.

The selectivity index is defined as the ratio of the two clearances:

$$SI = \frac{U\dot{V}}{P} IgG \times \frac{P}{U\dot{V}} T,$$

$$= \frac{U}{P} IgG \times \frac{P}{U} T$$

In this way, the actual volume of urine is ignored, the only measurements required being the blood and urine levels of transferrin and of IgG. The measurements are performed by immunodiffusion in commercially available plates of agar containing anti-T or anti-IgG serum. The plates are sold with six wells. Twelve additional perforated wells of identical capacity (8 to 10 μ liter) are provided. The six median wells are filled with six different concentrations of antigen, prepared from a standard solution. The 12 other wells are filled with the urine or plasma samples to be studied, with no special preparation. The plates are incubated for four hours at 37° C. The graph is constructed on semilogarithmic paper by plotting the diameter of the diffusion disks (on the abscissa) and the different sample concentrations (on the ordinate). The concentrations in the samples being tested can then be calculated.

Table 92. Correlations Between Renal Histology and the Selectivity of the Proteinuria in 60 Cases of Glomerular Nephropathy with Histologic Documentation

		Proteinuria and Index of Selectivity				
					Nonselective	
Type of Nephropathy	*Total*	Very Selective (0.01–0.09)	Selective (0.10–0.14)	Moderately Selective (0.14–0.19)	0.20–0.29	0.30
Nephrotic syndrome with minimal glomerular lesions	21	16	2	1	1	1
Segmental and focal hyalinization	11		2	1	6	2
Membranoproliferative glomerulonephritis	10		2	2	2	4
Endocapillary and extracapillary glomerulonephritis	6			1	2	3
Extramembranous glomerulonephritis	4	1	1	2		
Nephrotic syndrome with endocapillary proliferation	2	1				1
Miscellaneous*	6				2	4

*Three cases of Alport's syndrome, and one each of amyloidosis, congenital nephrotic syndrome, and severe unclassifiable nephropathy.

The graph of the standard solutions is usually linear. However, at low concentrations (30 mg./100 ml. for T, 50 to 90 mg./100 ml. for IgG), the correlation between the diameter of the diffusion disk and the concentration is no longer linear. This is the principal limitation of this technique because very often the urinary levels of T and IgG are below these limits.

Results

Our experience of this technique is summarized in Table 92.

The proteinuria of nephrotic syndromes with minimal glomerular lesions is nearly always very selective, and the converse is true as well: very selective proteinuria is virtually confined to this condition.

The proteinuria of glomerular disease, whether the lesions are hyaline or proliferative, is never very selective.

In the few cases of nephrotic syndrome with minimal glomerular lesions in which the proteinuria was not very selective, we have nearly always found resistance to treatment.

TECHNIQUE OF NEEDLE BIOPSY OF THE KIDNEY

Needle biopsy of the kidney is possible even in small children. The technique is the same as that used in adults.

Preparation of the Patient

Intravenous urography is essential to show the presence of both kidneys, their size and morphology, and the absence of any abnormality of pelvis or calyces. It is also very valuable as a guide to the biopsy site by a well centered film superimposing the picture of the kidney on the skin markers. This film must be taken in the same position as that used for the renal biopsy: ventral decubitus with the head resting on folded arms and a small pillow under the upper abdomen. The skin marker is placed over Petit's triangle, and its position is indicated with marking ink.

It is important to make a careful study of bleeding and clotting factors before performing renal biopsy. Any defect in hemostasis is a contraindication to biopsy.

If the child is hypertensive, the diastolic blood pressure must be brought below 80 mm. Hg by suitable therapy.

Equipment

Many types of needle can be used. One of the most satisfactory is the Vim-Silverman needle as modified by White for pediatric use by the addition of a small adjustable stop.

A disposable needle of the Travenol type has the advantage of allowing perfect cutting, but there is no pediatric version of this type of needle, and certain precautions are necessary if it is used in small children.

Technique

After premedication with phenobarbital or diazepam, the child is placed lying face down, with a small pillow under the upper abdomen and his head resting on his folded arms.

The bone landmarks, iliac crest, twelfth rib, and spine are marked with a skin pencil, and the puncture site is chosen with reference to the radiopaque skin mark and its projection on the picture of the kidney. The elective site is the outer border of the lower pole. A vertical line is drawn about 1 cm. outside the line of the calyces; puncture medial to this line is dangerous. These preparations are unnecessary if an image intensifier is available.

After infiltration with local analgesia, the depth of the kidney is determined by a needle of the lumbar puncture type; respiratory movement is transmitted to this needle as soon as its tip enters the kidney. Then, through a tiny incision made with the point of a knife, the renal biopsy needle is introduced to the previously measured depth. Next, with two rapid movements, the two parts of the biopsy needle are plunged into the kidney to a depth that depends on the size of the child.

The needle with the specimen enclosed is removed and the child is kept in bed and under observation for 24 hours.

The fragment of renal parenchyma must be fixed immediately. The best fixative for light microscopy is Dubosc-Brasil solution. Immunofluorescence study, essential for the diagnosis of most glomerular nephropathies, requires special preparation of the fragment, and the specimen should be kept at $-70°$ C. until the time of examination. Special fixation methods are needed also for electron microscopy.

Complications

Hematuria may sometimes occur. In most cases, there is only slight discoloration of the urine for one or two days. Rarely, bleeding may be more severe, with clots in the urine and renal colic; in such cases, hemostatic drugs such as epsilon aminocaproic acid (EACA) must never be used. If bleeding is very severe, transfusion may be required.

Perirenal hematoma is also unusual unless there is some coagulation defect. In this context, it is important to emphasize the danger of renal biopsy during heparin therapy. Heparin therapy must not be undertaken for at least 10 days after biopsy. These complications are very rare in our experience. In over 250 cases of needle biopsy, we have had only one instance of major hematuria and one perirenal hematoma as a result of beginning heparin therapy too soon after biopsy. The hematoma recovered spontaneously.

Index

Page numbers in *italics* refer to illustrations;
(t) indicates tables.

437